The Economics of Disability:
International Perspectives

Published by
Rehabilitation International
in cooperation with the
United Nations

A publication of the Rehabilitation International Project on International Perspectives on the Economics of Disability: Project Director, Susan Hammerman; Research Assistant, Stephen Maikowski; Publication Design, Barbara Duncan. This publication was made possible in part by Grant # G008005861 from the National Institute of Handicapped Research, United States Department of Education, Washington, D.C.

Contents

"The most valuable resource any country has is its people."

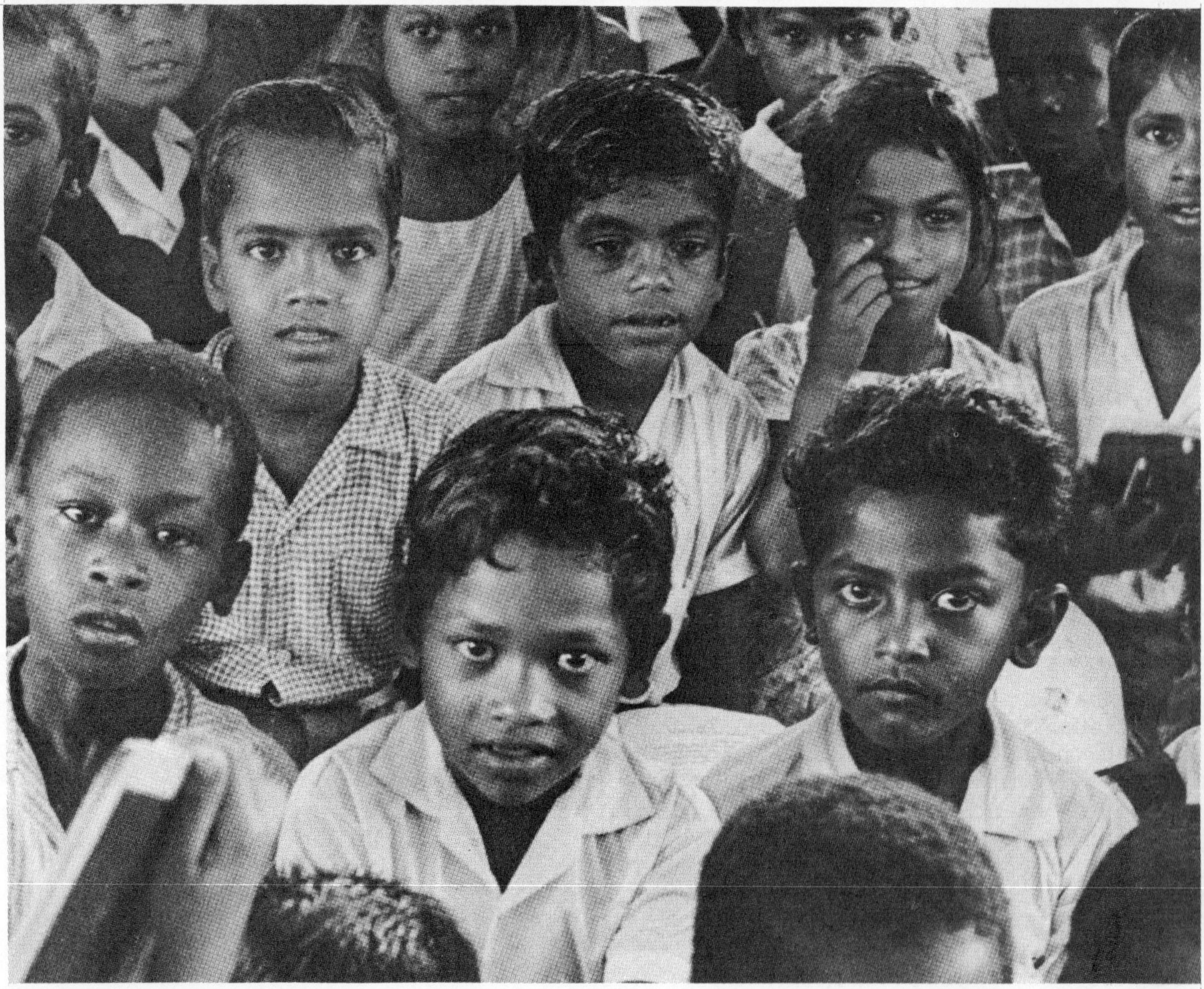

The World Bank, World Development Report, 1980

Preface

We are grateful to Rehabilitation International for securing funds for printing this report on the work of the Expert Group organized by the United Nations Centre for Social Development and Humanitarian Affairs on "Socio-economic Implications of Investments in Rehabilitation for the Disabled", held in Geneva in December 1977.

The increasing and unsatisfied demands for rehabilitation services worldwide, in particular in developing countries, represent a serious social and humanitarian problem. Without medical, prosthetic, educational and vocational services, the social integration of disabled persons encounters insurmountable obstacles. Aware of the situation, the United Nations and United Nations specialized agencies are involved in a number of activities dealing with the rights of disabled persons and the various services needed to overcome the obstacles. The proclamation of 1981 as the "International Year of Disabled Persons" by the United Nations General Assembly constitutes a major source of strength for such activities.

The Expert Group Meeting was a part of the United Nations activities in this field. Its report shows clearly that investment in well-organized, efficient rehabilitation services not only helps disabled persons to become active members of society but also, in the final analysis, leads to savings to national economies, since rehabilitation means increased utilization of important human resources.

United Nations Centre
for Social Development
and Humanitarian Affairs

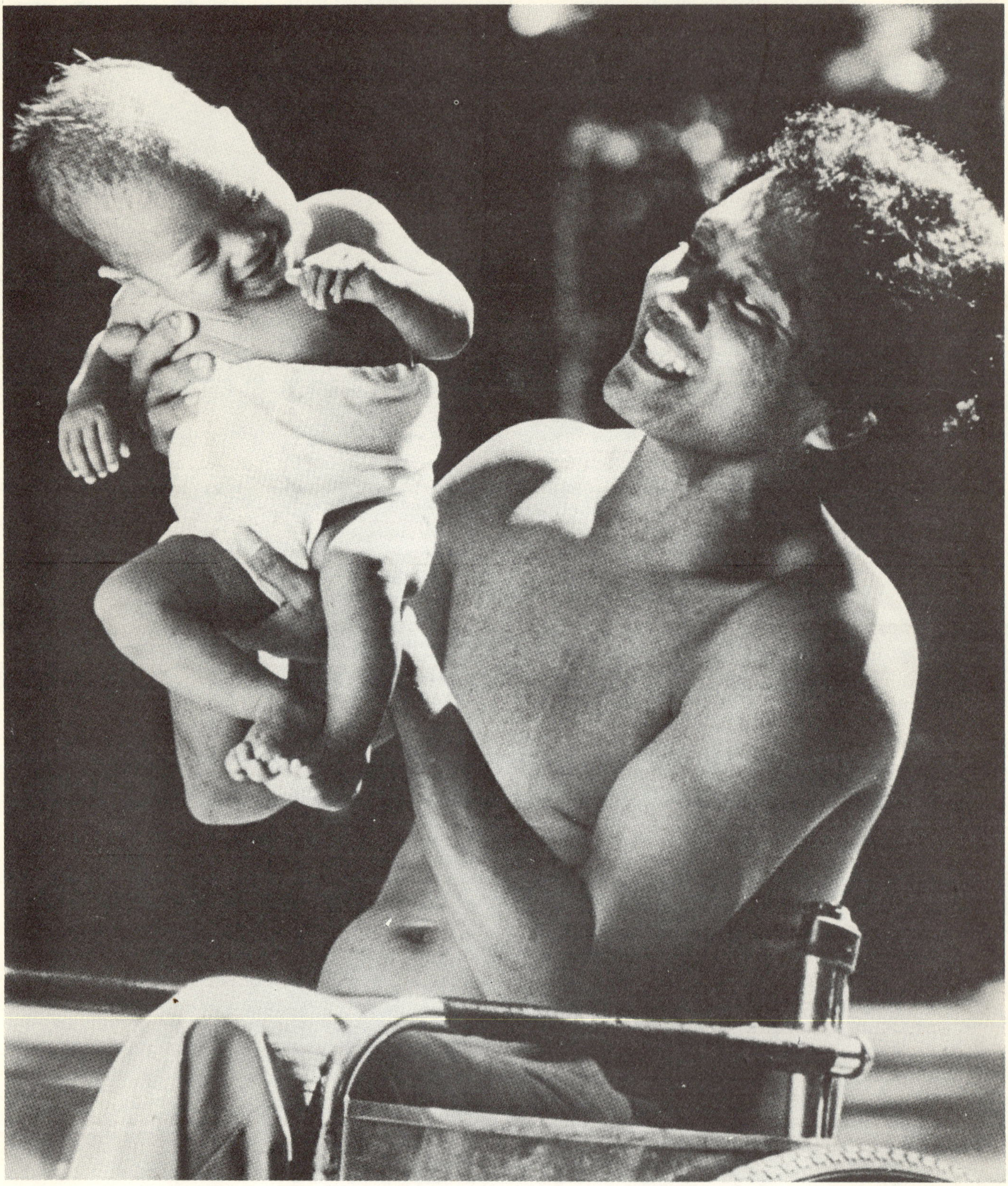

Foreword

Rehabilitation International is pleased to publish this important volume, The Economics of Disability: International Perspectives, as a contribution to the global effort involved in the International Year of Disabled Persons in 1981. Assisting as it does in the amplification and dissemination of the results of a United Nations study and expert group meeting, the book testifies to the dedication of Rehabilitation International to cooperation with the United Nations. We are grateful to the U.N. Centre for Social Development and Humanitarian Affairs for its initiative in investigating this critical subject, and for its agreement that this publication be issued.

Dissemination of the information contained in these pages, information that is essential to an understanding of the issues involved in solving the problems presented to society by disability, is in keeping with the aims of the Rehabilitation International Charter for the 80s. This document, a statement of global consensus about the policies and priorities for disability prevention and rehabilitation in the 1980s, is another contribution of R.I. to the International Year.

The publication of this book is the culmination of a long process of cooperative effort between the United Nations and Rehabilitation International. Starting with a study of the subject carried out by Susan Hammerman, the R.I. Assistant Secretary General, at the request of the U.N., it has proceeded through experts meetings of the United Nations and of Rehabilitation International, and the accumulated information and insight are assembled in this volume. We are deeply grateful to the individuals who have contributed to the process, to the institutions they have represented, and to the authors who have authorized use of excerpts from their works.

Particular gratitude is expressed to the United States National Institute for Handicapped Research for its understanding of the importance of the material presented in this volume and for the support that has made publication possible.

Norman Acton
Secretary General
Rehabilitation International

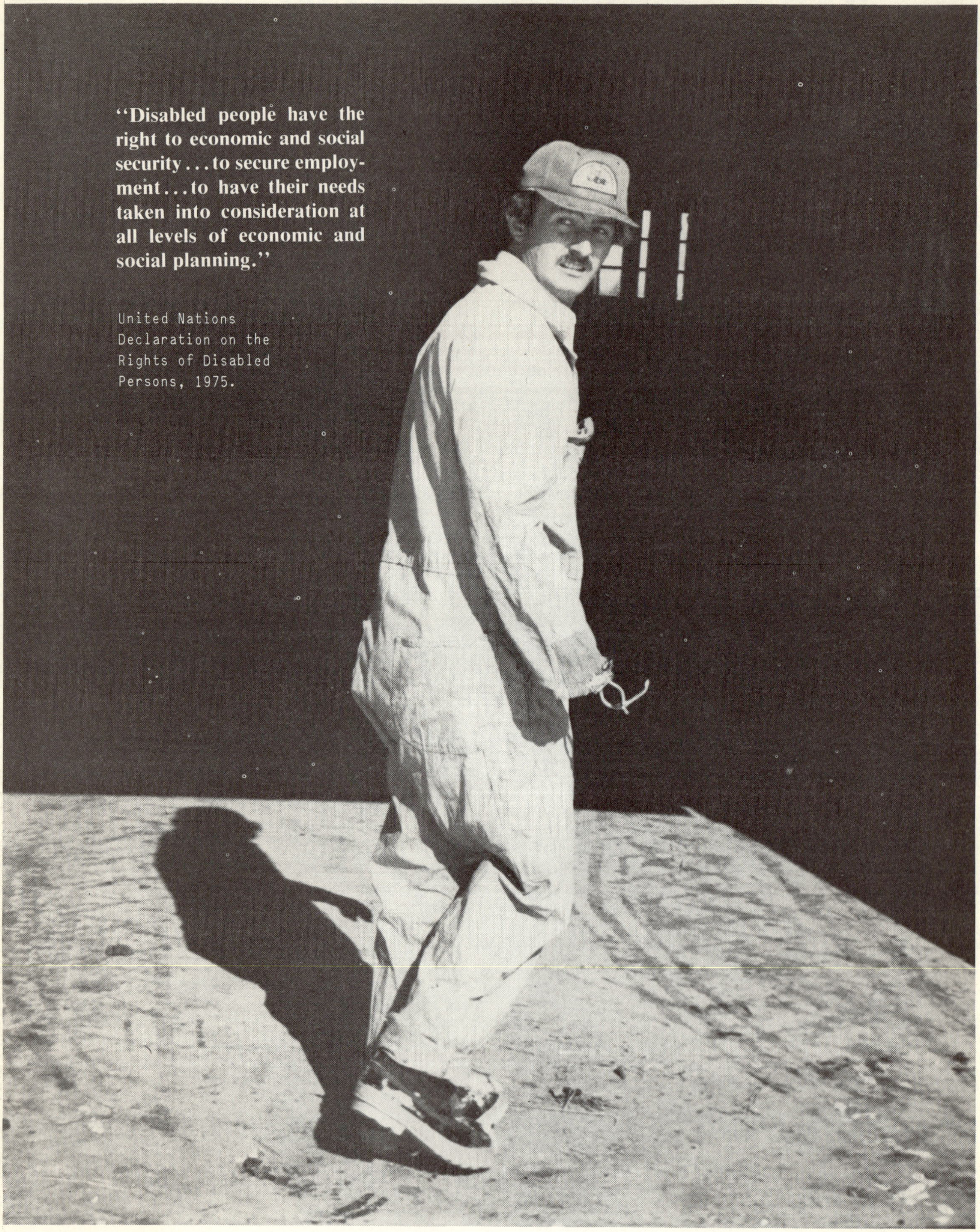

"Disabled people have the right to economic and social security . . . to secure employment . . . to have their needs taken into consideration at all levels of economic and social planning."

United Nations Declaration on the Rights of Disabled Persons, 1975.

Introduction

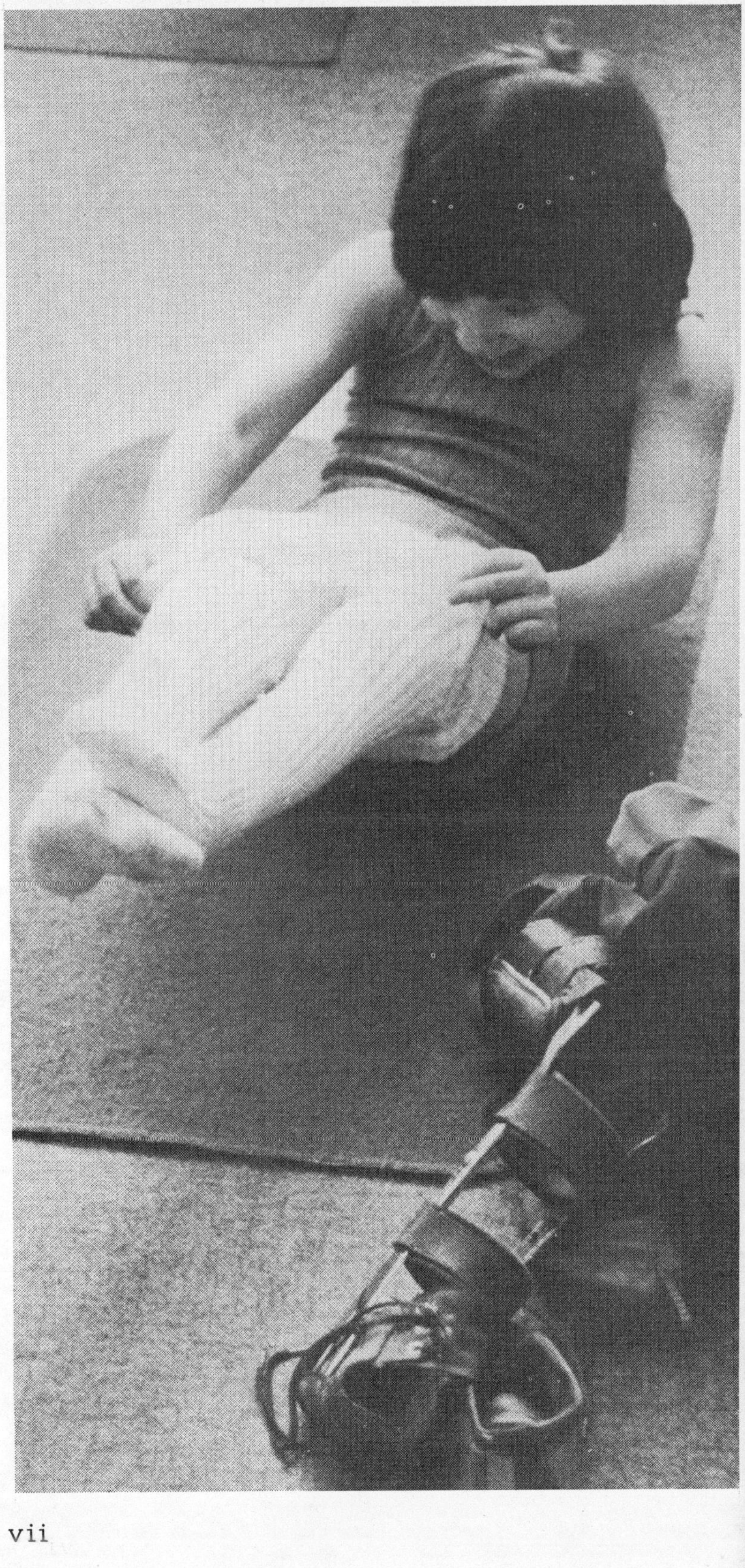

The Economics of Disability: International Perspectives contains within a single volume three component parts: the report of the United Nations Expert Group Meeting on the Socio-Economic Implications of Investments in Rehabilitation held at the Palais des Nations in Geneva, December 1977; excerpts from the United Nations study Rehabilitation for the Disabled: The Social and Economic Implications of Investments for this Purpose (No. E.77.IV.11) upon which the Expert Meeting was based, and, annotations from additional references which highlight with case studies and empirical data many of the concepts and issues cited in the United Nations documents. The annotations are included pursuant to the recommendation of the United Nations Expert Group that a bibliography of references be published to illustrate "why disability and its prevention should be of concern to all."

Taken as a whole, the volume is intended to encompass for policy makers and all others concerned with the impact of disability upon society the full range of issues included within the economics of disability prevention

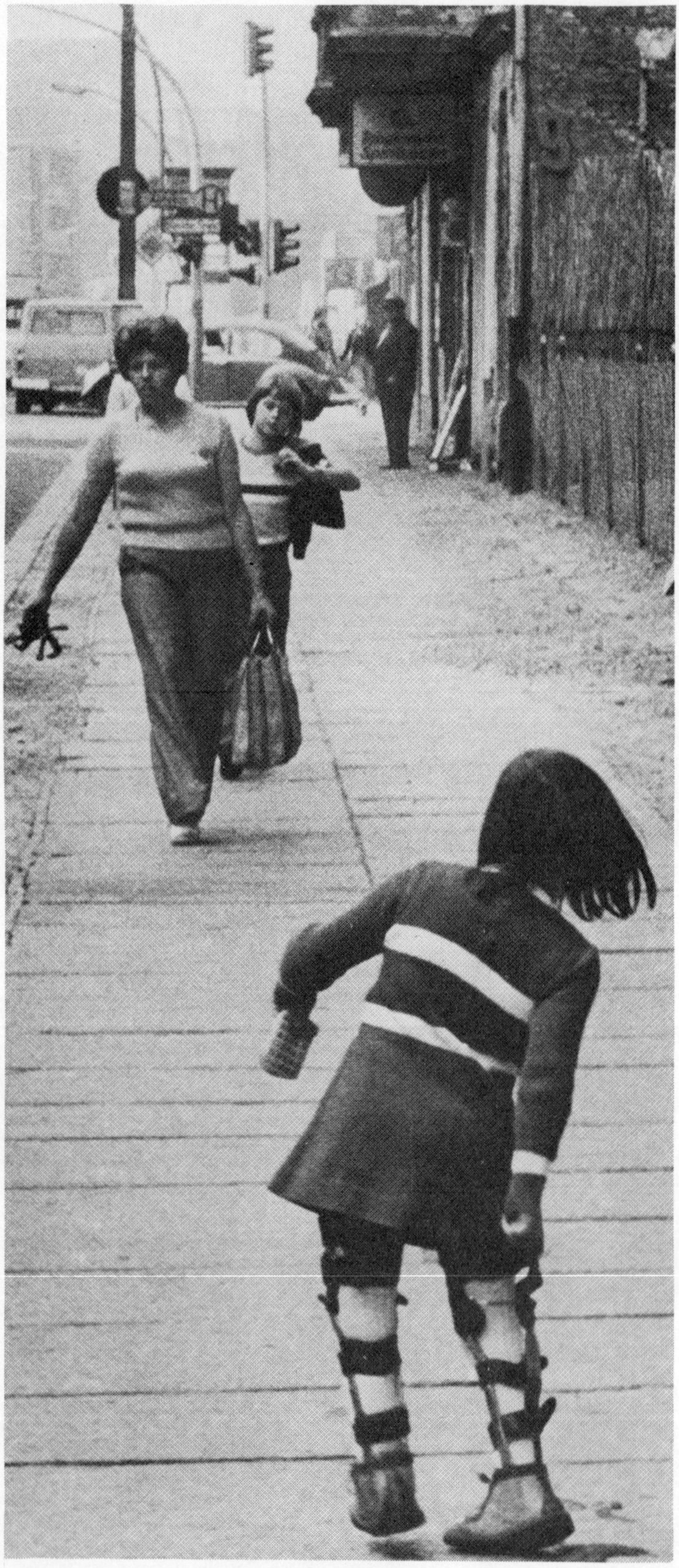

and rehabilitation: the economic and social costs of disability, the concepts and implications of cost/benefit analyses, the labor market and social benefit system issues. For the purposes of the present volume, the concepts have been divided into separate chapters. In life, of course, they are interwoven and interdependent.

In 1974, the Council of World Organizations Interested in the Handicapped, a federation of 40 non-governmental organizations working in consultative relationship with the United Nations, proposed a need for more information on the economic and social costs to society resulting from disability and on how the reduction of those costs would fit into more general economic and social development. In 1975, the United Nations Department of Economic and Social Affairs commissioned a research study on this subject which I had the privilege to carry out for Rehabilitation International. Officials of the United Nations, the International Labor Organization, the United Nations Educational, Scientific and Cultural Organization and the World Health Organization as well as those of many international and national non-governmental organizations provided information and background studies for the project. The preoccupation at that time was to answer the question so frequently posed by government officials to advisors who were assigned to help them develop services for disabled people: "How can we afford to develop rehabilitation and disability prevention measures when so much else must be done and these programs are so costly?"

Since then, the international community has come to realize that the causes of physical, mental and sensory impairment may be similar throughout the world but their consequences will vary in terms of the disability experienced by people in their daily lives and in terms of the handicap they experience as a result of societal expectations and attitudes. The nature and implications of disability will vary according to the socio-economic circumstances of each nation and the provisions which it makes for all of its members. Disability is a problem which exists in relation to society and which each society, therefore, has the capacity to reduce and to control.

The present volume is a tribute to the growth in our understanding. It takes into account the fact that disability is now internationally recognized as a creator of costs to society whether or not rehabilitation services exist, and the awareness that the more a society recognizes and deals with these costs, the greater will be the overall economic gain. Of greater importance, it illuminates the fact that people are the most precious asset of any nation. A society which shuts out any segment of its people from full participation and contribution is indeed an impoverished society.

Susan Hammerman
Assistant Secretary General
Rehabilitation International

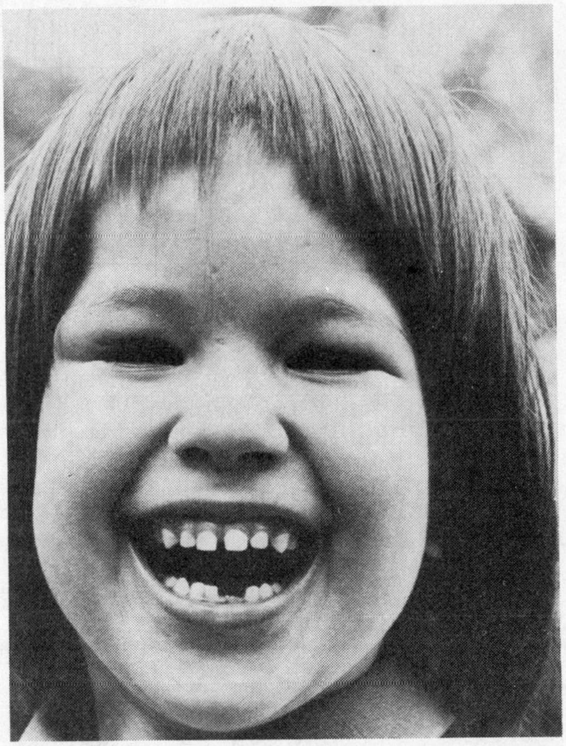

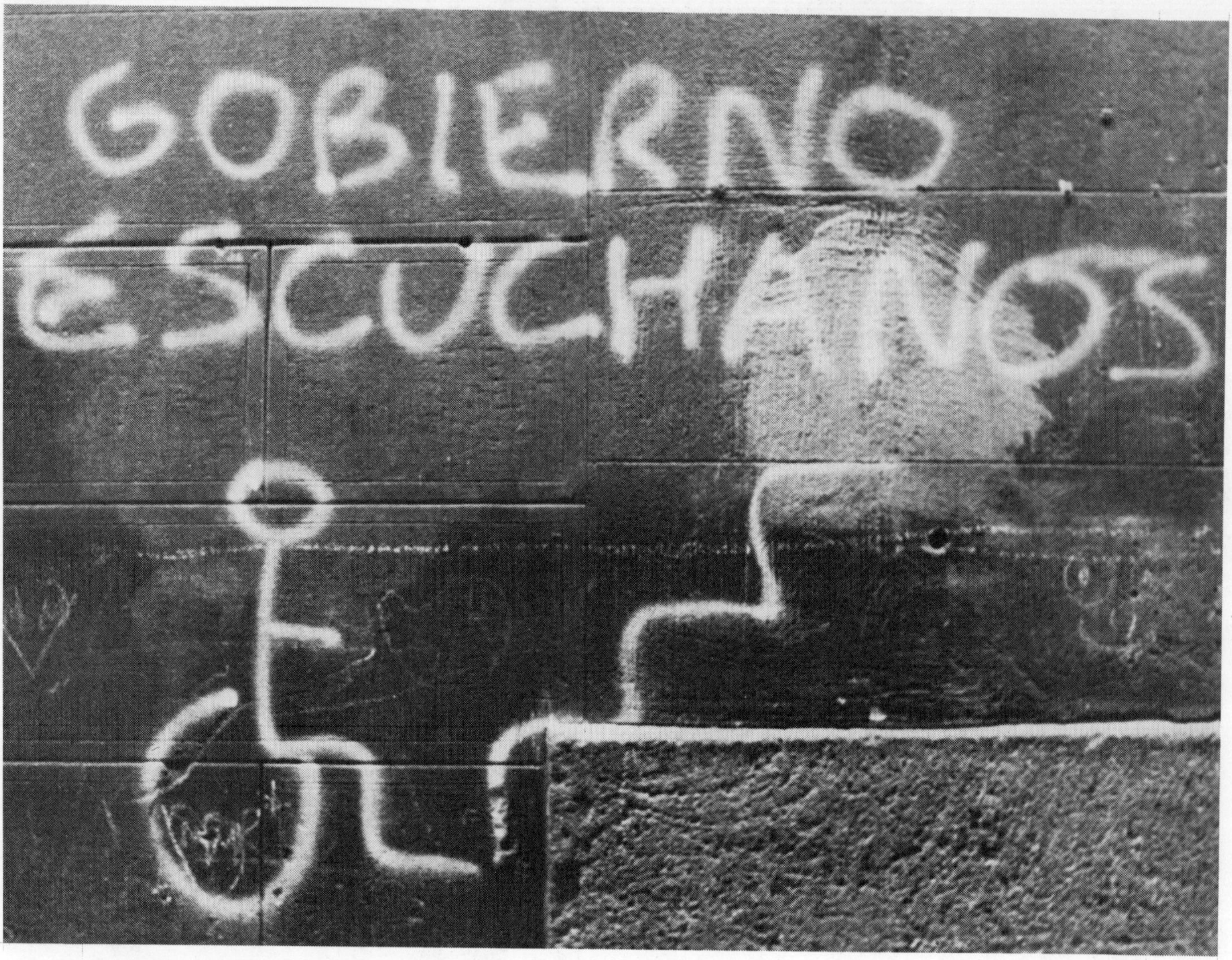

Graffiti in Spain, "Government, Listen to Us!"

The United Nations Expert Group Meeting on the "Socio-Economic Implications of Investments in Rehabilitation for the Disabled," was held December 1-9, 1977 in Geneva. The meeting was attended by the following experts appointed by the Secretary-General: Miguel A. Aguilera (Guatemala); Jonas Bedford Amoako (Ghana); Manuel-Angel Garcia Viso (Spain); Susan Hammerman (United States of America); Avideh Shashaani (Iran); Helga Ulbricht (German Democratic Republic); and the following experts appointed by the Council of World Organizations Interested in the Handicapped and representing different member groups of the Council: John Noble; A.I. Simkins; and Rosli Stahel. Representatives of the International Labor Office, the World Health Organization, the United Nations Educational, Scientific and Cultural Organization, the International Social Security Association and the International Institute for Rehabilitation in Developing Countries also attended. The following officials were elected: Jonas Amoako as Chairman, Manuel-Angel Garcia Viso as Vice-Chairman and Susan Hammerman as Rapporteur.

United Nations Expert Group Meeting on the Socio-Economic Implications of Investments in Rehabilitation for the Disabled

December 1-9, 1977
Geneva

INTRODUCTION

1 The work programme of the United Nations Centre for Social Development and Humanitarian Affairs for the biennium 1974-75 contained a research project on social and economic implications of investments in rehabilitation services for disabled persons. Mrs. Susan Hammerman, Assistant Secretary General of Rehabilitation International, was contracted in 1975 to carry out this study as consultant to the United Nations. Her study was published in 1977.

2 In it the consultant had reviewed existing documentation and experience from 16 countries concerning costs and benefits of rehabilitation service delivery. She had identified substantial gaps in available data on the magnitude of actual rehabilitation services costs and uncovered many areas of difficulty in assessing the social and economic benefits deriving from such services. She had also noted the absence of documented experience from developing countries in this regard.

3 One of her recommendations was that the United Nations should convene an expert group to further explore some of the problems on which sufficient data could not be gathered for the above study. The recommendation was approved and a United Nations expert group convened from December 1-9, 1977 at Geneva to consider the findings of the study and, in particular:

(i) the economic benefits of rehabilitation in developing countries and rural areas,

(ii) investments in rehabilitation in relation to improved methods of service delivery,

(iii) the effects of disability upon the productivity of family members and dependents of the disabled, and

(iv) methods to assess the non-monetary/economic benefits of rehabilitation.

4 The expert group was expected to produce a report on the subject which, it was considered, would be of value to rehabilitation services planners at the national level as well as to those concerned with technical assistance activities in this field.

5 The group agreed that it should discuss, in particular, the following principal items:

I. Assessment of investments in rehabilitation services.

II. Measurement of socio-economic implications of disability (within the community, particularly in developing countries).

III. Comparison of the costs and benefits of rehabilitation services provision.

I. Assessment of Rehabilitation Services

6 The Expert Group recognized the great difficulty in defining the costs of rehabilitation service provision. Some costs may be measured exactly whereas others cannot. Many of the actual costs of rehabilitation services may be met within the general social, health, educational and vocational services of a nation. The question "costs for whom?" needs to be answered. The burden of rehabilitation service costs may be borne by society as a whole, by sectors and institutions within the society or by the individuals and his or her family members. The costs may be transferred from one sector of society to another; usually the people who incur the costs differ from those who bear them.

7 The Group, agreeing with a previous United Nations Expert Group, agreed that rehabilitation is a social concern and that its aim is to enable the disabled person, restricted in his or her physical or mental capacity, to take an active part in the life of the community and to participate with all members in the development of society. It was suggested that rehabilitation services should utilize a comprehensive range of medical, educational, social and vocational techniques to reduce the consequences of disability. Extension of rehabilitation services and realization of its goals also depended on the availability of economic resources and on policy decisions as to their use.

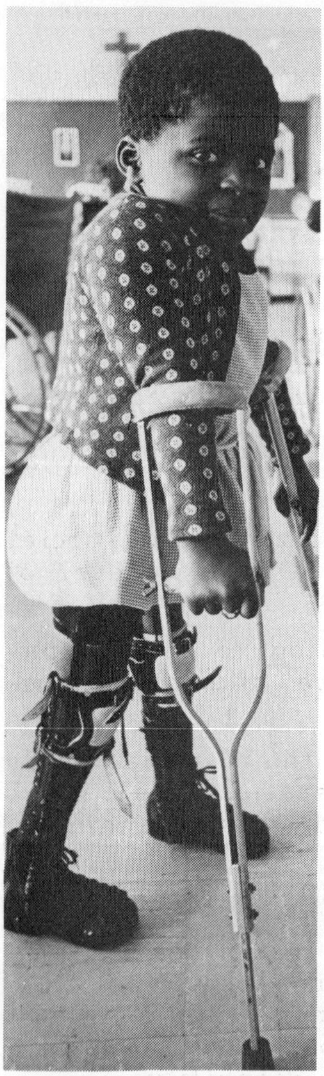

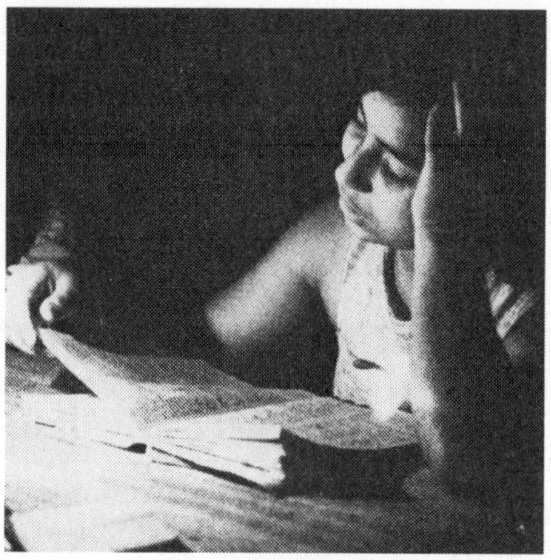

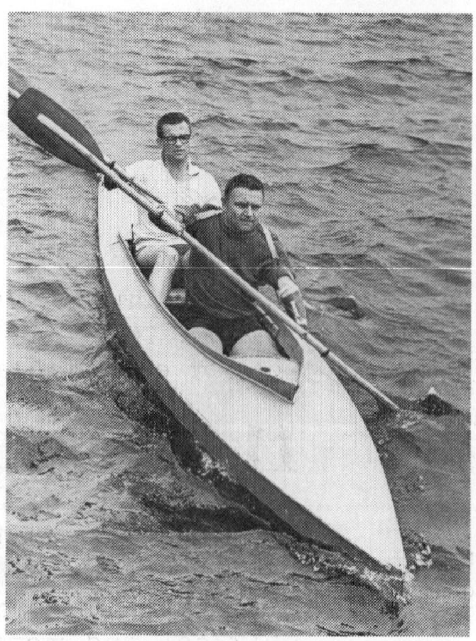

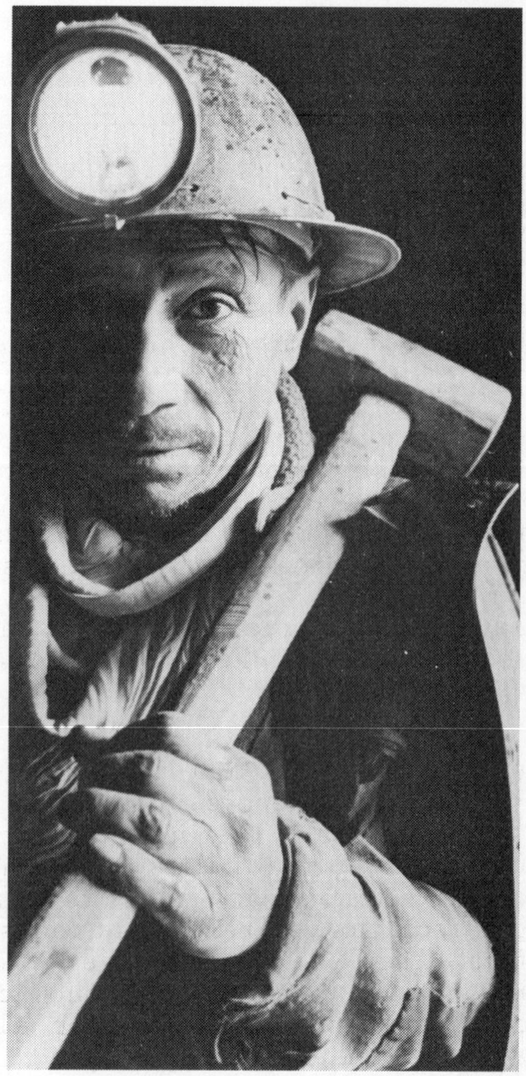

"Rehabilitation services should utilize a comprehensive range of medical, educational, social and vocational techniques..."

"the right to services to hasten . . . social integration"

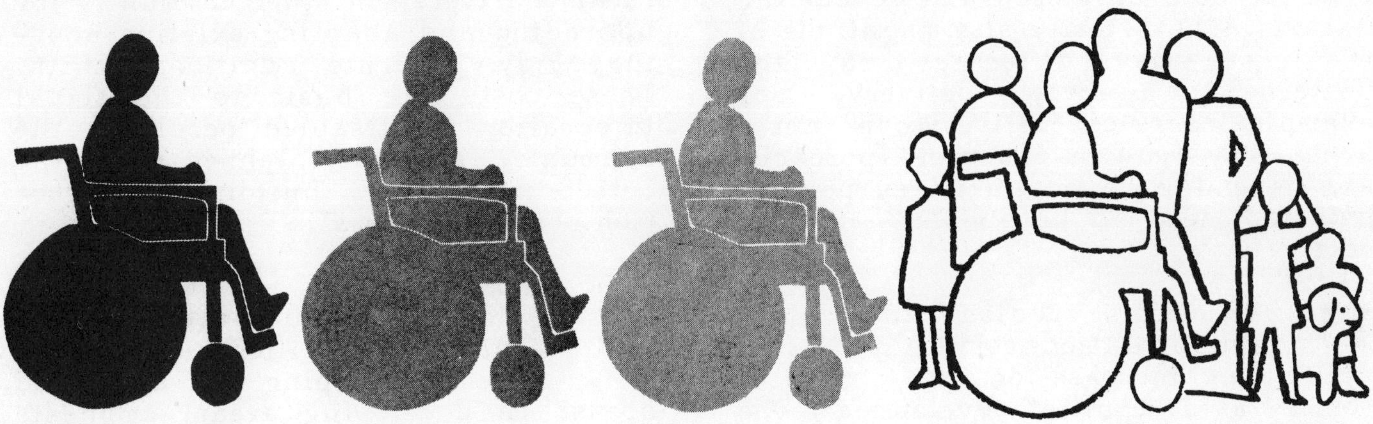

Some of the problems of disability were intractable with only limited solutions possible; rehabilitation might only defer the most severe consequences.

8 The Group was of the view that rehabilitation services should be integrated in the whole country in order to promote the process of integration, not only by acceptance of the basic idea but also through its implementation. As far as possible, the general social policy should assure the rights of all people to work, to be educated, to receive health care and social security when unable to work.

9 Rehabilitation services for disabled people should, as far as possible, be included within the normal responsibilities of each sector of the social policy. This is to prevent the isolation of rehabilitation services from other social actions and to foster recognition of the socio-economic implications of such services for all other aspects of the social policy.

10 Disabled people, children, youth, adults of working age and older age groups, have the same rights as other members of society as specified in the "United Nations Declaration on the Rights of Disabled Persons" and these include:

the right to services to develop their capabilities to the maximum and to hasten the process of social integration;

the right to economic and social security, and to a decent level of living;

the right, according to their capabilities, to secure and retain employment;

the right to have their special needs taken into consideration at all stages of economic and social planning.

11 It was recognized that all nations vary in the degree to which they have realized achievement of their social policies, including protection of the rights of their citizens, especially those with physical and mental disability.

MEASUREMENTS IN DIFFERENT ECONOMIC SYSTEMS

12 Developed versus developing economies. The Group agreed that the basic costs of rehabilitation (see paragraph 21) are of the same type for both developed and developing nations. The priority and magnitude of the costs may differ as may the patterns of service delivery. For example, service delivery in rural areas may require different approaches, depend more on auxiliary personnel and need to be simpler and less costly.

13 The costs of disability and of rehabilitation service provision may increase for some groups in society as a result of development. The disabled aged, displaced from traditional family structures, may require more intensive community services. It was reported by the representatives of WHO that severe disability, related to traffic and work accidents and to occupational disease, was increasing. Pollutants in the air and water may also create additional disabling conditions. Infants with congenital disability may survive birth as a result of improved medical care. Needs of people with mental disorders may increase as traditional social support systems change or deteriorate.

14 Development may also increase the expectations of disabled people for service and may result in a greater sensitivity by the general population to the problems of the disabled and their needs. Thus actions such as removal of architectural barriers in the community or upgrading and adapting existing housing, may generate additional costs. These costs are basic to the social integration of disabled people in the community and, if planned from the outset in all new building construction, can be minimal.

15 Priorities for utilization of resources may differ sharply between developing and developed areas. In developing areas, emphasis on the development of industry and agriculture and of a basic infrastructure of health, transport, communication and education facilities may prevent expenditure of resources on social services, in particular rehabilitation services.

16 In developed countries where the service sector of the economy is expanding, higher wages paid to more productive service workers may bid up the costs of securing rehabilitation personnel. This situa-

"Priorities for the utilization of resources may differ

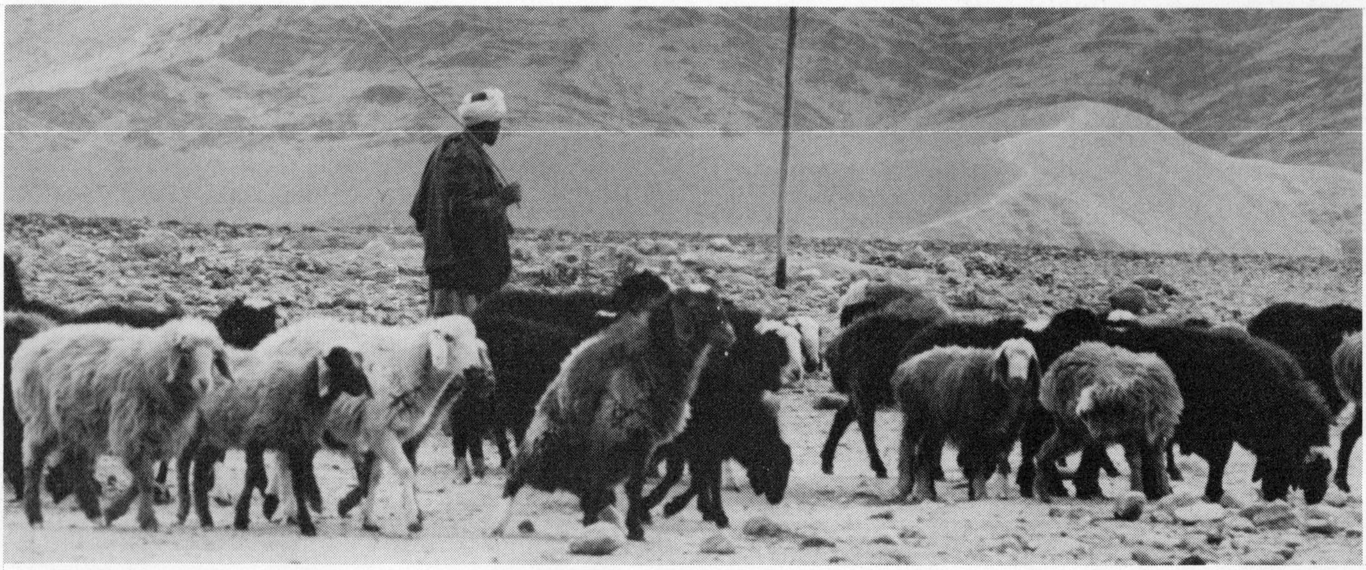

tion will inflate the costs of caring for disabled people and create a need for higher budgetary outlays to keep up with the demand for rehabilitation services. In effect the demand for rehabilitation services competes with the demand for many other types of service in the economy.

GENERAL VERSUS SPECIFIC COSTS OF REHABILITATION

17 The meeting recognized that many of the basic components of rehabilitation service provision may be encompassed by the general systems for health care, education, vocational training and placement, transportation and social services, available within a nation to all citizens. When such services are available for the entire population, the "excess costs" of special service adaptations for the disabled may be estimated with some accuracy.

18 It is very difficult to assess the proportion or amount of the general system expenditures ("common costs") which are utilized by the disabled. Even if such a calculation could be made, its value for use in a cost/benefit comparison is questionable, and could be very confusing for planners.

19 Particularly in developing countries where general service systems are not yet well developed, as well as in less-developed regions of developed countries, planners tend to overlook or discriminate against the needs of disabled people on the basis of giving first priority to the development of systems that will benefit the greatest number of people. This may have the effect of keeping disabled people and their families amongst the lowest strata of society, socially and economically. The necessary facts on the need to integrate services for the handicapped within all general systems from the very outset of planning need to be brought to the attention of national planners and those responsible for the formulation of social policy.

DEFINING THE BASIC COSTS OF REHABILITATION SERVICES

20 The Group divided the specific costs of rehabilitation service provision, whether or not monetarized, into five basic categories. The first of these categories, "special services and case expenditures", has associated with it costs that may be classified by reference to four remaining categories. The five basic categories of specific rehabilitation costs are as follows:

sharply between developing and developed areas."

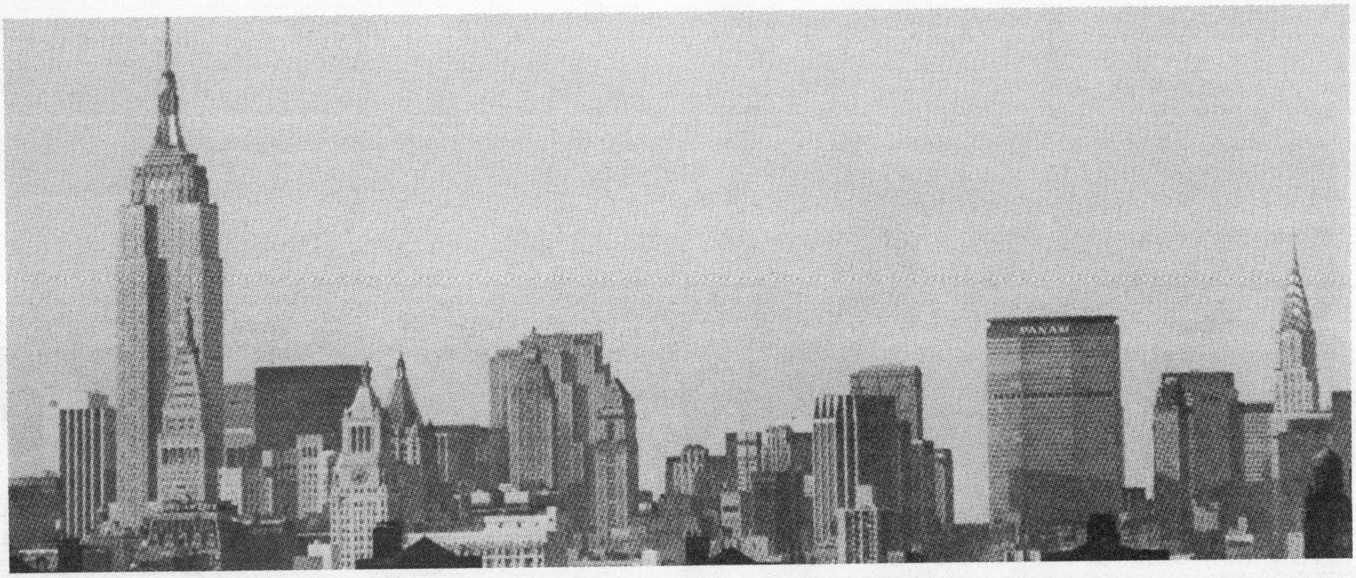

(i) special services and case expenditures;

(ii) administrative salaries and overhead expenses for maintenance and upkeep of facilities and equipment;

(iii) facility development, professional training, first purchase of equipment research development;

(iv) income loss and foregone earnings or work by disabled persons themselves while receiving rehabilitation services;

(v) social costs - the value of resources that would have been available for other uses had special and/or general services not been rendered to disabled persons by both formal organizations, such as voluntary societies, religious organizations, chartered social groups and/or associations of disabled people, and informal structures, such as parent groups, village leaders, family members, and individual volunteers.

21 The basic costs of rehabilitation service provision for disabled people may be incurred through special services integrated within existing general service systems or through special services in specially provided facilities. Examples of basic rehabilitation services that incur expenditures are listed below. They apply to both developed and developing countries and include special services provided both within general systems and within special facilities and programs.

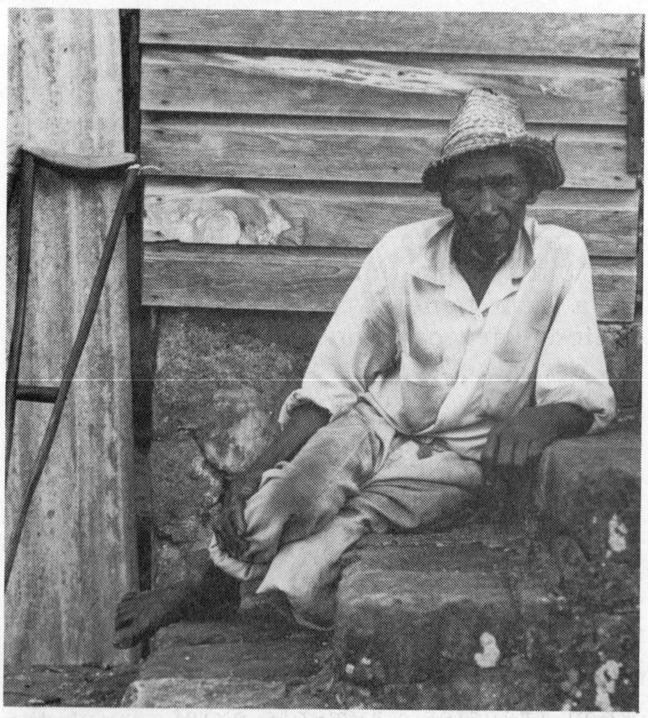

"Disability will often lead to poverty."

A) FOR ALL GROUPS OF THE DISABLED:

(i) Specialized health services rendered as a part of general health and hospital care or by special hospitals, e.g. hospital bed care, specialized medical care, including surgery and post-surgical treatment; psychiatric services, social nursing and counselling in the hospital, diagnostic services of all kinds, including psychological measurement, work capacity testing.

(ii) Counselling offices requiring specialized staff and documents or other communication media for imparting information.

(iii) Technical aids, special equipment and adaptive devices, and assistance in performing activities of daily living at home.

B) FOR CHILDREN:

(i) Creches, for weekly or continuous nursing, and day nurseries, together with specialized staff, buildings and equipment.

(ii) Kindergartens and homes for disabled children of pre-school age, together with specialized medical and educational provisions.

(iii) Hospitals for disabled school age children and youth, together with special educational and vocational training programmes therein.

(iv) Resource centres, classes and schools for physically and mentally handicapped children.

(v) Institutions or centres for the vocational training of disabled children who are unable to attend regular institutions offering similar training.

Services for the young and

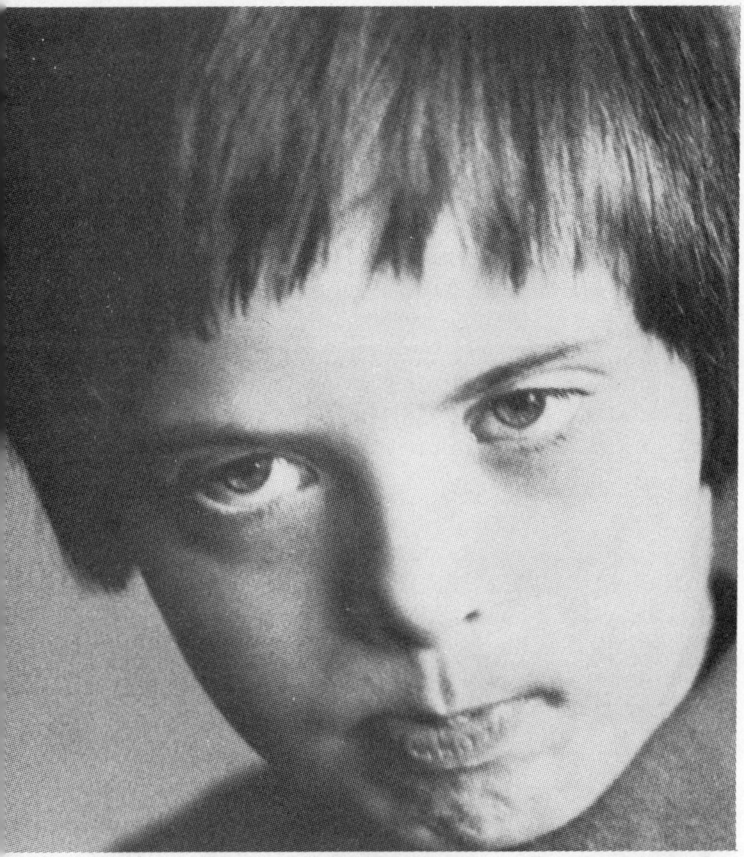

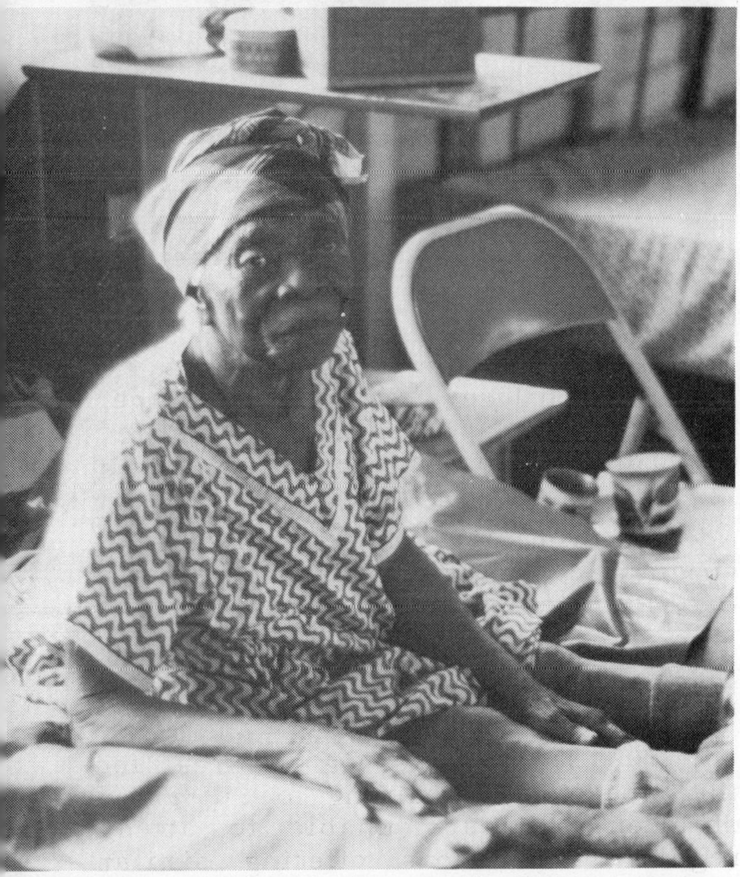

for the old.

C) FOR ADULTS:

(i) Centres for vocational training and retraining.

(ii) Employment programmes in the ordinary work place and in sheltered work places.

(iii) Preferred housing (e.g. lower floor flats and/or in close proximity to the work place) or adapted housing for adults and families with disabled members.

(iv) Adapted transportation to assist the disabled to be mobile in the community and to commute to work.

D) OTHER:

(i) Publicity campaigns to alter community attitudes towards the disabled.

(ii) Expenditures to remove architectural barriers in public buildings, including schools of all levels, hotels, walkways above and below streets, railway stations, etc.

(iii) Subsidies from governmental or other sources to enterprises which employ the disabled or to encourage disabled worker co-operatives.

22 Social costs are very difficult to quantify with present methods of economic analysis. Researchers have made various estimates to explain how social costs multiply the other basic costs of rehabilitation and add to the overall total costs. The exclusion or inclusion of social costs in a cost/benefit analysis of rehabilitation services, and the method used to estimate such costs, can radically influence conclusions about the productivity of investments in rehabilitation.

23 Transfer payments, income maintenance payments such as short-term sickness benefits and disability pensions, represent the transfer of wealth from one sector of society to another, a redistribution of the already existing wealth in society. When transfer payments exist, they are not included in the basic costs of rehabilitation service provision within

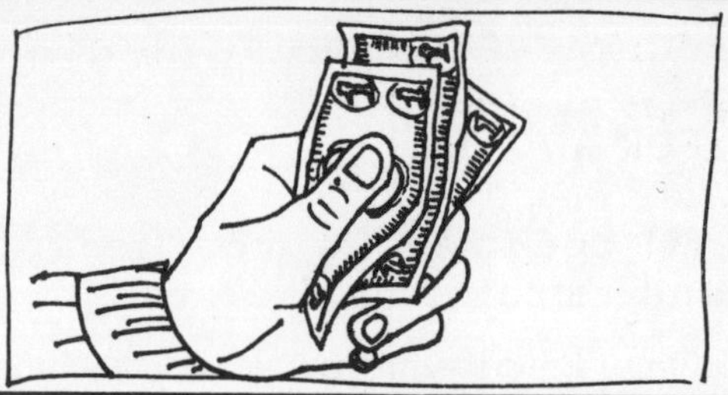

the cost/benefit assessment model. Transfer payments do have, however, important social and political implications depending upon how redistribution of income is perceived by the society. In socialist countries, these payments are treated as costs and are planned in the State budget.

24 The availability of transfer payments may alter the effectiveness of rehabilitation service provision and in this way affect the costs of services. In some cases, they may act as an incentive to the disabled person to undertake rehabilitation measures, and they may serve as a basic support for the disabled person's family, freeing other members of the family to return to active productivity. In other instances, they may serve as a disincentive to a return to as full and active a life as possible.

ECONOMIES IN REHABILITATION SERVICE PROVISION

25 The Group identified many factors related to the effectiveness of rehabilitation service provisions which could either increase or decrease the basic costs of such services. These include:

(i) The capability of the rehabilitation system to actively involve the disabled person in the rehabilitation process and to enhance his or her self-motivation.

(ii) The exclusive use of highly qualified personnel without involving auxiliaries, aides, volunteers or members of the community, or the use of unnecessarily sophisticated equipment and techniques to deliver services.

(iii) The creation of cumbersome administrative systems and/or institutions geared to meeting the needs of the system rather than those of the disabled person; the lack of procedures - economic and administrative - to maintain and utilize existing services adequately.

(iv) The quality and quantity of services provided in both rural and urban regions to different groups in the disabled population with varying production capabilities and in activities of varying production potential.

(v) The integration of the components of the rehabilitation process for each disabled person and the relative effectiveness of each component (medical, social, cultural, vocational and educational) as well as the integration of the entire process into existing community systems.

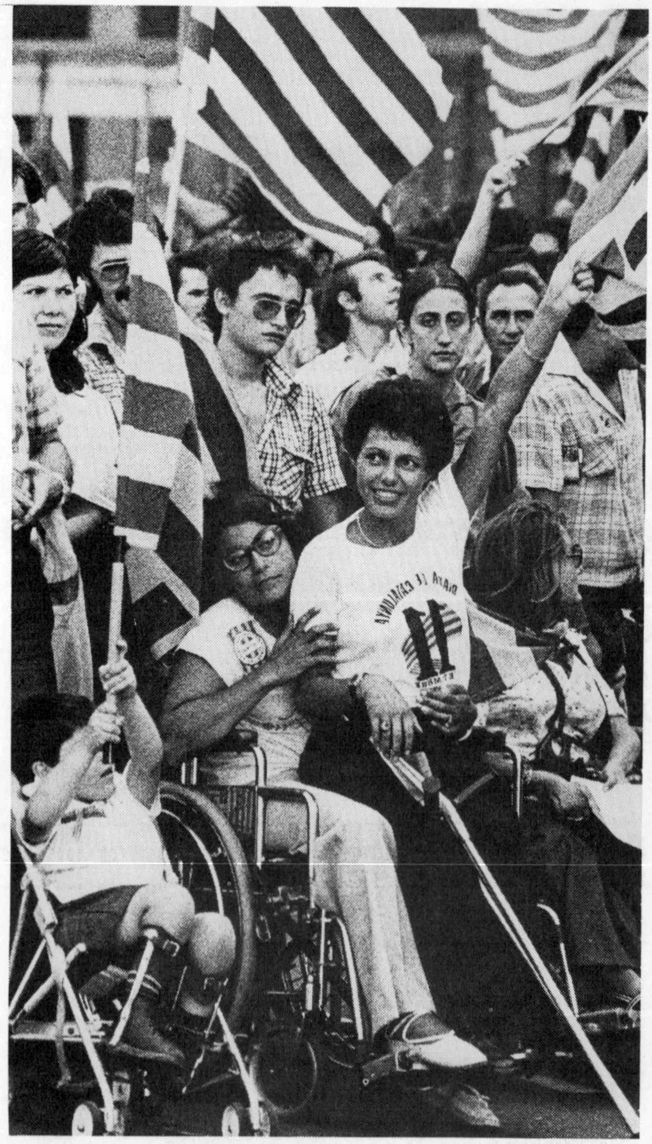

"to actively involve the disabled person..."

(vi) The comprehensive nature of the services provided and their continuity - to assure the maximum effect of initial investments in people and facilities.

26 Economies in the provision of rehabilitation services were emphasized as being of the greatest importance in any instance where resources are limited, particularly in developing countries.

27 It was agreed that the basic costs of rehabilitation service cannot be compared with the costs of disability prevention, since, among other things, it is impossible to measure the price of suffering avoided. It is the responsibility of rehabilitation specialists to help planners define the basic costs of rehabilitation services in their own countries on the basis of the kinds of services needed and the number of people needing such services. These costs will vary according to the situation and values in each country.

CHANGING PATTERNS AND REALITIES OF INVESTMENTS AND SERVICES DELIVERY.

28 The costs of rehabilitation services provision and the implications of disability for society as a whole will be dependent upon the developmental pattern of each nation, the quality of development and changing realities in delivery of educational, health, vocational and social services particularly as they relate to the delivery of rehabilitation services.

"It is impossible to measure the cost of suffering avoided."

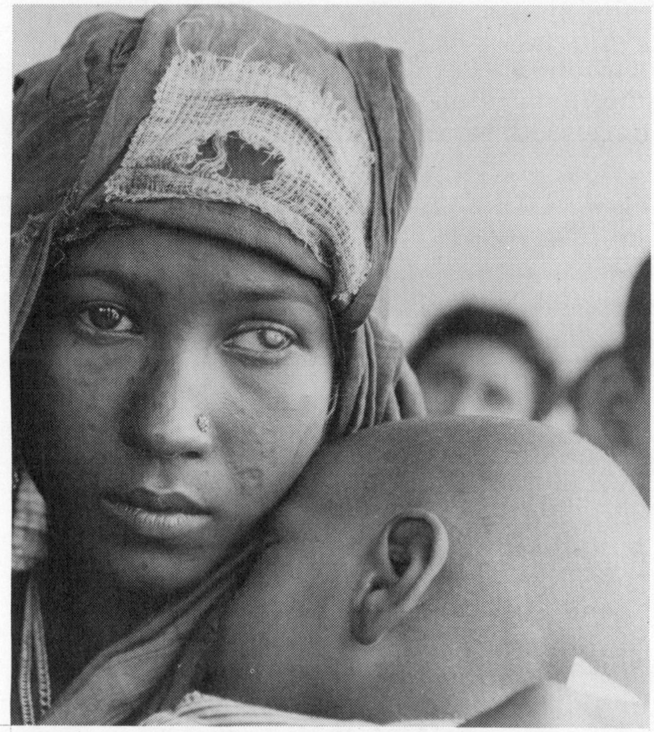

29 Investments in rehabilitation service delivery should, therefore, be examined in relation to:

(i) The overall type and condition of a nation's economy: market or centrally planned, an economy which is mainly developed, underdeveloped, or under-utilized; an economy characterized by full employment, massive unemployment or under-employment; an economy in recession or buoyant; an agrarian or industrially based economy;

Population growth is a major factor in consideration of service provision

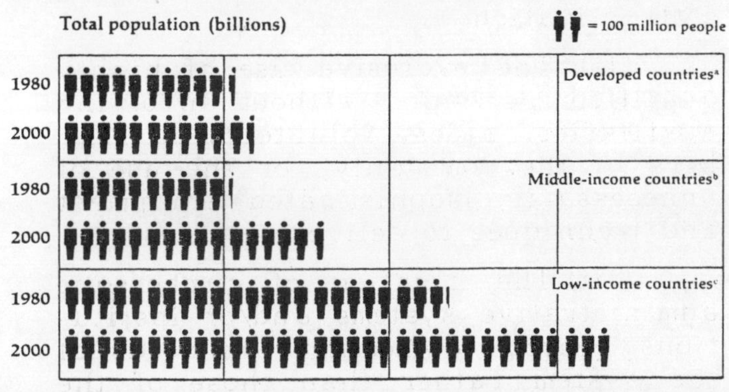

a. Includes Bulgaria, Czechoslovakia, German DR, Hungary, Poland, Romania, USSR
b. Includes Albania, Cuba, North Korea, Mongolia
c. Includes China

World Bank. World Development Report 1980.

(ii) the percentage of urban to rural population;

(iii) the availability of related education, health, vocational and social services and whether or not the nation was in a transitional phase in the provision of such services from the extended family to official provision;

(iv) changing demographic patterns which will alter the distribution and nature of facilities needed, e.g., advances in the proportion of the child population may increase the scope for vocational rehabilitation whereas advances in the proportion of the elderly may decrease it;

Population distribution by age, 1980

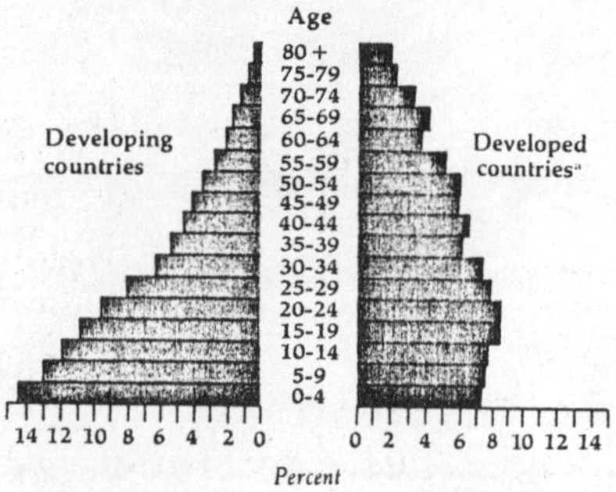

a. Include industrialized countries, the USSR and Eastern Europe.

World Bank. World Development Report 1980.

(v) changing patterns in the causes of disability which may also alter the distribution and nature of needed facilities, e.g., declining nutritional standards may increase disability related to malnutrition whereas improved education may reduce disability related to communicable diseases among children; increasing industrial and traffic accidents may introduce major new categories of orthopedic and neurological disability.

30 It was felt that where sufficiently developed education, health, vocational and social services existed, every effort should be made to integrate rehabilitation service delivery rather than to duplicate service delivery mechanisms, facilities and staff.

31 It was suggested that rehabilitation services should be planned to meet the assessed needs in a nation, not patterns or requirements transposed from other nations or areas. The service pattern should be tailored to fit the assessed needs of each area within the nation. Thus, for example, while vocational rehabilitation in an urban area may lead to a marketable skill, in rural non-monetarized economies it may more profitably be directed towards acquisition of useable skills for personal autonomy and independence.

32 The Expert Group recognized that the process of change never ends. Nations will vary in the degree of development achieved and in their place in the development process, but all nations must be cognizant of continuing changes in relation to the factors cited in paragraph 29 as they plan investments in rehabilitation service delivery.

33 The Group also identified the following factors more directly related to rehabilitation service delivery which can alter the pattern of service provision:

(i) the development of self-help organizations of disabled people and of family members, and the increased political action undertaken by such groups;

(ii) the creation of voluntary organizations for the disabled;

(iii) the availability of increasingly sophisticated services for technical assistance, detection, prevention and research related to disability, the possibility as well of over-mechanization and over-specialization in service delivery;

(iv) development of home service structures, reduced institutionalization, decentralized post-care services;

(v) increased public awareness of the needs of the handicapped, improved public attitudes toward the handicapped;

(vi) increased community involvement in rehabilitation efforts, removal of physical and social barriers to participation of disabled people in community life;

(vii) coordinated and collaborative service provision leading to comprehensive service delivery;

"changing attitudes towards the work of housewives."

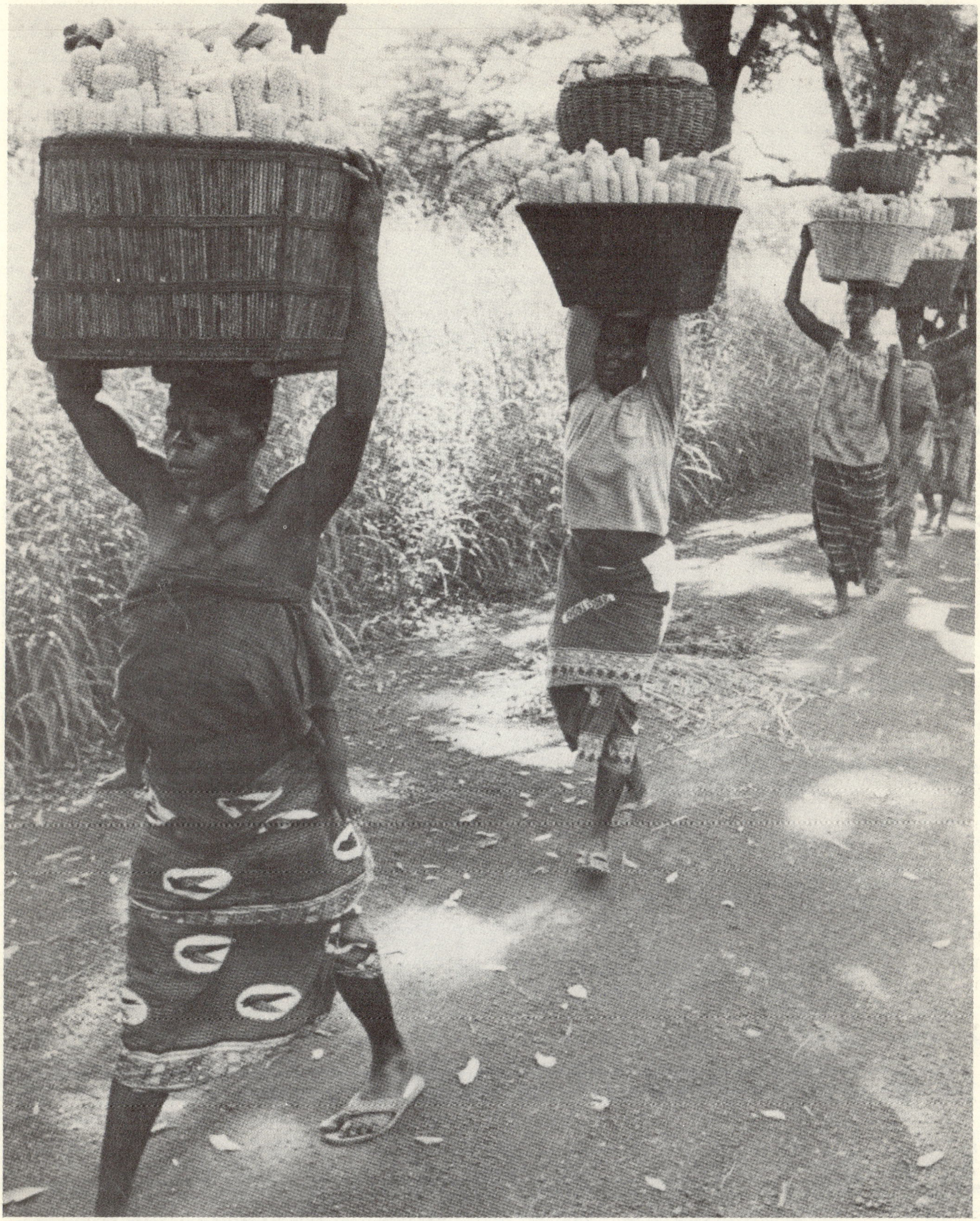

(viii) provisions of remunerative work for the disabled, changing attitudes towards the work provided by housewives;

(ix) increasing state assumption of responsibility for financing or providing services, extended coverage of social security systems, decreasing role of, or financing by, voluntary organizations.

II. Measurement of Socio-Economic Implications of Disability

General Principles

34 It was suggested that there is a need for terms applied to this subject to be defined, bearing in mind their relevance in both developed and developing nations.

35 Disability connotes a deviation from some societal norm. Such deviations or differences will be perceived differently in different cultures and under different socio-economic conditions. The specific definitions of disability will affect not only the measurement process but also the condition of the disabled individual in his or her society. It is easier to agree on a specific definition of the individual's impairment than it is to agree on a definition of functional limitations. This will differ from individual to individual and will be related in society to existing attitudes and services. Families will also differ in the way they regard the problem of the disability of one of their members.

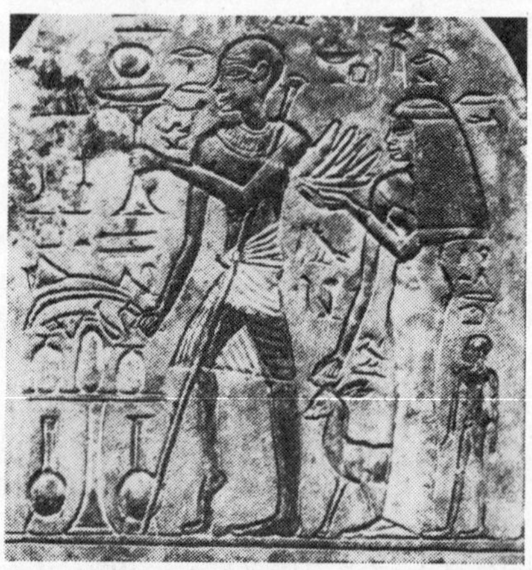

disabled Egyptian shown on stone tablet

36 Planners have been attempting to assess the costs of disability since earliest times. The laws of Hammurabi include estimations of disability compensation. It is important for planners to consider the impact of disability on development plans from the outset.

37 The costs of disability accrue regardless of whether or not rehabilitation services are available. One of the effects of rehabilitation is to reduce the costs of disability; for the individual and for society, however, in many instances disability creates irrevocable loss. The costs of disability must therefore be borne in some way within society, whether by the individual, by the State, by the family, by voluntary agencies or by some combination of all groups.

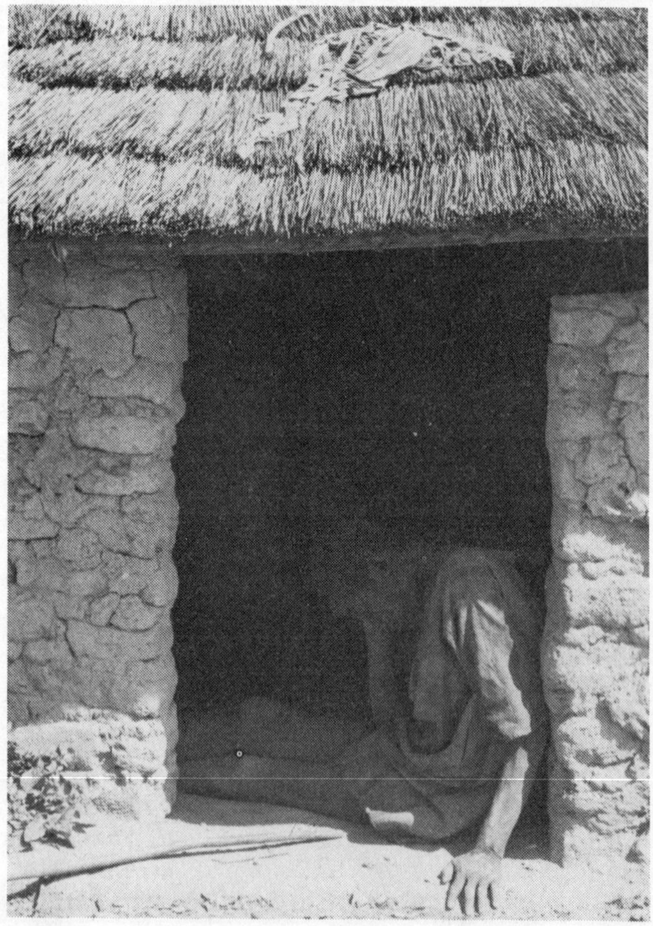

"The costs of disability accrue, whether or not rehabilitation services are available."

IMPLICATIONS FOR THE WORK FORCE, THE LABOUR MARKET AND INCOME DISTRIBUTION.

38 Loss of skill and experience. Disability can have serious financial implications for industry in terms of labour turnover and retraining of new workers. The volume of this loss is greater in the developed countries where a much higher percentage of disabled people will have previously received training and more has been invested in this training and their acquisition of skills. Nevertheless, the relatively small loss in the developing countries can be very serious where the skill in question is in short supply.

39 The disabled worker, with less flexibility than other workers, is more at risk of losing job skills when a change in employment situation occurs, when labour market conditions are altered or when new technologies are introduced. (Particular attention may be drawn to the disabled among migrant workers who, as a group, have been found to be "more exposed to disease and accidents than national workers in the same environment" and thus are often more at risk.) The loss of job skills through these factors can sharply reduce any gains achieved by rehabilitation investments for the disabled person.

40 Disability may force people to remain idle and be dependent on those working. In countries with unemployment or the likelihood of unemployment, the disabled may be relegated to reserve labour force status, be employed only when demand for labour is very high, be laid off as soon as demand falls and, generally, be given the least job security. Disability often confers low social status, affecting all of the person's relationships and, particularly as far as the work force is concerned, with employers and colleagues. The precise implications of disability for the individual depend on his or her sex, age (stage in the life cycle), marital status, whether there are family dependents and family size, extent of his or her social network, socio-economic group and whether he or she is an employee or self-employed.

"Disability may force people to remain idle and be dependent on those working."

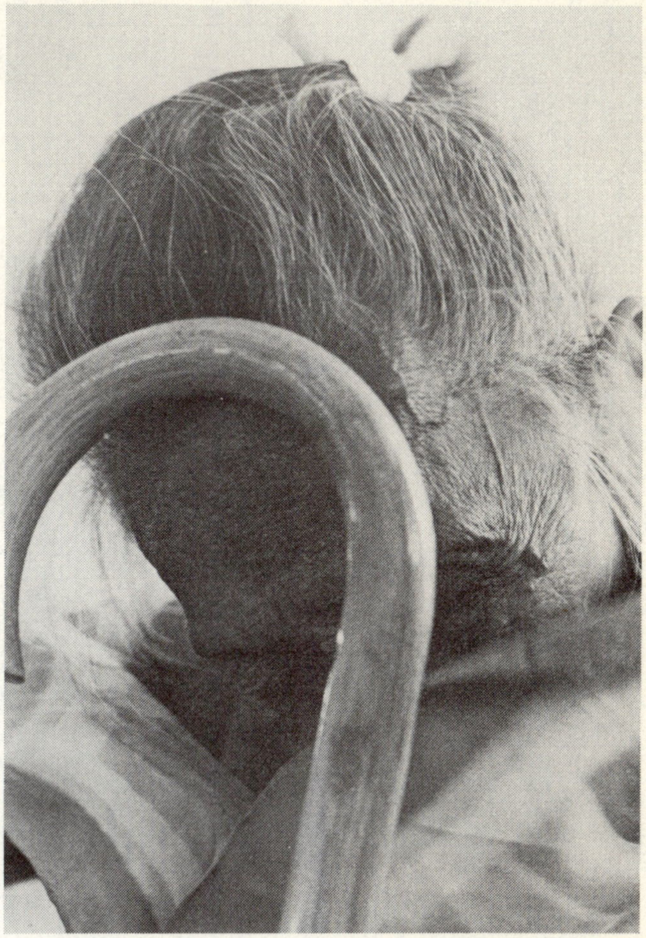

41 Disability may produce secondary effects on the work force participation of those close to the disabled person. When these effects are taken into account, a large proportion of the working population may be found to be adversely affected by disability, certainly much more than the 10% of the population generally recognized as having mental or physical disability. On the basis of the average family size, the proportion of the population thus affected by disability could be at least 25%. Productivity may also be affected by secondary emotional disturbance, stress and other psycho-social problems that lead to an increase in work accidents and lessened output.

"the proportion of the population affected could be 25%"

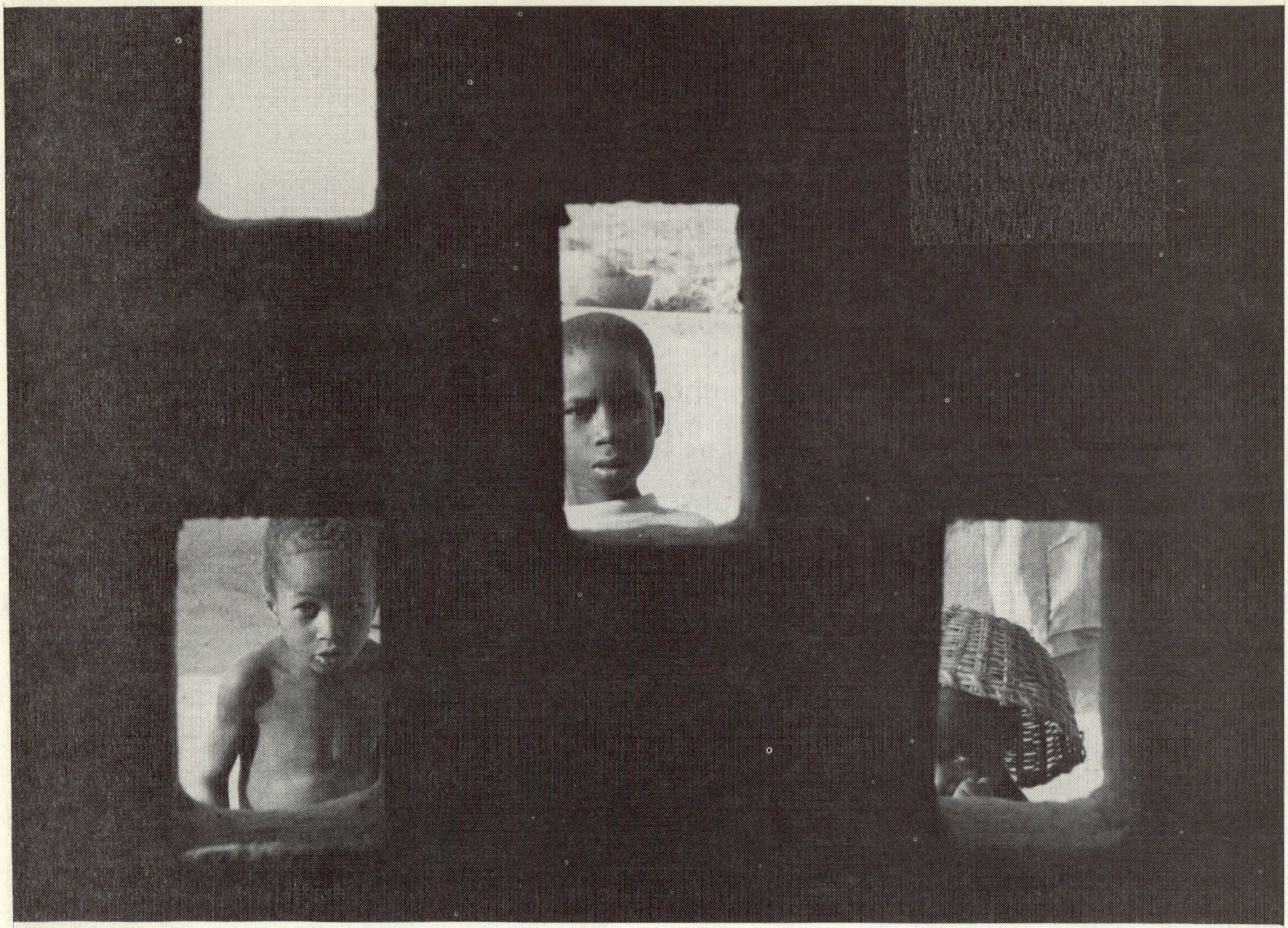

42 The implications of disability will also depend on certain characteristics of the country: whether there are effective guarantees in labour legislation for workers who become disabled, whether enterprises wish to or are able to circumvent this legislation, the existence and extent of social security legislation, and access to health care, to rehabilitation and to subsidized or sheltered employment.

43 The costs of disability will be greatest where nations are in need of an increased active work force. Disability may reduce the active work force capability of a nation with a resultant effect on the support of the social benefit system. Thus, for example, many industrial countries are willing to pay older workers and the disabled costly pensions to encourage them to leave the labour market and create places for new workers. In some industrialized nations with aging populations and increased numbers of disabled persons, there is a trend towards reduced numbers of active workers supporting each recipient of social benefits. In other nations, the population in younger age groups is increasing. These trends have long-term effects of the financial bases of social benefit schemes. In developing countries with normally low rates of employment, planners may erroneously conclude that it is unnecessary to include the disabled in the labour policy.

44 The Group considered the possible relationships of a policy of "preferential access" to jobs for disabled people and the displacement of able-bodied workers from the labour market. This is of particular importance in situations of under and unemployment. From some economic investment points of view, it can be argued that the most productive members of society should have the first opportunity to be employed. Such an argument will be related to the value placed by each society on productivity. Alternatively, it was agreed that disabled people should receive preference in obtaining jobs and training as a matter of social equity since they are more at risk of failing to become productive on the basis solely of their own resources.

45 Emphasis was placed on the possibility of creating job opportunities for the disabled without detracting from the existing opportunities for the non-disabled. In developing countries, for example many opportunities for setting up new industrial handicraft and agricultural activities exist and can positively contribute to national growth.

46 Income distribution. Disability will often lead to poverty or disruptive change in economic status for the disabled individual and for his or her family, creating a more unequal distribution of income in society. The effect on the distribution of income between households may be doubly adverse: the disabled person loses his or her income from work, and the need to care for the disabled person may cause his or her spouse or some other family member to stop working.

47 The adverse implications of disability for the distribution of income will be less serious:

- where rehabilitation is generally available and operates in conjunction with labour legislation which e.g. may ensure continued employment in the original workplace or with government supported employment schemes;
- where social security exists (although this may not be very effective where only a minority of the population is covered and where that minority is far from being the least well-off in general, where levels of protection vary and are very low (e.g. below poverty level) for some of the groups covered and where the level of protection depends on the cause of the disability (e.g. whether or not

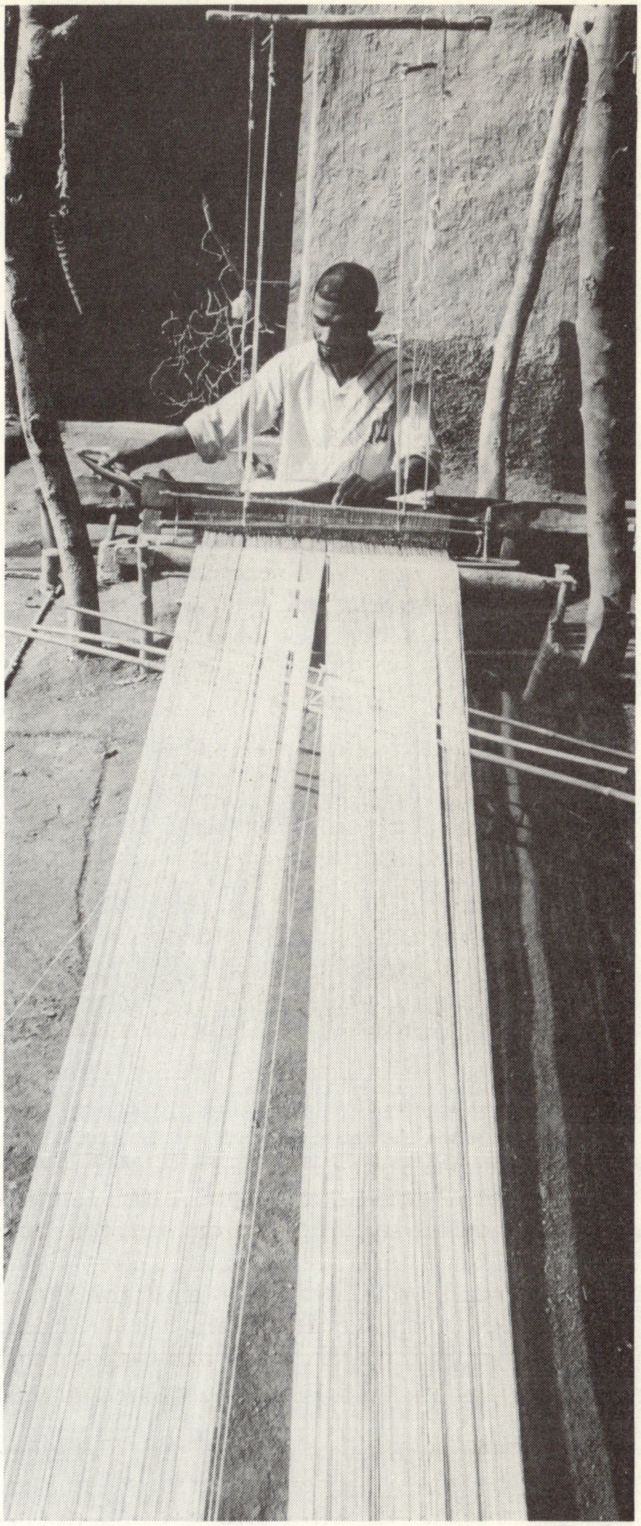

"the possibility of creating job opportunities for the disabled without detracting from opportunities for the non-disabled."

from industrial injury) rather than on its consequences);

- where health and social services are available locally and free of charge.

48 For the rural population in developing countries, the need to travel to the cities for treatment will not only act as a drain on any remaining income, but may use up the entire savings of a family.

49 Measuring the implications. It is conceptually possible to measure many of the effects of disability on essentially economic areas such as the work force and income distribution. The following sorts of data would be useful:

- absolute number of disabled,
- the incidence of disability in different age groups,
- data on the kind and degree of handicap,
- percentage of the disabled who leave the work force entirely and do/do not receive an invalidity pension,
- labour force participation rate of the disabled vs. non-disabled,
- employment rate of adults in households with a disabled member vs. that of adults in households without such a member,
- household income data, comparing households with and those without a disabled member,
- percentage of the disabled who never enter the work force,
- prevalence, especially life-time prevalence, and the incidence of disability.

50 Variables which condition the effects of disability may also be measured, e.g. the number of places provided for individuals in rehabilitation; vocational training possibilities in general compared with some measure of the number of places required; the percentage of the work force covered by social security.

Chart 1

Hypothetical Interrelations between Social Benefits of Rehabilitation that do not Contribute to Return to Paid Employment

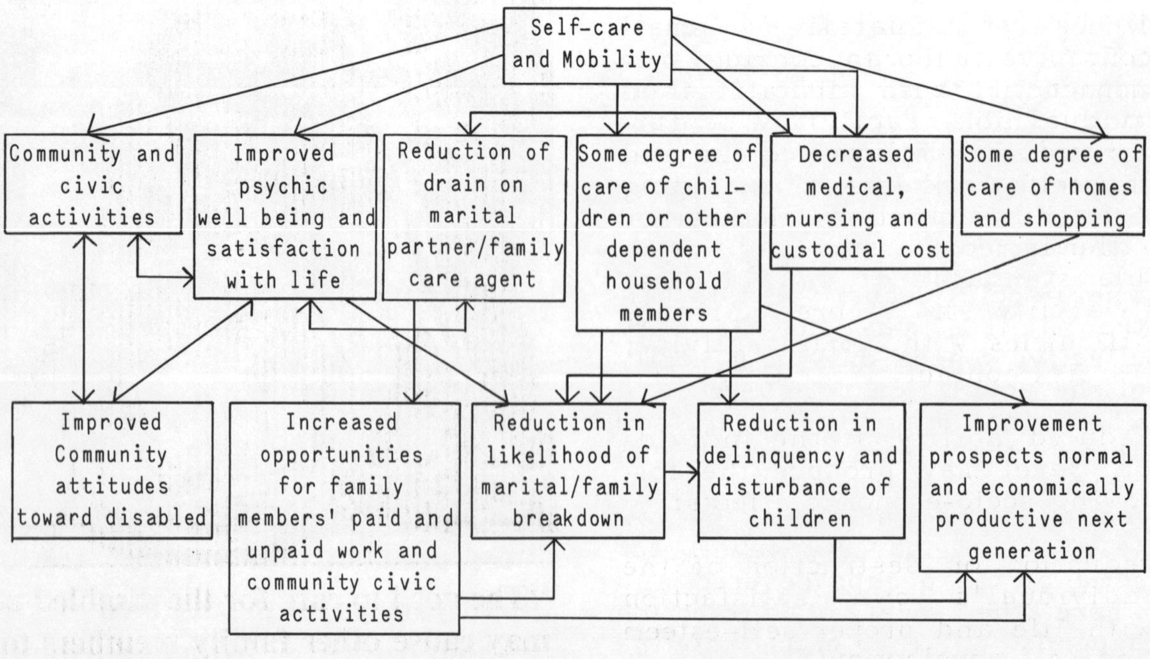

IMPLICATIONS OF DISABILITY FOR FAMILY LIFE AND PRODUCTIVITY, SOCIAL SERVICE AND HEALTH SERVICE CONSUMPTION

51 Chart I illustrates the social implications of disability as related to four levels of society:

(i) the individual

(ii) the family

(iii) the local community (e.g. village)

(iv) the wider (national) community.

52 Disability may limit an individual's ability for self care whether for reasons of physical, sensory or mental handicap: the inability unaided to wash, dress and do hair; feed himself/herself; use a toilet; change posture (e.g. from sleeping to daytime posture) and move about within the home and outside, to carry out a vast range of activities from getting an object that is just out of reach, through getting to the fields or to fetch water or milk for the household, to the complex mobility of industrialized/urban living (driving a car, using public transport, having access to shops and public buildings).

53 It is a comparatively small conceptual step to consider the impact of these limitations on the individual's own activities of daily living: reduced ability to clean and clothe himself or herself, including making/ fetching/ washing clothes, or to keep the immediate surroundings to acceptable standards of sanitariness; reduced ability to secure/ prepare food; difficulties with sexual activity; reduced social contact.

54 Reduced ability at the individual level may produce the following socio-economic effects:

- reduction or destruction of the individual's own satisfaction with life and proper self-esteem and self-development;

"Children may face reduced opportunities for social integration and learning experiences."

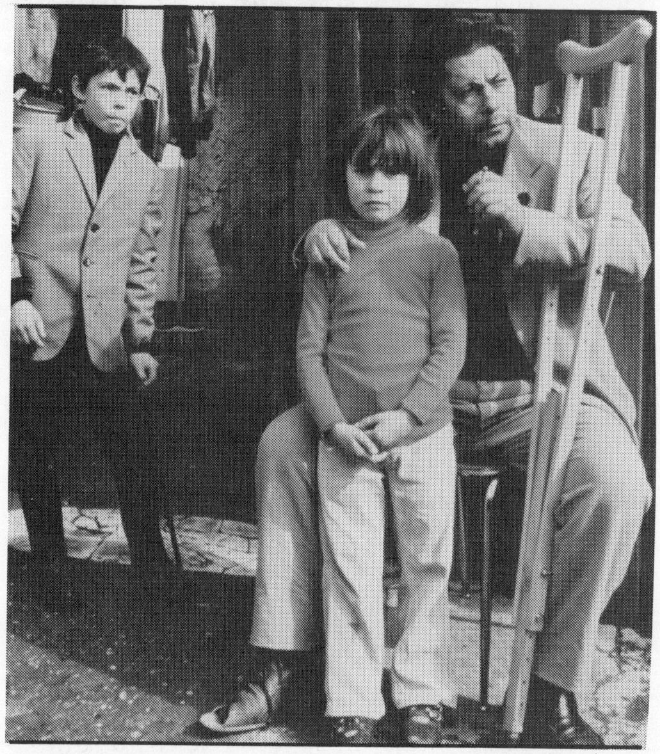

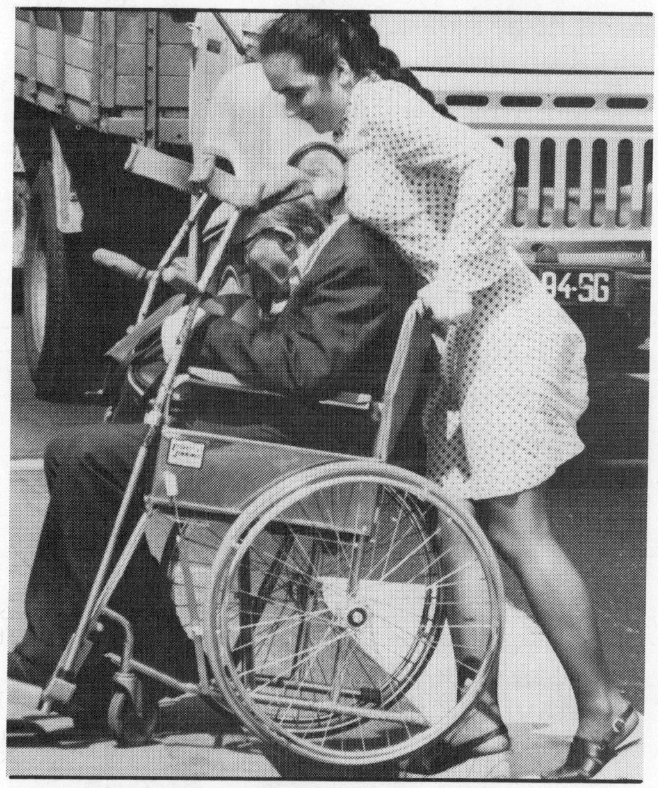

"The need to care for the disabled person may cause other family members to stop working."

- increased personal stress, both physical and emotional, for marital partners and family members, whether or not they themselves are the care providers, and demand for attendant and/or "nursing" care;

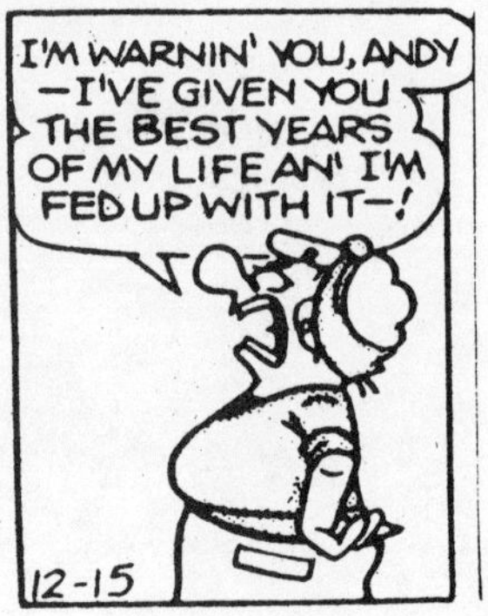
I'M WARNIN' YOU, ANDY —I'VE GIVEN YOU THE BEST YEARS OF MY LIFE AN' I'M FED UP WITH IT—!
12-15

- reduced ability to care for children or undertake household tasks;

- reduction of the time and energy available to others of the household and friends for work activity inside or outside the home, paid or unpaid;

- reduction of the social contribution/interaction of the individual: loss of friends, loss of educational opportunity, reduced chances of forming a marriage and family of his or her own (this may differ for men and women, and according to different social settings);

- reduction of the status of the family in the community, possibly making it the focus of fear or aversion in the local community;

- rejection of the individual by the family as a result of the above effects leading to expensive institutionalization which may, in turn, lead to added chronic dependency and possible loss of all prospects for rehabilitation.

55 When consideration of the activities of daily living is extended to the whole range of social and economic activities which may be involved in management of the household, including the care of children or other dependent persons, it is clear that the implications of disability may include the likelihood of family or marital breakdown and reduced opportunities for the children to take part in normal social interaction or learning situations whether in terms of formal education or traditional skills. It may create a need for children to require professional care or institutionalization or lead to delinquency in the next generation and/or reduced earning capacity from those children when they grow up.

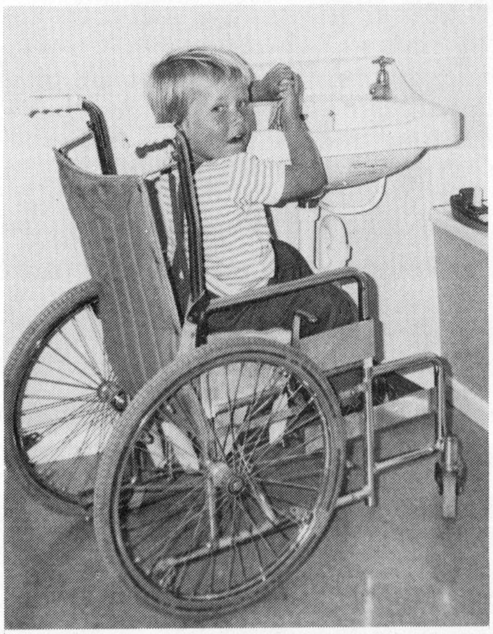

"Disability may limit an individual's ability for self-care."

56 Measurement tools exist for virtually all of these factors. It is suggested that planners in developing countries should acquaint themselves with some of the batteries of measures developed in industrialized countries, selecting those most appropriate or most adaptable to their own circumstances. Such use should be within the context of an overall project design which would minimize built-in bias.

57 Examples of measurement tools include:

(i) Psycho-metric measures for such factors as satisfaction with life. Simpler measures, e.g. the amount of time spent complaining, are sometimes also quite valuable.

(ii) Measurement of activity limitations in terms of time. A time-diary could be very valuable to measure the precise way a handicapped person spends his or her time before and after rehabilitation, e.g. time spent lying in bed, using the services of others to fetch and carry or for personal care, complaining, etc. should all be significantly reducible. Simple symbol systems could be utilized, particularly when literacy is low.

(iii) Self-care activity measures in the form of a check list with an interview guide. These usually require very little training and are already in use in some industrialized countries.

(iv) Measures of housewife disability in relation to the normal range of activities expected in a given socio-cultural background.

(v) Behavioural check lists of other types. A prepared list could be filled in with the assistance of family and neighbours as well as using observations and the handicapped person's own response to give a full picture. It should be done by people familiar with the local socio-cultural background.

58 Difficulties of attracting trained staff to rural posts in developing countries and retaining such staff in rural positions were recognized. The use of aides selected and trained from each local community was suggested. Specialized workers with a wider background of medical and social work training would be needed to periodically supervise such local aides and maintain liaison with specialized facilities in the urban areas.

59 A form of negative measurement was recognized, in that it is possible to examine what happens to individuals, families and their communities when no rehabilitation is provided. In those societies where adequate rehabilitation resources exist, where there is full capability to provide needed services, and where the effects of the services provided are fully understood, examination of a control group denied services would not be possible on ethical grounds since the rights of the individuals in the control group would be infringed upon for experimental purposes. No society has as yet achieved such a total capability to provide and to understand the effects of its rehabilitation services. In those developing countries or in other situations where resources simply do not yet exist on the scale required to serve all, it may be possible and could be ultimately valuable to send into the areas not receiving rehabilitation services observers who would record exactly what happens. A carefully matched comparison could then be made with similar cases receiving rehabilitation. Pictures and case histories on such a basis could have more impact than many statistics.

"Disability may reduce the active work force capability of a nation, with a resultant effect on the support of the social benefit system."

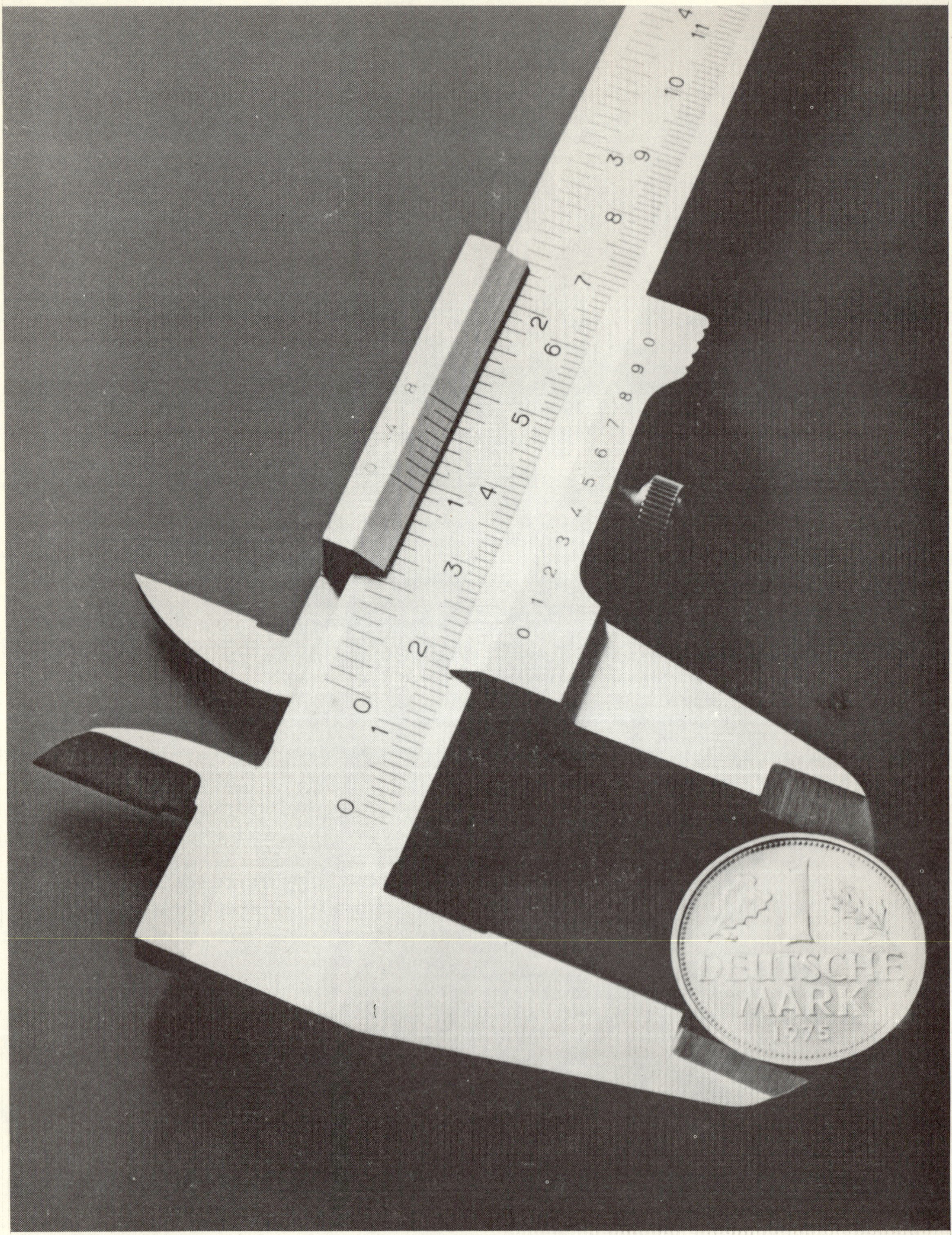
DEUTSCHE
MARK
1975

III. Comparison of the Costs and Benefits of Rehabilitation Service Provision

COST BENEFIT ASSESSMENT AND ITS VARIABLES

60 Cost-benefit analysis is an economic assessment procedure which attempts to evaluate the advantages and losses to society of a given policy or action or of a series of alternative policies and actions. It requires the ability to measure the effects in economic units which are comparable. Important variables exist in cost/benefit assessment methodology which limit its application to social phenomena, in particular to disability and the delivery of rehabilitation services. These variables may be structural and methodological.

61 Methodological variables. Some examples of methodological variables in cost-benefit analysis considered by the meeting included:

- the sampling technique used to identify disabled people: questionnaires, self-selection, random sampling;
- the definition and type of disability;
- the method of measurement, e.g. of determining wages before and after rehabilitation;
- the comparability of data collected from different sources;
- the perspective of the analysis: costs and benefit to whom - society, the individual, the institution;
- the characteristics of the sample population: e.g. age, sex, and educational differences;
- the choice of discount rate.

62 The choice of discount rate can strongly influence the outcome of the cost-benefit assessment. It represents the "opportunity" cost of having spent funds for one purpose which might have been used for some other pupose. It takes into account the risks associated with the investment, the present value of future uses of the alternative investment and the range of uncertainty as to future benefits. Because so little is known about risks and foregone opportunities, economists apply a range of discount rates which produces a wide range of cost-benefit ratios.

63 Structural variables. Some factors which may be considered as structural and which can alter radically the outcome of the cost-benefit analysis include:

- the quality and extent of rehabilitation service coverage;
- the extent of awareness in society of the availability of rehabilitation services;
- the placement of service costs within various levels of the social service system and the shifting of costs between levels;
- the availability of income transfers as an alternative to paid work;
- community attitudes towards not working.

Cross national research may be complicated by the presence of structural variables between nations which may not exist within a single nation.

64 To the extent that rehabilitation investments and/or proposals for allocating scarce resources for rehabilitation purposes are subject to the test of economic efficiency, cost-benefit analyses of rehabilitation services can be strategic in guiding investment decisions, provided that they are valid.

65 Measurement of the concepts of benefits and costs, however, will be likely to require quite different techniques in developed and developing countries. In applying cost-benefit analysis to developing countries, it will be necessary to shift the emphasis of case service costs to unpaid services rendered on behalf of handicapped persons. Developing countries, as a result of their economic situation, will probably have to seek a catalytic effect from small budgetary allocations of cash. This may take place by spending to unleash the unpaid services of informal groups and family members themselves on behalf of the handicapped with the objective of helping the handicapped achieve greater independence. In this regard, these unpaid services, released perhaps by small cash expenditures, would be part of the social costs of rehabilitation since they consume the real resources of time and energy of persons in the community who could have put this time and energy to an alternative and potentially more productive use.

66 The major problems of applying cost-benefit analysis to rehabilitation services in developing countries are:

(a) to specify how budgetary expenditures are to be used to stimulate unpaid services of families and members of the community on behalf of handicapped persons;

(b) to link, via "cause-and-effect" models, the unpaid services intervention to the expected rehabilitation outcomes;

(c) to make operative whatever concepts of benefits and costs are consistent with the form of rehabilitation intervention selected;

(d) to implement the study design that will permit collection of data according to the operational definitions of benefits and costs.

67 The problems of applying cost-benefit analysis to rehabilitation services in developed countries are the same, except for the emphasis on measuring benefits of unpaid work and the costs of unpaid services. These may be more prevalent in developing countries. If the decision is to proceed with a cost-benefit analysis because it is felt budgetary decisions will be favourably affected, then rehabilitation planners must take great care to think through carefully and systematically what means they are going to adopt to achieve specified rehabilitation results. Once the model of rehabilitation intervention, with cause-and-effect specifications as hypotheses, has been set forth, it will be necessary to develop the appropriate measurement and accounting system to capture the costs of intervention and the benefits along as many dimensions as are relevant and/or feasible.

68 Limitations of the Cost-Benefit-Method. The meeting recognized that cost-benefit analysis is only a tool, and it is one tool among many in assessing the impact of rehabilitation services or in deciding which segments of the disabled population should receive services. The greatest danger of misuse lies in any decision to exclude the disabled, or particular groups of the less productive disabled, from service provision on the basis of a cost-benefit analysis. The other serious limitation is that the analysis may not fully take into account non-monetary values such as changes in capability for self-care, the satisfaction of working, the stimulation and benefits of education. Nor can the cost benefit model indicate the value placed by disabled people on different aspects of the rehabilitation services they receive.

69 Even the designation of monetary values is relative. The same amount of money will mean different things to different people in different circumstances as will the same amount of costs and benefits mean different things in different societies. It is important for rehabilita-

"Nor can the cost-benefit model indicate the value placed by disabled people on the services they receive."

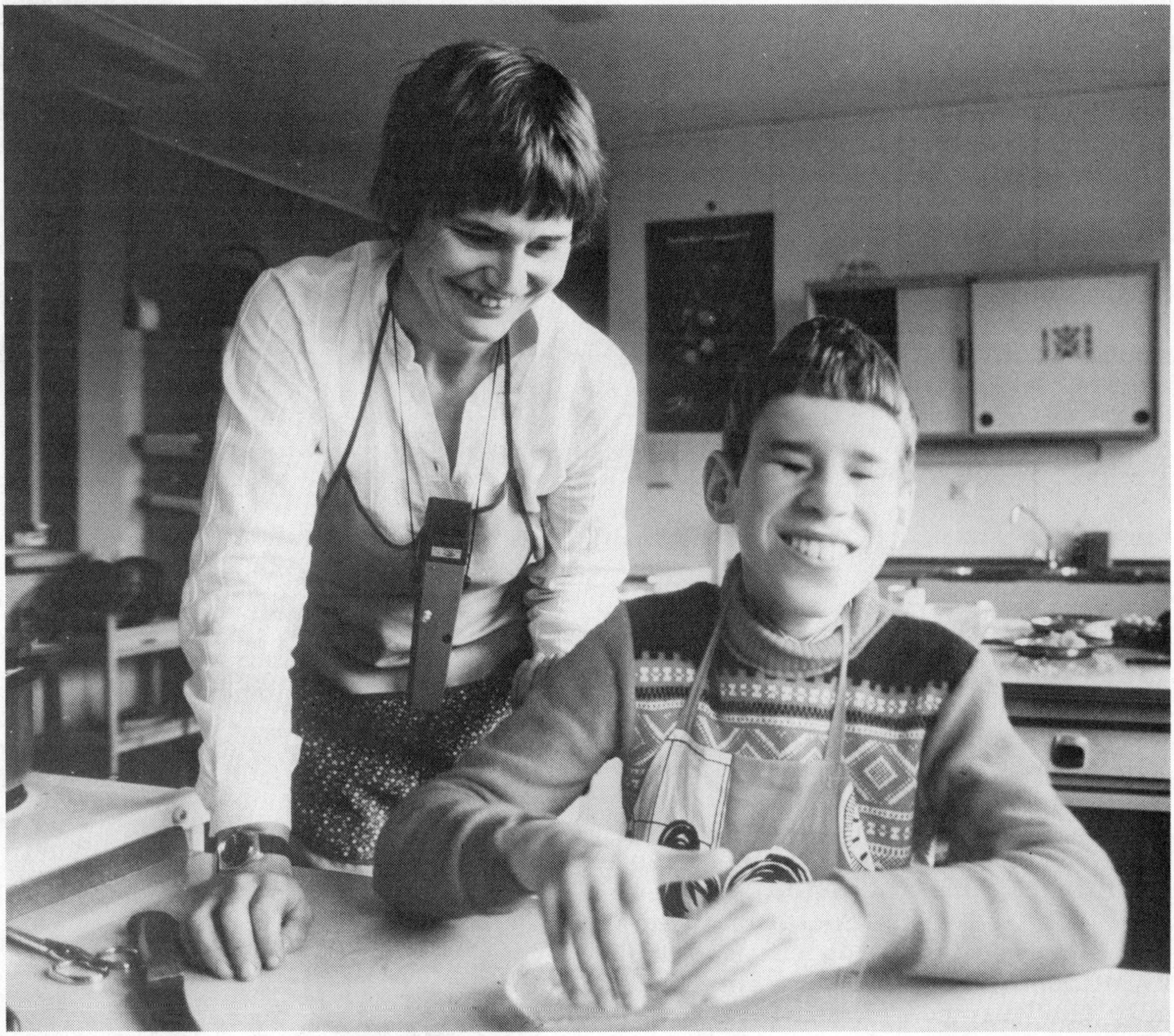

tion service providers to describe fully all of the moral, social and monetary benefits of rehabilitation, since these constitute its value in reality.

70 Invalid analyses, when discovered, create backlash. If cost-benefit analysis of rehabilitation does not yield a net social gain, it may call into question the particular form of rehabilitation that is brought under scrutiny. The finding of a net social cost argues for discontinuation or alteration of the particular form of rehabilitation investment being analyzed, not for elimination of the whole enterprise. Once this fact is understood by policy decision-makers, the possibility of negative findings may be somewhat less threatening. Nothing can make those whose interests can make those whose interests are fixed in a particular form of rehabilitation investment which has been found wanting feel better about the negative cost-benefit analysis received. If, however, the form of rehabilitation found wanting is the only way of channelling resources to the disabled according to some existing standards of social equity, the cost-benefit analysis should not countermand continued investment in that form.

71 If the case for rehabilitation expenditures can be made without recourse to the "cost-benefit" argument, then it makes no sense to spend scarce resources trying to conduct a cost-benefit analysis.

72 Development of an intervention plan. To the extent that budgetary authorities are reluctant to invest in rehabilitation because they have no evidence of the benefits and costs, rehabilitation planners might argue for pilot projects subject to cost-benefit measurements to prove their point. At times, this approach has won conditional approval for small initial rehabilitation investments in developed countries. It might also be useful to argue simultaneously for balanced investments in rehabilitation and in prevention of disability. Both are needed.

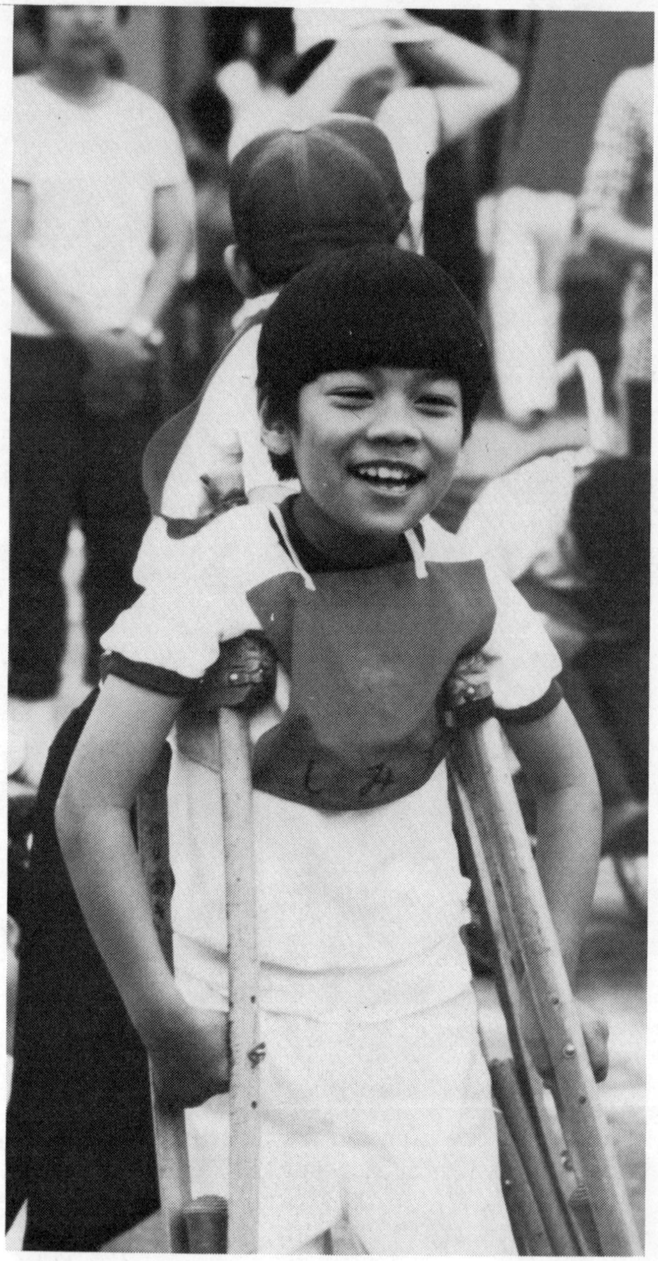

73 It is very important that budget authorities and policy makers at the highest level be made a part of the rehabilitation planning process. Their contribution should not focus on the technical means of achieving specific rehabilitation outcomes, but on the outcomes which they value enough to invest in initially and, if the cost-benefit analysis is positive, in the future. Once the outcome criteria are specified, rehabilitation planners will have to develop the model of intervention which they think will optimize the desired rehabilitation outcomes, subject to budgetary constraints.

74 Towards the end of the intervention planning process, it may be useful to utilize social research consultants to develop the measurement tools and study designs necessary to assess the concepts of benefits and costs consistent with the form of rehabilitation intervention selected. The study design must be adapted to the requirements of the intervention model, in the broadest sense of an "action system" linking all levels of organizational and personnel inputs to individuals and families and communities. Every effort must be made to insure the scientific integrity of the study design and its control of all variables except the one being manipulated and examined. This is to minimize inference concerning the cause-and-effect relationships between rehabilitation results and the particular form of rehabilitation chosen for study.

75 The accounting system for capturing the benefit and cost concepts selected will require custom tailoring. Developing countries necessarily will adopt rehabilitation interventions of "action systems" that reflect their unique characteristics. The schemes which have been devel-

in rehabilitation and in prevention of disability. Both are needed."

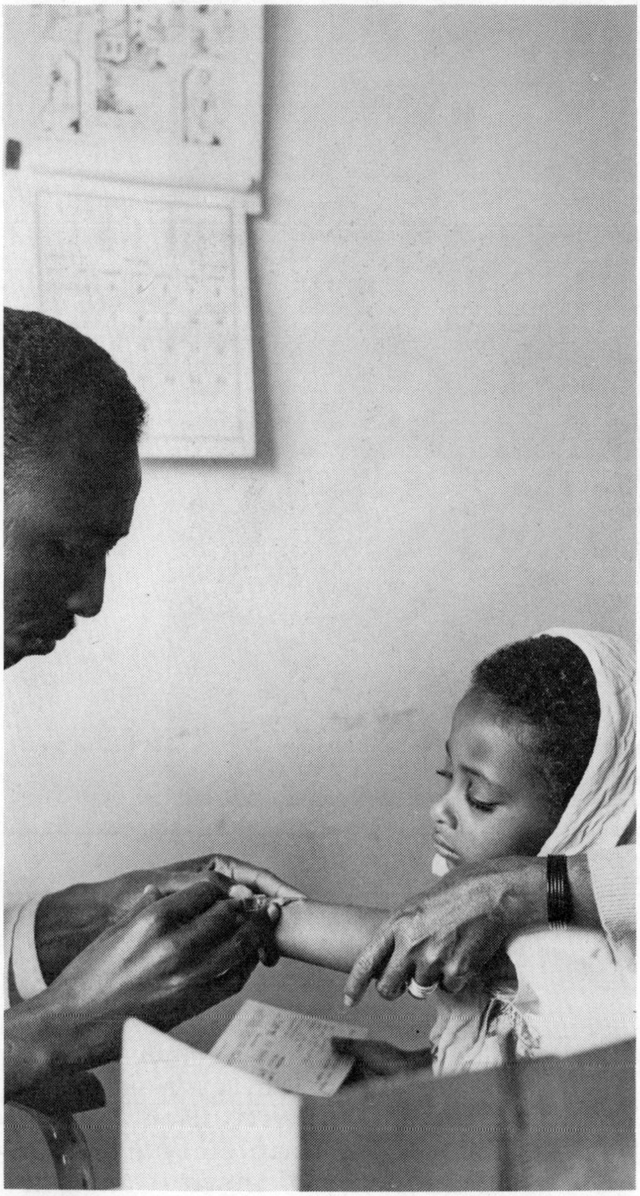

theless will infringe on "nature" and create some degree of artificiality. This is the price that must be borne to achieve documentation. Documentation includes not only the concepts of benefits and costs, but also the characteristics of the rehabilitation intervention that is eventually carried out. "Paper" plans have a way of shifting when tried under actual field conditions. Planners will want to understand what actually happened compared to what was planned, and whether or not it worked.

oped for the conduct of cost-benefit analyses in the developed countries should be examined for possible applicability in developing countries.

76 In no case should the developing country's form of rehabilitation intervention be unduly pushed out of shape to accommodate a cost-benefit accounting scheme. Instead, the accounting scheme of approximate utility, if there is one, should be shaped to fit the dimensions of the desired rehabilitation action system. Any accounting scheme never-

RELATIONSHIPS BETWEEN ECONOMIC AND SOCIAL GAINS AND REHABILITATION

77 It is difficult to demonstrate the link of cause and effect between rehabilitation service provision and the various beneficial outcomes already specified in this report. Many of the benefits may derive from the general structure of society itself, making the causal relationship ambiguous. As cited in paragraph 74, it is also most important in any cost-benefit study design to avoid inference of cause and effect relationships when the nature of the rehabilitation intervention is not precisely known. Rehabilitation services for the disabled may demonstrate many types of changes in human behaviour; the possibility for measurements of these changes has already been described (see paragraph 57).

78 Some of the major potential modification in social behaviour possible for disabled people as a result of rehabilitation include:

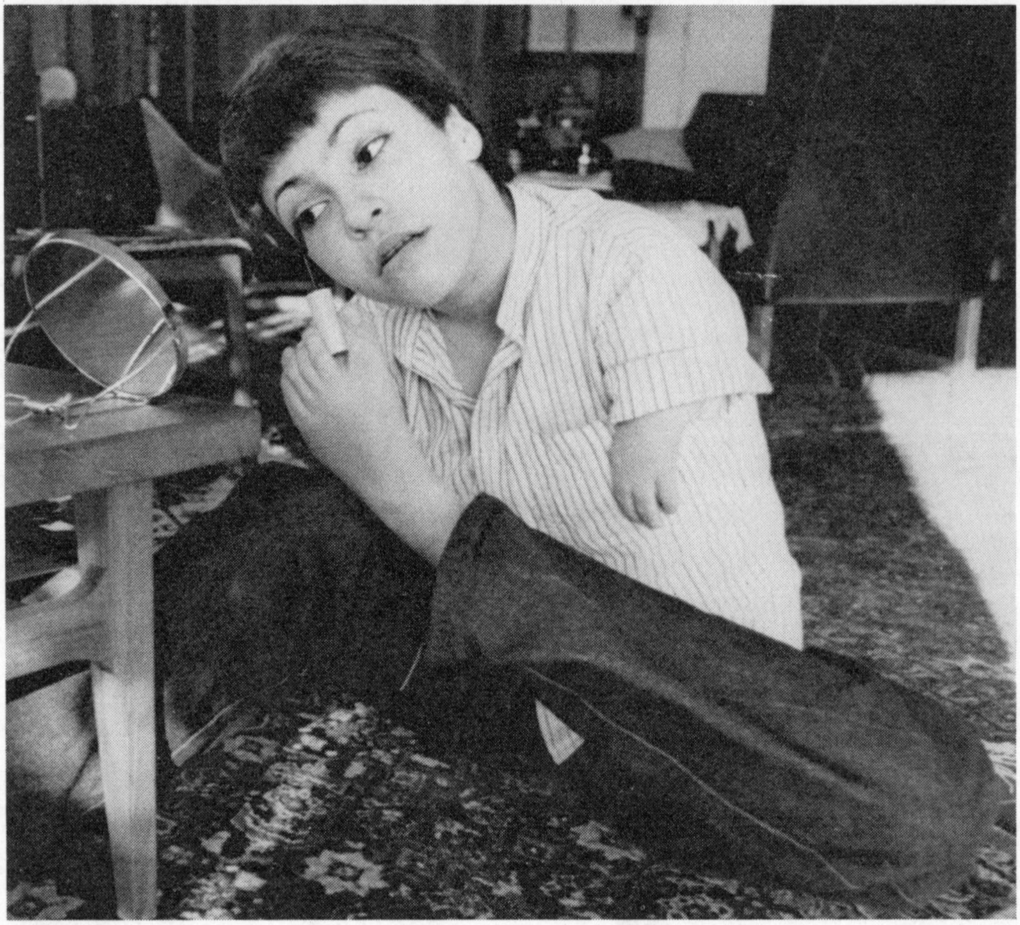

"Increased self-care and activities of daily living."

- improved self care and activities of daily living; even if remaining homebound, the disabled individual can reduce his or her demands for attendance/nursing/fetching/carrying;
- increased self-esteem and self-development;
- increased contribution to household management and serving in an advisory/ counselling/ service function in the community, especially where there is a basis of respect for such service, e.g. caring for children while parents are at work or at the market, undertaking home industry activities such as weaving, assembly and basketwork;
- reduced marital stress and increased possibilities for establishing marriage and family ties.

79 In addition, community attitudes towards the disabled may improve, other members of the family with a disabled member may be freed for economic activity and demands for costly institutionalization may be reduced or completely eliminated, particularly if institutions are adapted to family needs, e.g. to provide night care or day care for disabled people otherwise living at home.

80 As far as work and income are concerned, rehabilitation aims to rectify the adverse effects of disability, notably by:

- restoration of the disabled person to a useful role in the work force, thereby ensuring an income for him or her and his or her household and contributing to community and national development;

- raising the low social status of the disabled individual - improving, in particular, social relationships with colleagues and employers;

- integration or re-integration of the disabled in the community (and as one example, helping them better to articulate their needs through trade unions and political channels);

- mobilization of people in the community to become involved in rehabilitation efforts; such communal involvement may help to produce a healthier society and promote the general well-being of all of its members, particularly, by increasing their capacity to accept and deal with disability.

81 It is most important to avoid dehumanization of the rehabilitation process. The human bond which must exist between the rehabilitation service provider and the rehabilitation service recipient must be retained. In this way, only, can the full socio-economic potential of the rehabilitation services offered be achieved. In no instance should the humanitarian values of rehabilitation be overlooked nor should its capability to alter the lives of people be ignored.

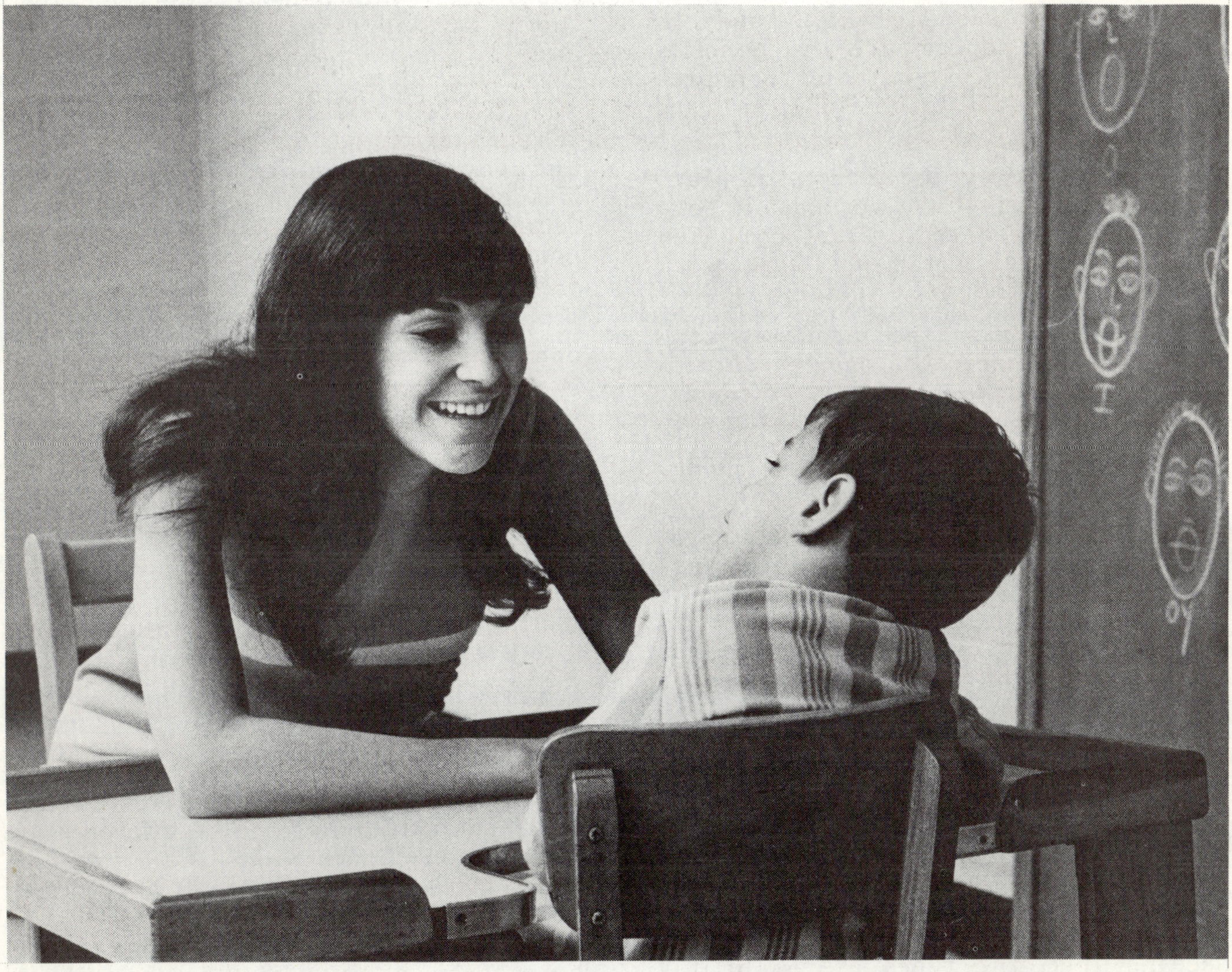

"The human bond between service provider and recipient must be retained."

Recommendations for Action

82 The Expert Meeting agreed there is a need to look for such new approaches to disability problems as may result in rehabilitation services fulfilling the requirements of both social equity and economic efficiency.

83 It was recommended that collaborative research should be undertaken by developed and developing countries to compare rehabilitation services of a similar type provided under varying conditions and to learn where economies can be obtained in achievement of the range of possible rehabilitation outcomes. Specifically, the following was suggested:

(i) replication of a study carried out in Sweden which used a control group to compare the benefits obtained with provision and non-provision of rehabilitation services (see also paragraph 84);

(ii) to study the effects of placing severely disabled workers in segregated sheltered employment compared with placement in the sheltered work departments of normal industry;

(iii) to study the problems confronted by different categories of disabled workers with totally different conditions of life and the relationship of these differences to rehabilitation service outcomes.

84 With regard to the first proposal it was noted (see paragraph 59) that it may not be possible to establish research control groups made up of individuals who do not receive rehabilitation services or who receive less than adequate services when denial of such services would constitute an infringement on their rights and existing entitlements. Such control groups could only be established ethically when sufficient resources did not exist within the nation or community to extend equitably to all of the disabled people needing them the types of rehabilitation service under examination.

85 It was further suggested that study/demonstration projects be initiated in a selected number of developing countries, the main objective of which would be to obtain information, presently unavailable, on disability and the delivery of rehabilitation services with particular emphasis on rural areas and ways in which rehabilitation may be provided through inexpensive and innovative methods employing appropriate technology and reaching larger numbers of disabled persons while avoiding unnecessarily lengthy periods of time spent in the rehabilitation process, and that further study be made of the values placed by disabled people on the various elements of rehabilitation services and the benefits derived from them; further research be carried out on:

(i) the effects of disability and rehabilitation services on the economic and emotional conditions in the families of the disabled, particularly with regard to the productivity of the non-disabled family members;

(ii) the effects of rehabilitation services on the children and dependents of disabled people, with regard to their health and educational development and their potential productivity;

(iii) the effect of disability on the active base of work force support for social benefit systems, particularly in developing countries;

(iv) the effect of unemployment and under-employment on labor policy towards the disabled in both developing and developed nations.

86 In this connection, the Expert Meeting recommended to the Second International Conference on Legislation Concerning the Disabled, which was held in January 1978, in Manila, the Philippines, that it consider the need for establishing a legal base for a policy which would promote in the private, as well as the public sector of any nation, the importance of keeping disabled people integrated in their prior work situations pre-disability to the maximum degree possible.

87 The International Institute for Rehabilitation in Developing Countries, located in Tehran, Iran, as a part of its mission to promote and develop methods for the low cost delivery of rehabilitation services, might consider:

- initiating research to prepare and follow simultaneously pilot projects and alternate models in various developing countries so as to make it possible to promote the exchange of national experience and mutual inspiration in the field of rehabilitation.
- evaluating its own success or failure in carrying out its mission over a specified period of time, to serve as the basis for modifications in its approach or policy, should this be necessary, and to serve, perhaps, as the basis for considering establishment of similar Institutes in other developing regions of the world.

88 The Expert Group agreed that further emphasis should be given to the need for a rehabilitation worker who can integrate services for the disabled client at some level in the rehabilitation service delivery system, possibly at the local community level. Such a worker would assure that the services provided would be comprehensive, effective, and economical. Special training of such personnel, who would retain ongoing responsibility for coordination of the client's total program, was recommended. Guidelines for the functions and qualifications of such a general rehabilitation auxiliary worker were proposed by a Rehabilitation International Expert Meeting in 1969 and could serve as the basis for further examination.

89 The Expert Group recognized that the prevention of disability and increased efforts in this regard would be directly relevant to economic assessment of the effects of disability and rehabilitation service provision in the future. This did not fall within the terms of reference of the Group, but it was agreed to be a subject area of great importance for further study.

90 Finally, the Group suggested that the possibilities should be explored of preparing useful public information materials tailored for both the general public, social planners, and for government decision makers to inform them, within the context of socio-economic investments in rehabilitation, about:

- the fundamental problems related to disability;
- the negative impact of disability on national development and well being, and
- why disability and its prevention should be of concern to all, and that a bibliography of references relevant to its discussions and to the United Nations study on this subject be published.

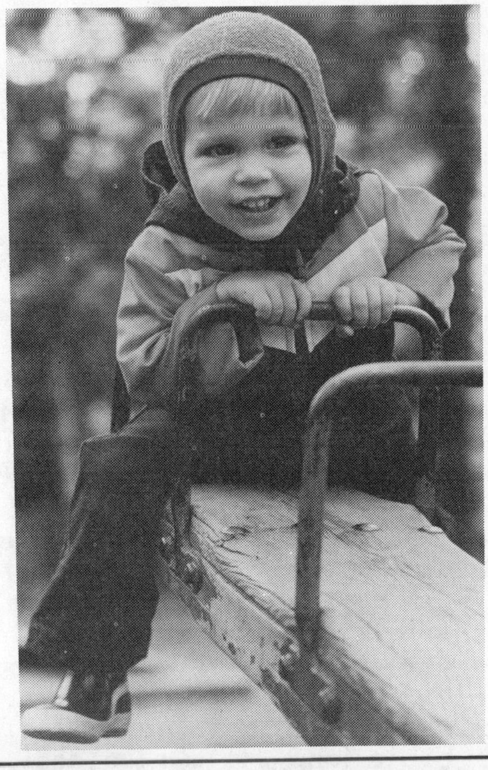

"Disability and its prevention should be of concern to all."

I. DISABILITY AND REHABILITATION: THE CONCEPTUAL FRAMEWORK

The sections of each chapter set in a one column format are excerpts from the United Nations report *Rehabilitation for the Disabled: The Social and Economic Implications of Investments, for this Purpose,* New York, 1977. Additional references appear in a two column format.

A. DEFINITIONS AND PREVALENCE OF DISABILITY

In general, disability -- the limitation in an individual's capacity to perform activities which are generally accepted as basic components of daily living, such as self-care, social relations, and economic activity, according to his or her age, sex, and social role, as a result of some physical or mental impairment -- is recognized as being the result of not only a physical or mental functional limitation but also of the individual's adjustment to it.

At least 10 percent of the population of any country suffers from some form of mental or physical disability, the most prevalent forms being physical impairment, chronic illness, mental retardation and sensory disabilities. There are more than 400 million disabled people in the world. (1975. See page 32 for current estimates.) The World Health Organization, in a recently completed estimation of the causes of disability and the number of disabled people in the world, found non-communicable somatic diseases and malnutrition to be the main causes of disabling conditions, with large proportions of the problem also identified as being caused by trauma and injury, communicable diseases including poliomyelitis, trachoma and leprosy, and congenital diseases. The WHO study concluded: "There can be no doubt that the problem is large enough and sufficiently widespread to justify interventions in all countries."1/

The number of disabled people in the world is increasing, and predictions of future growth suggest that factors such as increased longevity, improved social conditions and medical care, industrialization and urbanization, as well as a deteriorating world food situation, will accelerate the increase in the magnitude of the problem.

Additional References on Definitions and Prevalence of Disability:

World Health Organization. International Classification of Impairments, Disabilities, and Handicaps. Geneva: W.H.O., 1980.

This report defines the different dimensions of the consequences of disease: impairment, disability, and handicap. These distinctions permit policy makers to focus on the potential contributions of medical, vocational and social rehabilitation. It is also designed to promote uniformity in the concepts and terminology related to disability, and enhance the comparability of data.

Impairment. "In the context of health experience, an impairment is any loss or abnormality of psychological, physiological, or anatomical structure or function...Impairment is characterized by losses or abnormalities that may be temporary or permanent,

"In 1975 people throughout the world suffering all types and degrees of disability numbered an estimated 490 million (12.3 percent of the world population); by the year 2000, their number will reach an estimated 846 million (13.5 percent). Whereas in 1975 more than three-quarters of this population lived in developing countries, by the year 2000 more than four-fifths of all disabled people will live in these countries."

John H. Noble Jr., "Population and Development Problems Relating to Disability Prevention and Rehabilitation," 1981.

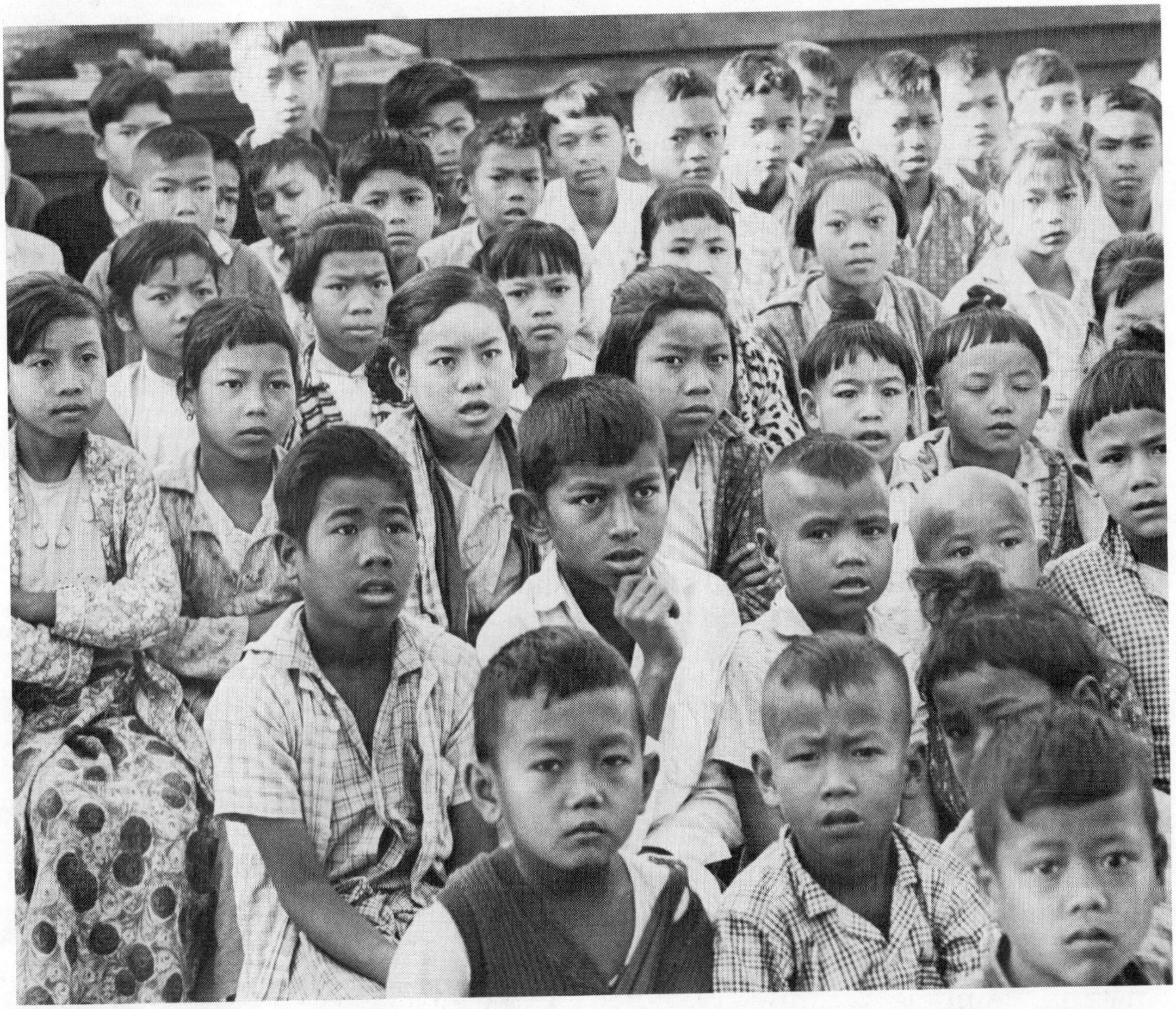

and that include the existence or occurence of an anomaly, defect, or loss in a limb, organ, tissue, or other structure of the body, including the systems of mental function. Impairment represents exteriorization of a pathological state, and in principle it reflects disturbances at the level of the organ."

Disability. "In the context of health experience, a disability is any restriction or lack (resulting from an impairment) of ability to perform an activity in the manner or within the range considered normal for a human being...Disability is characterized by excesses or deficiencies of customarily expected activity performance and behaviour, and these may be temporary or permanent, reversible or irreversible, and progressive or regressive. Disabilities may arise as a direct consequence of impairment or as a response by the individual, particularly psychologically, to a physical, sensory or other impairment. Disability represents objectification of an impairment, and as such it reflects disturbances at the level of the person...Disability is concerned with abilities, in the form of composite activities and behaviours, that are generally accepted as an essential component of everyday life. Examples include disturbances in behaving in an appropriate manner, in personal care (such as excretory control and the ability to wash and feed oneself), in the performance of other activities of daily living, and in locomotor activities (such as the ability to walk)."

Handicap. "In the context of health experience, a handicap is a disadvantage for a given individual, resulting from an impairment or a disability, that limits or prevents the fulfilment of a role that is normal (depending on age, sex, and social and cultural factors) for that individual...Handicap is concerned with the value attached to an individual's situation or experience when it departs from the norm. It is characterized by a discordance between the individual's performance or status and the expectations of the individual himself or of the particular group of which he is a member. Handicap thus represents socialization of an impairment or disability, and as such it reflects the consequences for the individual--cultural, social, economic, and environmental--that stem from the presence of impairment and disability...Disability arises from failure or inability to conform to the expectations or norms of the individual's universe. Handicap thus occurs when there is interference with the ability to sustain what might be designated as "survival roles."

The sequence can be presented graphically as follows:

Impairment ⟶ Disability ⟶ Handicap

The global picture 1.1

WORLD INCIDENCE OF DISABILITY
(in millions)

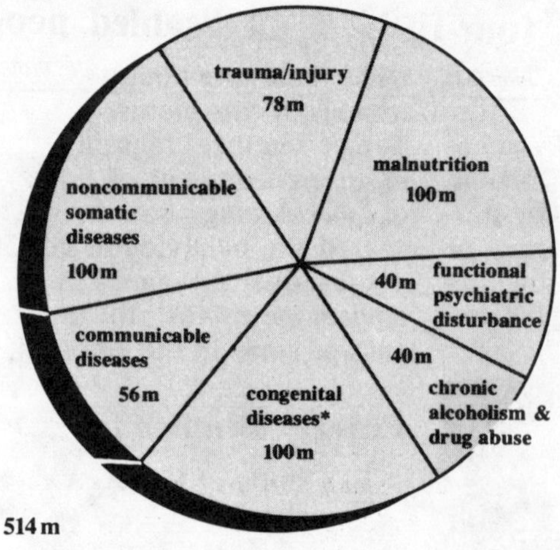

Total = 514m

The accepted minimum estimate of the magnitude of the disability problem is that at least one in ten children is born with, or acquires, a physical, mental or sensory impairment. The data are very incomplete; estimates rise to 15 or 20% depending on definitions used and conditions included.

* eg: back disorders, heart conditions, epilepsy, arthritis, etc.

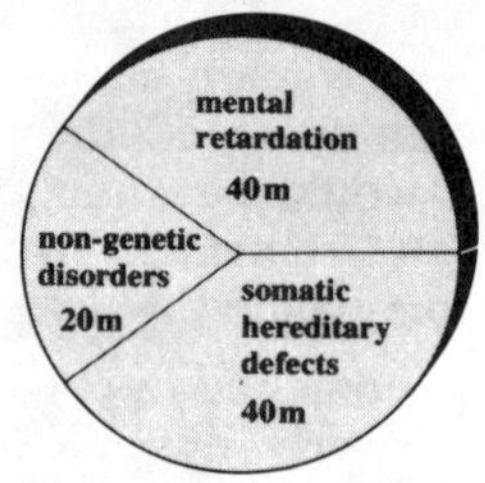

CONGENITAL DISEASES

Definition: diseases existing at, and usually before, birth, regardless of cause. Somatic hereditary defects: physical imperfections genetically transmitted from parent to offspring, eg clu foot, cleft-lip, spina bifida, blindn ss, deafness, muscular dystrophy, genitourinary malformation, cyctic fibrosis. Non-genetic = non-hereditary disorder.

COMMUNICABLE DISEASES

Definition: diseases which can be carried from one person to another, directly or indirectly. Where people live in a deprived social environment and in insanitary conditions, as in poor, densely-settled urban areas, the risk of contracting a communicable disease rises considerably.

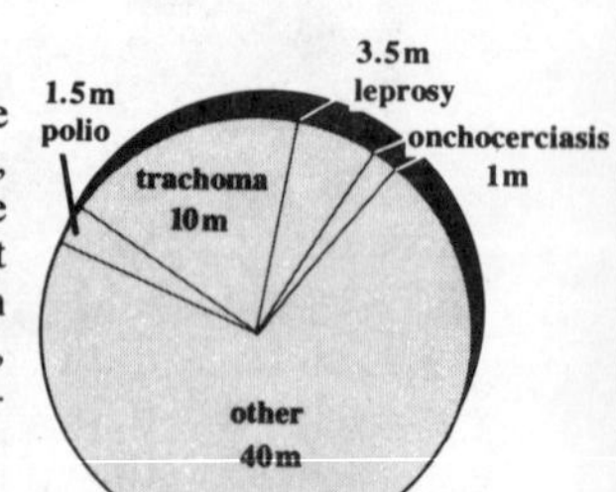

Source: UNICEF NEWS, Issue 105, 1980.

There is no simple linear progression though. "One can be impaired without being disabled, and disabled without being handicapped." The external environment, such as an absence of physical barriers or family support, can mediate an impairment and not result in a handicap.

Haber, Lawrence, D. "Some Parameters for Social Policy in Disability: A Cross National Comparison", Health and Society, Summer 1973, pp. 319-340.

Social planners, in order to develop a disability policy which allocates scarce goods and services efficiently, must identify the size and scope of the disability problem. This is largely a function of the definition of disability; it may be defined as "the pattern of behaviour arising from the loss or reduction of the ability to perform expected or specific role activities because of a chronic disease or impairment". Yet each agency, program and service group within a nation will define disability and develop criteria for the evaluation of the degree of disability which reflect the goals and objectives of the particular organization.

1.2
Prevalence of disability, handicap, limitation, or impairment in five countries

Study population	Percent of specified population
U.S.A., 1966 (age 18-64)	
Disabled	17.2
Severe	5.9
Occupational	4.9
Secondary	6.4
Australia, 1968 (age 15-64)	
Chronic limiting condition	8.4
Denmark, 1961-62 (age 15-61)	
Physically handicapped	6.5
Great Britain, 1968-69 (age 16-64)	
Impaired	3.9
Handicapped	1.2
Israel, 1965-66 (men age 14-64, women age 14-59)	
Vocationally handicapped	2.9

Source: Haber

To underline the problems entailed in comparison of the results of disability prevalence studies, of two disability surveys undertaken in the United States in the 1960's, one survey found approximately twice the disability prevalence levels as the other. The disability criteria for men was the same, but study methods differed, and for women both the criteria and methods differed. Estimates for "partial disability" were also twice as high in one study.

If the prevalence of disability varies substantially when the same definitions and measurement methods are used in one country, when different populations are studied, with different study criteria and different research methods, comparisons of prevalence rates among populations or nations become difficult at best.

In reviewing the rates of disability prevalence in the United States, Australia, Denmark, Great Britain, and Israel, the estimates range from a high of 17.2 disabled persons per 100 population aged 18-64 in the U.S., to a low of 1.2 handicapped persons per 100 population aged 16-64 in Great Britain. Given the relative homogeneity of the population of the U.S. and Great Britain, the large differences in the rates of disability call into question the usefulness of cross national comparisons especially of developed to developing nations.

The five studies used five or more different concepts and criteria for limitation, ranging from the Israeli criteria for "vocational handicaps", the Australian definition of a "chronic limiting condition", and "adults whose limitations affect their ability to work" in the U.S. The definition in Britain focused on personal care ability, and the study in Denmark excluded those with mental disorders. Each of these definitions excludes a segment of the population with disabilities.

The methodologies employed also result in different findings. For example, "the use of screening questions directed toward chronic diseases and impairments and asked of household or proxy respondents has been found to be conducive to understatement,..and chronic conditions are substantially under-reported". The Australian study, for example, found that 24 percent of the New South Wales population (age 15-64) had a chronic condition or impairment, whereas a U.S. study reported that 60 percent of the U.S. population aged 17-64 had a chronic condition. Although the percentages differed, the five studies agreed that the disabled or handicapped tended to be older, less educated, and less skilled than the non-disabled or the lesser disabled.

Krute, Aaron and Mary Ellen Burdette. Chronic Disease, Injury and Work Disability: 1972 Survey of Disabled and Non-Disabled Adults. Report # 10. Washington, D.C.: United States Social Security Administration, 1978.

The United States Social Security Administration 1972 Survey showed that an estimated 15.6 million adults aged 20-64, or 15 percent of the total non-institutionalized population of those ages, were disabled as a result of some chronic condition or impairment. Yet more than three times as many reported that they suffered from one or more chronic health conditions. For every disease group, older persons were more likely to suffer from a chronic condition or impairment and more likely to be disabled as a result. White persons were somewhat more likely than blacks and other minorities to report one or more chronic conditions, but less likely to be severely disabled.

Netherlands Central Bureau of Statistics. The Physically Handicapped in the Netherlands - 1971/1972. The Hague: Staatsuitgeverij, 1976.

This study found that out of the total Netherlands population of 5 years of age and older, 8.7 percent (more than one million persons) appeared to be physically handicapped according to the definition used for the survey. (Physically handicapped was defined as those persons who have one or more functional disorders to at least a certain degree). The majority of the physically handicapped differed not only as regards to age, sex, province of residence, but also as to the type of their functional disorder, its cause and the degree of severity.

The chance of becoming handicapped increases with age. Of those between 5 and 24 years of age, about 2 percent were physically handicapped; for those 75 and older this percentage was over 35. Up to an age of 55 the study found no marked difference between men and women. For older persons differences started to occur. They are probably caused by difference in mortality pattern, and differences in physical strain. Most striking was the marked increase recorded for men aged up to and including 64. The percentage of physically handicapped persons was lower in rural municipalities than in urban municipalities.

Nagi, Saad Z. Disability and Rehabilitation: Legal, Clinical, and Self-Concepts and Measurement. Columbus: Ohio State University Press, 1969.

The magnitude of the problem of disability in the United States can be expressed in terms of the

"Most physical limitation occurs amongst people aged 50 years or more and stems from causes quite different from those most commonly associated with disability in the school-age population."

Office of Health Economics, Physical Impairment: Social Handicap, 1977.

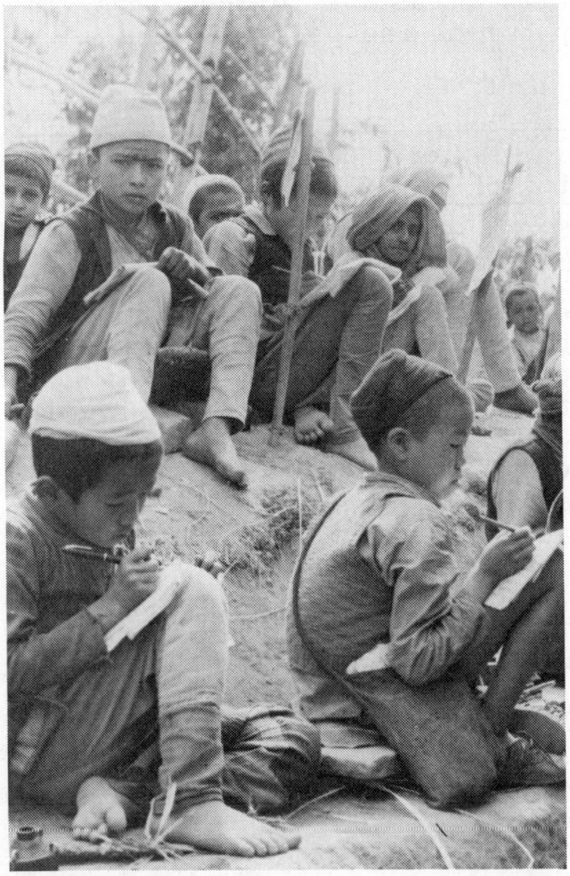

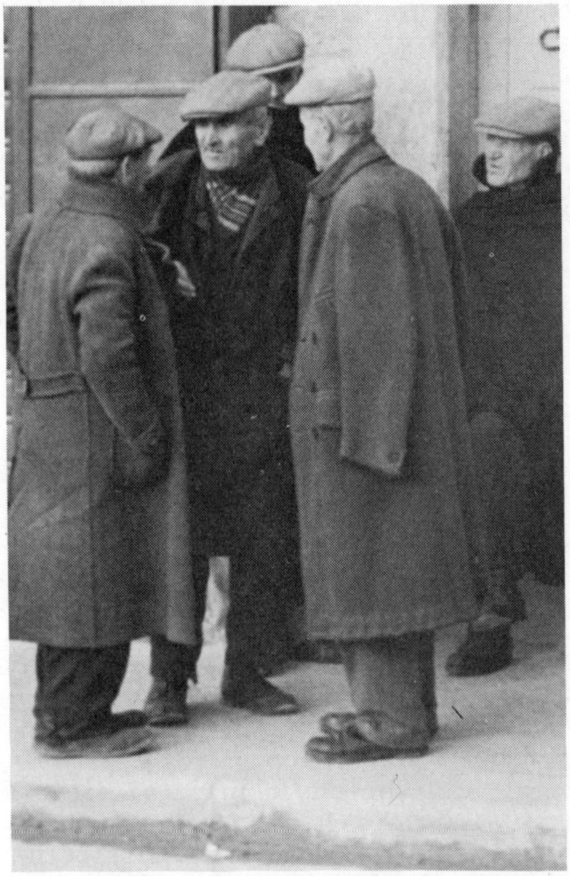

number of individuals and families affected: one in ten adults of working age (18-64 years) cannot work, or is limited in the amount or type of work possible. The programs designed to prevent disability and rehabilitate the disabled are based on policies shaped by specific concepts of disability, and methods of measuring disability.

The concept of disability "typically refers to inabilities precipitated by injury, disease, or other forms of deterioration in health conditions." However, disability must be distinguished from pathology, impairment, and limitation of activities--conditions that may or may not lead to disability.

Pathology is associated with the interruption in normal biological processes by infection, degenerative diseases, etc., and the mobilization of the defense mechanisms of the body. Impairment "indicates a physiological, anatomical, or mental loss or abnormality, or both. Impairments do not necessarily involve active pathology"; e.g., abnormalities remain after the state of pathology has been eliminated.

Disability is a "form of inability or limitation in performing roles and tasks expected of an individual within a social environment...such as self care, education, family relations, recreation, economic life, and employment." Not all impairments result in disability, nor do identical impairments result in the same pattern of disability. The reactions of the disabled person, involving all personal characteristics and the social definitions of the impairment, are key factors in the relationship between impairment and disability.

A handicap is defined as a "limitation in function at higher levels of activity--such as walking, climbing, lifting, bending, reaching, reasoning, seeing, or hearing."

There are three categories of variables that can be seen to influence the course of disability and the rehabilitation potential of disabled people: the characteristics of impairments, the disabled person's definition of the situation, and the environmental situation--family, health, the workplace and labor market possibilities, and the nature of services available. It is the interaction of all of these variables that determines the presence and severity of disability, and each of these variables needs to be reflected in the structure of services and benefits for disabled people.

Definitions and assessments of disability often emphasize limitations rather than the capacities or abilities of an individual. Existing disability programs tend to confuse impairment and disability; for example, benefits are often based on rates of compensation for anatomical losses (the impairment itself), rather than the effect of the impairment on earnings. Impairment is viewed as a "necessary and sufficient condition for disability."

An assessment of limitations in function, incorporating all of the categories of variables which are involved, "provide greater validity to disability assessment than measures based upon impairment and pathology."

Blaxter, Mildred. The Meaning of Disability. London: Heinemann Educational Books, 1975.

Disability and "normality" can be envisioned as points on a continuum, and the placement of a disabled individual on this continuum is a function of family and social environment, individual characteristics, cultural concepts of "normality", and clinical definitions of impairment. The definition of disability and the determination of client needs will in turn effect the provision of rehabilitation services.

There are a number of processes involved in defining someone as disabled and being defined as disabled. These consist primarily as the interaction of three sets of definitions: medical labels applied to a patient's condition, the administrative categories of service agencies, and self definitions.

Medical labels are of great importance, since they "name and legitimize a condition involving physical impairment." These may diverge from the patient's perception of the problem, and from administrative definitions of the impairment or disability. The administrative definitions are often rigid, arbitrary, and based on stereotypes. They are determined by the history and structure of the service institution. The behaviour of the disabled person will also depend on his or her

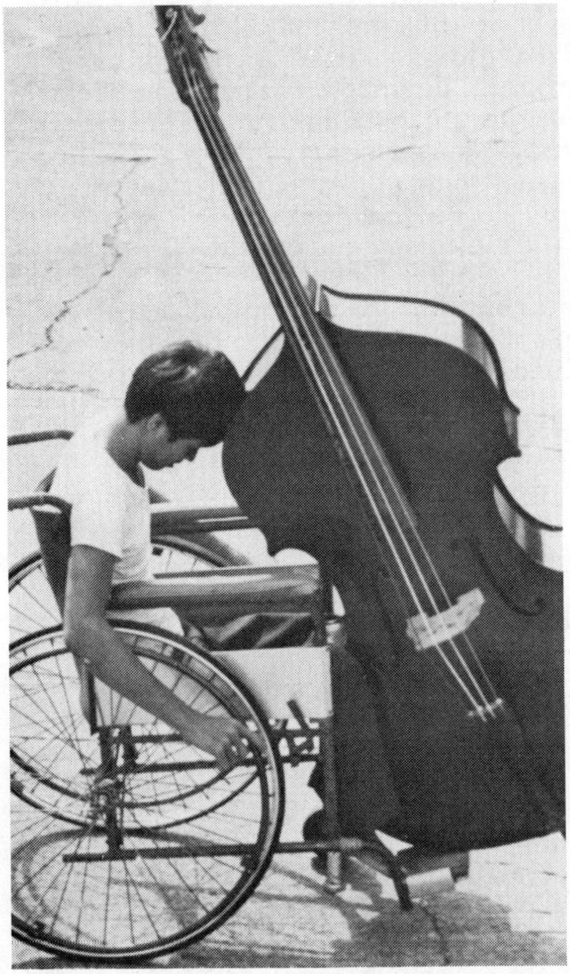

own definition, a definition that is influenced by the medical and administrative definitions, and constantly recreated during the rehabilitation process.

The shortcomings and contradictions of these definitions will affect the income, employment, and family/social life of disabled people. Assessment of disability and need must be based on functional measures, such as individual characteristics and social factors, rather than on so-called "objective" clinical or administrative definitions.

Sainsbury, Sally. Measuring Disability. London: Social Administration Research Trust, 1973.

The identification of the number of disabled people in a population is partly a question of the definition of disability. The procedures utilized to identify and assess a disability are also employed in the allocation of services and benefits to disabled people. A wide variety of procedures and definitions will result in a great disparity in treatment of different categories of disabled people.

In order to determine the equity of a program for disabled people in the U.K. it is necessary to consider the concepts of disability which underlie the social security and social services systems.

There are two main concepts of disability incorporated into the social welfare system in the U.K. Physical and financial independence is the first concept. The distribution of social benefits to those in need is based on four different principles: a means tested assessment of need, the assessment of earnings from full time work in the normal occupation, assessment of employability, and the principle of payment to meet certain unspecified needs. The manner in which these principles are applied in the assessment of the degree of disability and need reflect the political, social and economic interests that determine the functioning of the benefit system.

There is a great deal of ambiguity in each of these principles; how can there be one standard to judge the "employability" of a disabled person given the different definitions and measurements of disability. Sickness benefits are determined by "incapacity for work", yet this is a status that depends on the interaction of the physical requirements of the job and the state of health of the employee.

The second primary concept of disability is compensation for loss of limb or faculty, which is a function of the cause or origin of the injury (e.g. in the course of employment versus criminal injury, etc.). In order to qualify for rehabilitation services, a disabled person must be one who, "on account of injury, disease, or congenital deformity, is substantially handicapped in obtaining or keeping employment, or in undertaking work on his own account, of a kind which apart from that injury, disease or deformity would be suited to his age, experience and qualifications." This definition is also vague and ill-defined.

Copeland, Lois S. Defining Disability: A Cross-Country Study. Washington, D.C.: U.S. Department of Health, Education, and Welfare, 1977.

Sharply rising costs have necessitated a critical reexamination of the basic definition of disability. This study examines how non-work-related disability is defined and measured under the social security systems in Belgium, France, the Federal Republic of Germany, the Netherlands, Sweden, and the United Kingdom.

The following shows the typical sequence of social security programs during the course of a disability: cash sickness benefit (first 26 or 52 weeks of sickness) -- invalidity pension -- retirement pension. The concept of invalidity generally applies to the state of persons whose capacity or ability for work has been reduced for a relatively long time. The six countries under study distinguish between short-term (sickness) and long-term (invalidity) disabilities.

Over the past several years, as a result of rapid economic and technological changes, the concept of invalidity has been liberalized to include prolonged unemployment and inability to cope with the work environment in cases of older workers. Defining invalidity is one of the major problems in drafting an insurance system. A liberal definition may permit more members to qualify for benefits and, consequently, increase program costs; a strict definition may have the opposite effect.

In contrast to the invalidity program in the U.S., some of the European systems use quantitative standards to measure invalidity in terms of loss of earning capacity. These systems compare the salary the disabled worker is capable of earning to what he would have been able to earn in his former occupation had he remained healthy. This is called a percentage of earning capacity. From this figure, the reduction in earning capacity may be derived. That reduction forms the basis for determining entitlement to long-term invalidity pensions under numerous invalidity systems.

Cash Sickness Benefits. Aside from satisfying the system's definition of disability, most cash sickness benefit programs require claimants to meet some kind of minimum qualifying period of contributions or to have some history of active labor force attachment prior to illness. The qualifying period for benefits varies from less than 1 month to 6 months or more. Benefits are calculated as a percentage of the worker's average earnings, often subject to a maximum amount, and may be increased by supplements for dependents.

Invalidity Pensions. There are basically two approaches to invalidity evaluation: Inability (1) to resume one's former or allied occupation--occupational incapacity (the Netherlands and West Germany)--and (2) to follow any occupation -- general invalidity (Belgium, France, West Germany, Sweden, and the United Kingdom)

Permanent incapacity for work can be defined as follows:

U.S.: "the inability to do any substantial gainful activity because of any physical or mental impairment which a doctor expects to result in death or which has lasted or, again, he expects to last for at least 12 months." S.G.A. means doing significant physical or mental work for which the worker is paid or may profit. It is a dollar measure, now set at $260 per month.

Belgium: "When an insured's physical or mental infirmities reduce his capacity to earn so that he is only able to earn one-third or less of that which a healthy person of similar age and with comparable training could earn in the same or similar occupation considering the claimant's vocational history."

France: "When an insured is unable to earn in any profession a salary more than one-third of the normal salary earned in the same region by similar workers prior to his stopping work or the date of the medical determination if premature aging is involved. The state of invalidity is evaluated considering not only the residual work capacity, the state of health remaining, his age and physical and mental abilities, but also his aptitudes and prior professional training."

Germany (FR): "(1) Occupational incapacity--When, as a result of illness or weakening of physical or mental powers, the insured's earnings capacity has been reduced to less than one-half that of a physically and mentally fit person with comparable training and equivalent knowledge and abilities. (2) General invalidity--When, as a result of illness or weakening of physical or mental powers, the insured is unable to work on a regular basis in the foreseeable future or is unable to work for significant earnings."

Netherlands: "When as a result of sickness or infirmity, the insured is totally or partially unable to earn what a physically and mentally healthy person with similar training normally earns by working either where the insured is employed or was last employed or at some nearby, similar place. A person who is incapacitated for work by <u>less than 15%</u> shall not be deemed to be incapacitated."

Sweden: "When a person's remaining capacity--considering the decline in his physical or mental powers-- to have an income from work corresponding to his energies and skills that can reasonably be expected of him in view of his training, previous employment, age, and living conditions, has been reduced by at least <u>one-half</u>."

United Kingdom: "When the impairment prevents the insured from engaging in any job which he might be reasonably expected to do, or for which he could be trained considering his age, education, work experience, his state of health, and other relevant personal factors."

Some systems may permit earning capacity to exceed that stipulated in the legislative definition in order to give pensioners incentives to work rather than lose his or her benefit rights and be forced to depend on disability benefits. For example, in order to counter possible work disincentives built into the system, regulations in France and Belgium that call for a two-thirds reduction in earning capacity for initial entitlement do not provide for pensions suspension or termination in cases of medical recovery unless the improvement results in residual earning capacity exceeding 50%. In the Netherlands, Sweden, and West Germany, which provide for more than one degree of invalidity, the rate of the pension is determined by the insured's ability to work and to earn.

B. REHABILITATION: GOALS, AVAILABILITY OF SERVICES, AND NATIONAL POLICIES

The Goals of Rehabilitation

The ultimate goal of rehabilitation has been stated to be attainment of "the maximum physical and psychological adjustment of each disabled person within the limits of his impairment; to enable him to live as useful and satisfying a life as is humanly possible."2/ For most handicapped people this can include employment in productive work. For others, it may mean only the restoration of a certain degree of functional ability. Being handicapped for certain physical or intellectual activities does not mean being handicapped for all activities.

"All human beings are born free and equal in dignity and rights" proclaims the United Nations Universal Declaration of Human Rights. "The handicapped person is an individual with full human rights which he shares in common with the able-bodied,"3/ stated the United Nations interagency technical working party which formulated United Nations activity on behalf of the disabled in 1950.

"Every citizen, the disabled no less than the able-bodied, has the right to basic economic security compatible with the standard of living in his community. Every citizen, the disabled no less than the able-bodied, has the right to set for himself his own life goals, with guidance if necessary, and to be provided the opportunity for developing to its maximum his intellectual and creative potential. Every citizen has the privilege and responsibility to be a contributing member of the community: the family circle, the immediate neighbourhood, the country to which he owes allegiance, or the world community" 4/ declared the Rehabilitation International Guidelines for the Future (published in 1972) when it was still apparent that the goals of rehabilitation remained no more than hopes and dreams for most of the world's disabled.

Rehabilitation is a comprehensive process. It is based upon the realization that the handicapped person must achieve emotional and social adjustment as well as physical adjustment to his or her particular circumstances and environment, and that all of the needs of the individual must be seen in the context of his or her relationship to the community. Effective rehabilitation services generally include four main components - the medical, educational, psycho-social and vocational - which, if provided in a comprehensive and coordinated manner, will help the disabled person to be reintegrated within the community. The necessary services staffed by qualified personnel may be provided in a variety of patterns and levels of technical sophistication depending upon the social and economic resources of the nation.

"the maximum freeing of the human spirit"

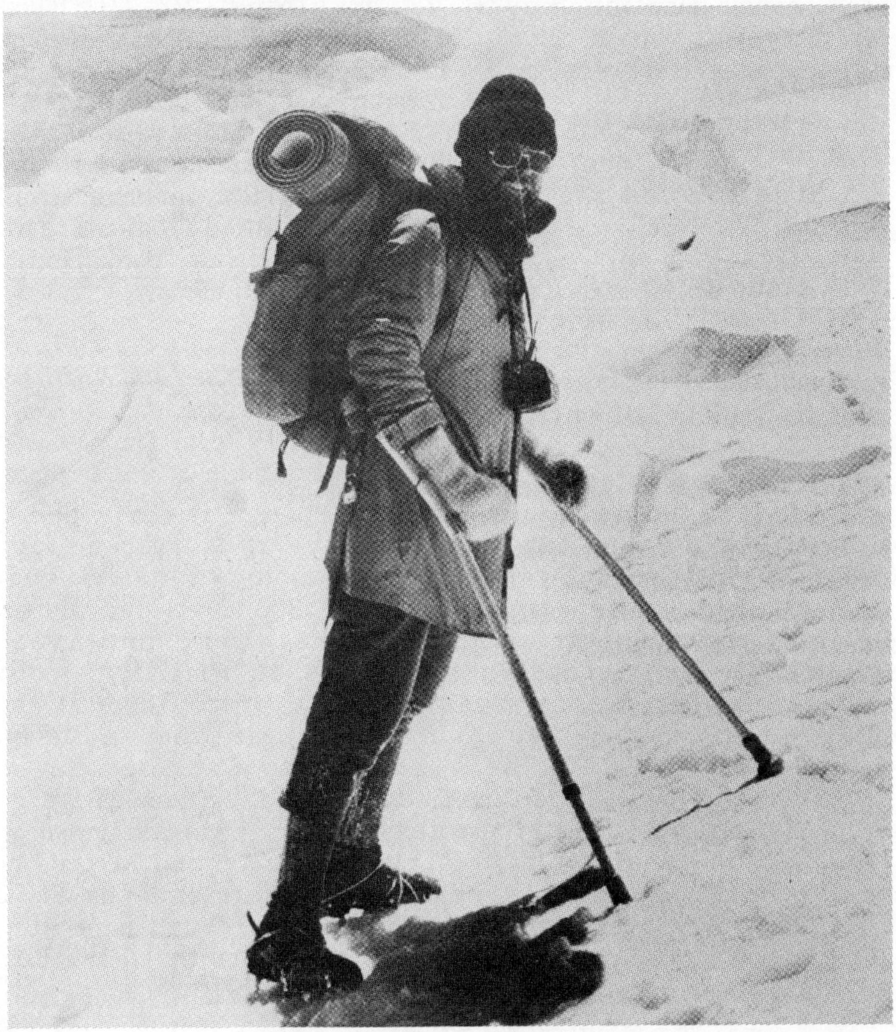

Norman Croucher of Britain, specialist in recreation for people with disabilities, has climbed the highest mountain in Peru and many other mountain ranges. He is a double amputee and has adapted his climbing apparatus according to his needs and aspirations.

There have been, within the past 30 years, remarkable developments in the technologies related to rehabilitation, and in the consequent capability to compensate for many of the major disabling conditions. New technologies have revolutionized diagnostic procedures, therapeutic practices, and the communication and processing of information. Bio-engineering has produced new methods to monitor a patient's vital functions, assess his tolerance of physical workloads and psychic stress, control prosthetic and environmental devices electronically. Ultrasonic and electronic equipment is helping the sensorially disabled to detect objects in the environment, and computer and space technology are being applied to a diversity of problems.

Only a small proportion of the disabled have benefited from the most innovative technological developments and, by and large, these developments have done little to remove the fundamental physical and social barriers which affect their participation in community life. People with an obvious physical or mental disability must still cope with the discriminatory and stereotyped attitudes of their non-disabled fellow citizens, and these attitudes are not generally well understood. Public education and awareness campaigns in many countries are just beginning to alter the problem. Architectural and other obstacles in the physical environment remain as formidable barriers preventing the re-entry of disabled persons into the community. These barriers restrict the use of public, recreational, religious and work facilities, and in many instances reduce any gains towards independence and self-development which rehabilitation may have stimulated. Mr. Wilf Race, leader of the United Handicapped Group of Ontario, Canada, has put the problem of architectural barriers into the following perspective:

> "Integration means much more than mere adaptation of physical facilities to meet the mobility requirements of the disabled. It means the opening of channels to allow for the totalization of the human experience according to the needs, aspirations, hopes and inclinations of each individual. It is the maximum freeing of the human spirit." 5/

Availability of Rehabilitation Services

An enormous gap exists between the number of disabled people in the world and the availability of services for them. A survey conducted by Rehabilitation International in 1968 suggested that there were at that time approximately 300 million persons in the world requiring rehabilitation services that were not available to them. In addition, it was estimated that at least 3 million people would be added to that number every year, taking into account population growth, increased longevity, increasing vehicular and industrial accidents, and other factors. In 1974 the World Health Organization estimated the need of developing countries for medical and paramedical rehabilitation staff to be 3.2 million trained professionals. This estimate was based upon an extension of rehabilitation services patterned after methods of comprehensive care provided in developed countries. The effect such a transfer of delivery system approach might have within a developing nation is exemplified by the following excerpt from the WHO Policy for Disability Prevention and Rehabilitation issued in 1976:

> "It was recently recommended that rehabilitation services be set up in the capital city of a country in Africa. The recommendation closely followed the conventional design of an institution in Europe or North America. It was then recommended that services be extended through the provision of a similar institution in the second largest city, then in the third etc. Figures for manpower needs (in 11 different occupations) and of patient turnover were provided for the first institute. When this plan was scrutinized, it appeared that if the entire health budget for the country were utilized solely for rehabilitation services, it would take 60 years to develop the necessary manpower, and about 200 years to provide the present needy population with the desired amount of care." 6/

It is widely hoped that as developing nations extend the availability of rehabilitation services for the disabled, they will avoid the errors of the industrialized nations that have preceded them in this development and not create systems of service delivery which are dependent upon extremely costly and highly specialized facilities and resources. It is obviously critical for developing nations to develop patterns of service which can be effective under conditions of very limited trained manpower and technical resources. Such nations may never be willing to afford the luxury of the un-coordinated and

The relationship between armament and development is still very much in the dark. The prospects which might open up if only part of the unproductive arms spending were turned to productive expenditure on development are only starting to dawn on people. The annual military bill is now approaching 450 billion U.S. dollars, while official development aid accounts for less than 5 percent of this figure. The military expenditure of only one-half a day would suffice to finance the whole malaria eradication programme of the WHO; for the price of one jet fighter (20 million dollars) one could set up about 40,000 village pharmacies.

Report of the Independent Commission on International Development Issues. North-South: A Programme for Survival, 1979.

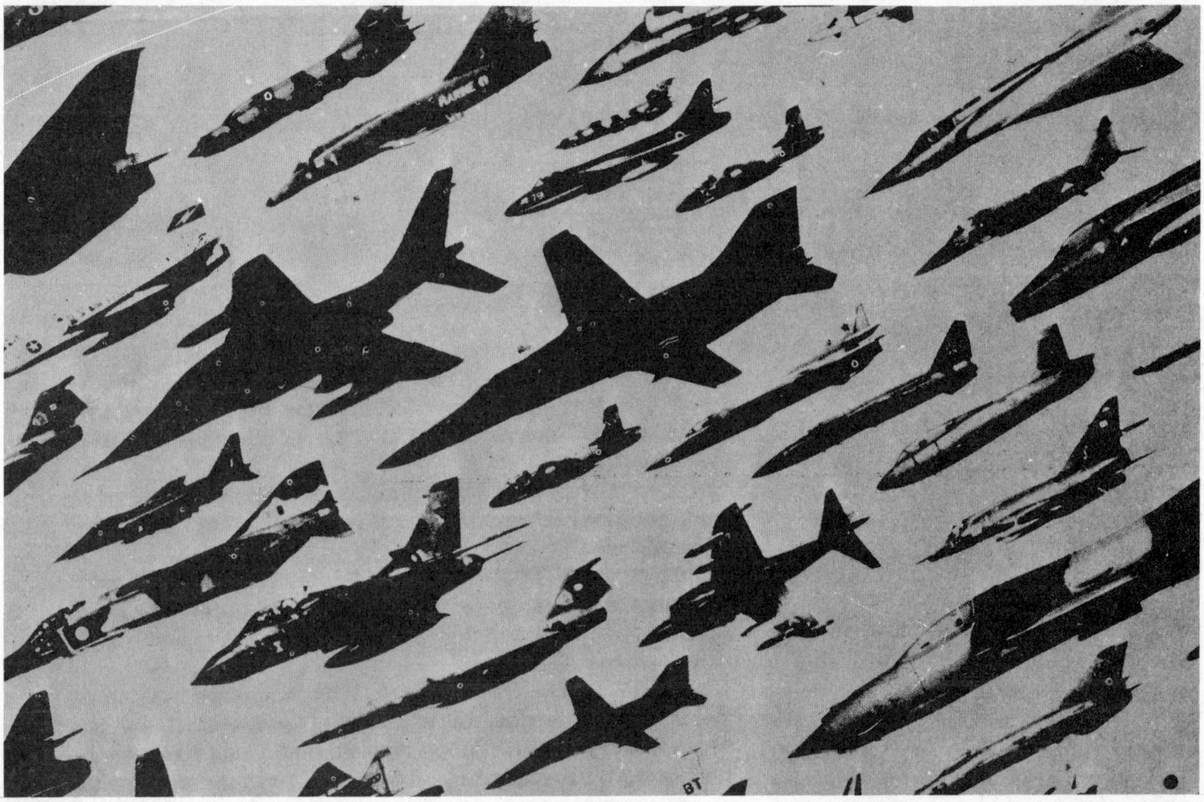

redundant service patterns that have become an incomprehensible maze for the disabled in many "advanced" nations. It is also becoming obvious that not even the most sophisticated and well-endowed nations can afford such patterns, as shifts in their population structures and changes in the global economic state reduce overall production capability. These issues, and the fact of an ever increasing gap between the availability of rehabilitation services and the need for them, led Rehabilitation International to convene in 1969 a meeting of experts on the Development of Rehabilitation Services in Relation to Available Resources. 7/ The experts concluded in part, that:

--Essential services can be provided with very simple buildings and equipment, and a high priority need not be given to the provision of elaborate physical facilities;

--It is possible to identify those medical, educational, social and vocational rehabilitation services which should be regarded as primary at the inception of a rehabilitation program and to create possibilities of progression, building on the primary services, to intermediate and advanced stages of service;

--Where fully trained personnel with currently accepted qualifications are not available in sufficient numbers, auxiliary personnel should be trained in institutions at which they work and through courses organized in the country or region. A progression of grades of auxiliaries may be established and, as far as possible, further training to reach full qualification should be encouraged.

Regrettably, these concepts have not yet been tested in a comprehensive rehabilitation program. While there are numerous instances of the successful utilization of simple facilities or of auxiliary personnel, no complete phased-development scheme has been established nor is it possible to estimate the effects such a scheme might have on reducing the costs of rehabilitation service delivery. The concept offers enormous potential for the future. It is most important that developing nations not be inhibited in their planning of rehabilitation services by the cost

1.3 THE CYCLE OF UNDERDEVELOPMENT

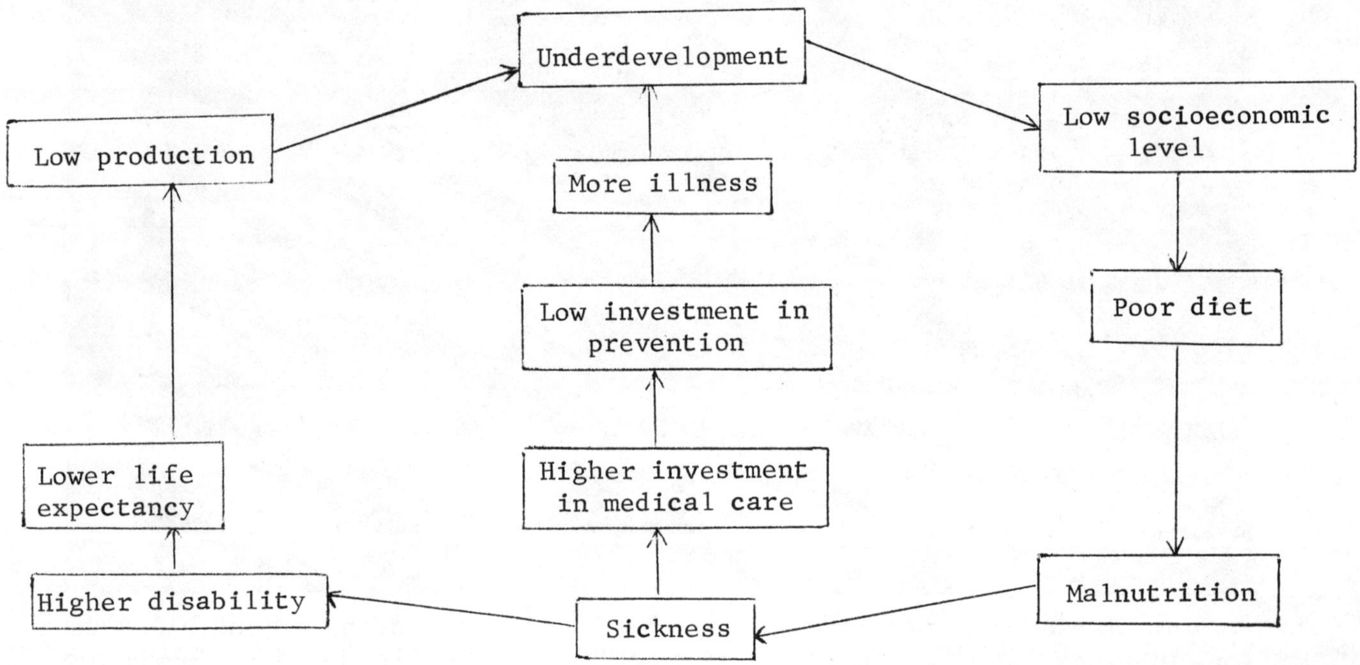

Source: Gaston de Mezerville. <u>Disability and Rehabilitation in Rural Costa Rica</u>, 1979.

patterns of the past. Experience in many nations has confirmed that it is not necessary to provide rehabilitation services according to a single pattern. It is not even to be recommended, nor is there any single level of expenditure which will be most effective within all of the possible combinations of social, political, cultural and economic conditions that exist throughout the world. According to present indications, nowhere in the world are the necessary measures being instituted to reduce the gap between available services and existing and predictable needs.

LOW COST TECHNOLOGIES FOR THE DISABLED

The kind of technical appliances that people in industrialized countries associate with rehabilitation for disabled people tend to be sophisticated and expensive. In many developing countries, thousands of paralysed people still crawl through lack of supports, and polio as a cause of paralysis is on the increase. In Uganda in 1960 the first orthopaedic workshop to make simple calipers was started at negligible cost. Calipers are used mainly to support the weakened lower limbs of people affected by polio. Those made in the industrialized countries are inappropriate for people living in rural Africa. Their complicated design and breakability does not withstand the rigorous lifestyle, and their expense puts them beyond the reach of all but a few. The calipers illustrated here are made by virtually unskilled craftsmen without screws, heating or welding, and cost one fiftieth of the price of an imported caliper. The crutches are another example of appropriate technology for disabled people.

Calipers

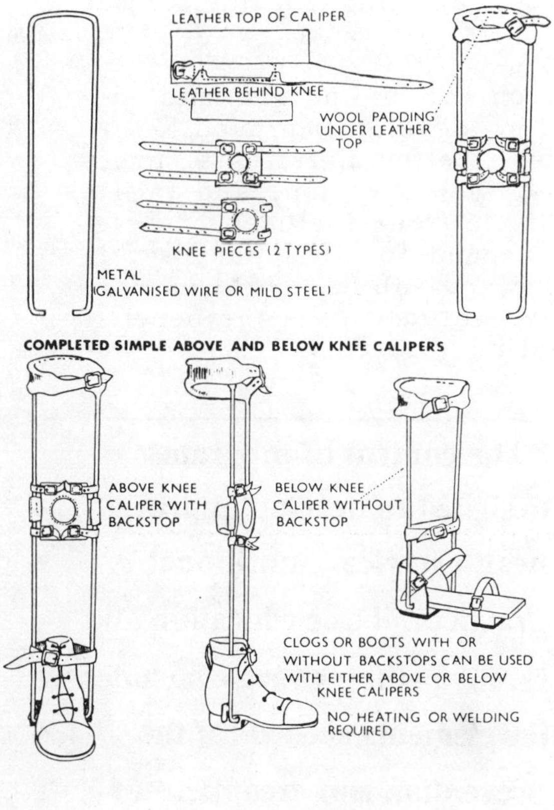

How to make simple crutches

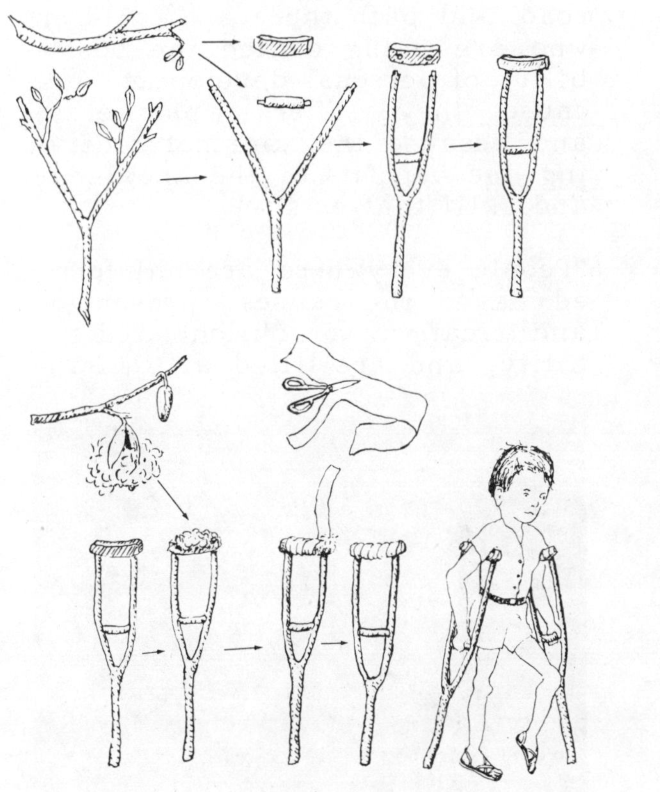

*From: **Donde No Hay Doctor** (Where There Is No Doctor) by David Werner*

Source: UNICEF NEWS, Issue 105, 1980.

Additional References on Rehabilitation: Goals, Availability of Services and National Policies:

United Nations Economic and Social Council. Childhood Disability: Its Prevention and Rehabilitation. Report of Rehabilitation International to the Executive Board of UNICEF. New York: United Nations Children's Fund, 1980. (E/ICEF/L. 1410)

"At least one in every ten children is born with or acquires a physical, mental, or sensory impairment--of 1.4 billion children under the age of 15 in 1975, 140 million were disabled; approximately 80 percent, or 120 million of these children are living in the developing world without access to rehabilitation services of any kind. Little or nothing is being done to prevent either the occurrence of impairment or its damaging consequences. One need only visit the villages of Asia, Africa, Latin America or the Middle East to learn that along every road and path there are children who are being denied the possibility of personal development because they suffer impairments, and because they are not receiving the benefits of the knowledge and skill that exist."

"People everywhere are uninformed as to the causes, prevention and treatment of childhood disability, and are filled with misinformation, superstition and fear about the subject...Resources that are allocated for the prevention and treatment of childhood disability by governments and others are, virtually without exception, being spent on high-cost projects which serve a relatively few children and ignore the great majority who are at risk of, or affected by impairment...Too often the programmes that are being financed, because of concepts drawn from models of limited relevance, are not providing optimum help to the children who are reached. They are rarely designed to make use of the resources available in the community and the family." "Preliminary findings of a study being carried out in Mexico by WHO/PAHO indicate that more than 80 percent of the disabled persons found in the communities studied can be helped by resources existing in the community."

"The content of programmes designed to develop improved health services, better nutritional practices, basic education, and family planning rarely includes the elements needed for this purpose; in practice, disabled children are usually excluded from the benefits of existing services."

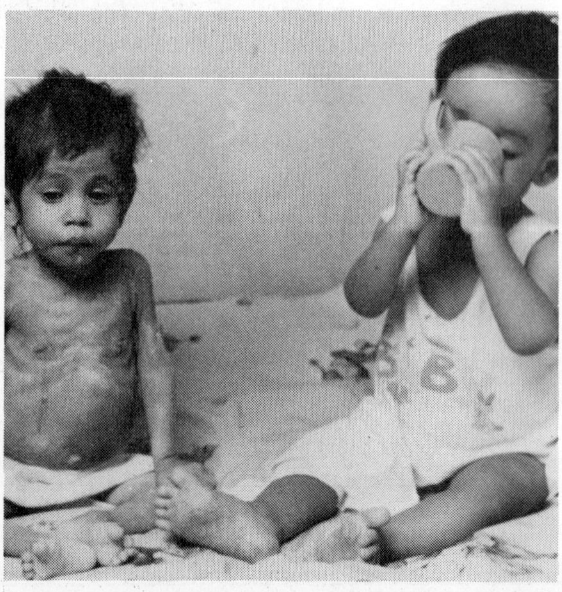

"The content of programs designed to develop improved health services, nutritional practices, basic education and family planning rarely includes the elements needed for the prevention and treatment of childhood disabilities."

Childhood Disability

A strategy for improvement of the current situation should concentrate on "primary prevention of impairment and on the early identification and appropriate treatment of conditions that can lead to permanent functional limitations. The components of these problems, and of their solutions, are so interrelated and interactive that the actions to be taken must be developed as parts of a continuum of prevention, care and treatment."

General national "health, nutrition, education, family planning and social welfare programmes...should be more responsive to what could be done in prevention and rehabilitation...The most important instrument for the implementation of the strategy is the family, since it provides the atmosphere, the support and the assistance most likely to foster normal child development...As most families depend in part on other members of the community and its institutions, the ideal target for this strategy is a composite of the child, the family, and the community."

Specific disability prevention and rehabilitation measures should include:

- the design of low-cost intervention techniques and appropriate technology suitable for community-level use;

- dissemination of procedures to instruct, motivate and activate family members in the disability prevention and rehabilitation process;

- the reorientation and training of primary health care workers and their counterparts in the fields of nutrition, education, social development and vocational adjustment.

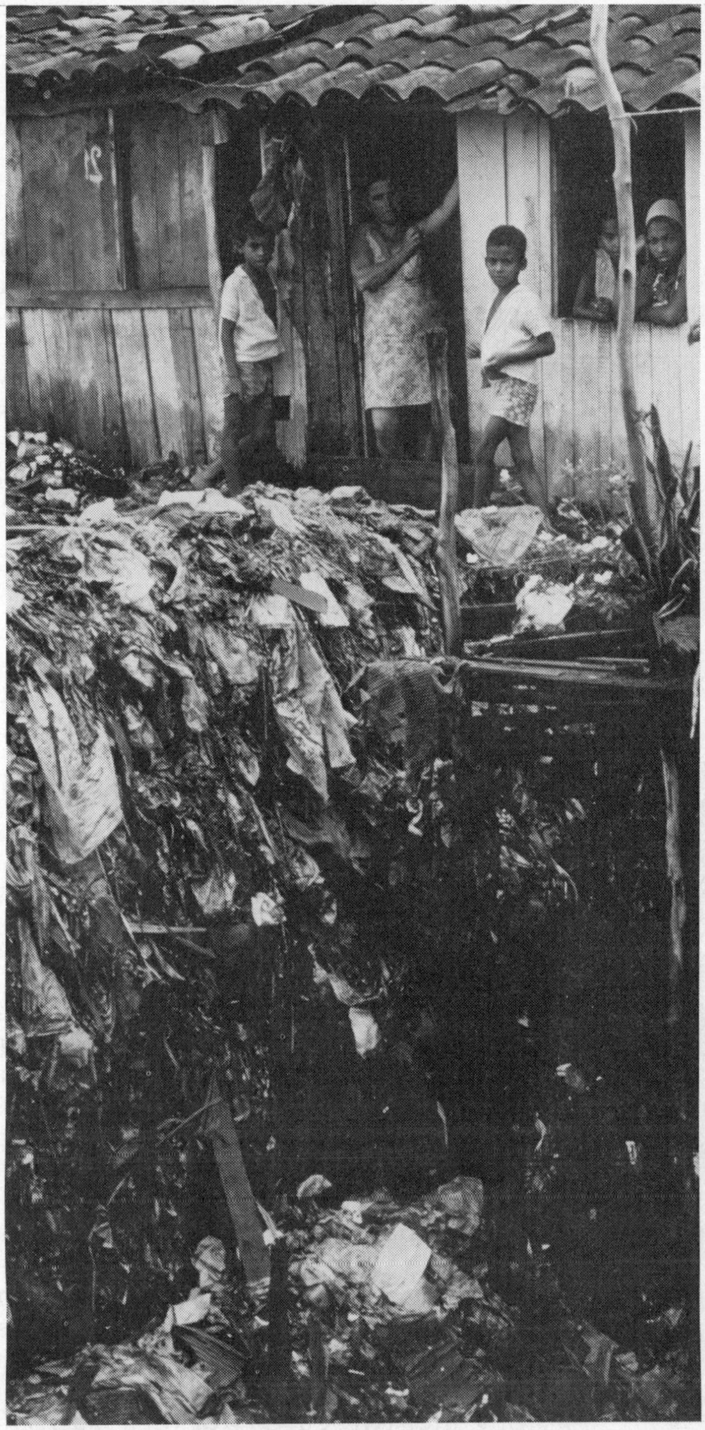

"Demographic factors may influence health at the community level as well as at the family level. Growth in population makes it more difficult to ensure safe or sufficient water supply, garbage disposal, and sanitation for the community. It increases the cost of providing adequately trained health manpower and medical facilities."

World Bank, Health Sector Policy Paper, 1980.

Djukanovic, V. and E. P. Mach, eds. Alternative Approaches to Meeting Basic Health Needs in Developing Countries. A Joint UNICEF/WHO Study. Geneva: World Health Organization, 1975.

"The tendency has been to create relatively sophisticated health services staffed by highly qualified personnel, in the hope of expanding them progressively as resources increased until the entire population was covered. The outcome has been quite different. The services have become centered largely in the cities and towns, are predominantly curative in nature, and are accessible mainly to a small and privileged section of the population...In many developing countries over half of the national health budget is spent on health care in urban areas, the home of no more than a fifth of the total population."

"Most health care delivery systems have failed to make care accessible and acceptable to the people who need it...As the acceptance of many health measures may involve a change in living habits, the community itself must decide on the measures, help in carrying them out, and evaluate their success...Organizing the delivery of health care so that part of it 'belongs' to those it is designed to serve has enormous advantages. Local resources can be tapped and the community's view of the nature of the system can be radically changed. Primary health care workers can be recruited from among the villagers and be trained in or near the village, so that they truly belong to the people. Education and training programmes, both undergraduate and post-graduate, at home or abroad, are frequently irrelevant to or fall short of local health needs and aspirations."

For example, in the Peoples Republic of China, each person is expected to participate wholeheartedly in community public health measures, the organization of medical care, and the conduct of all aspects of his or her personal life, including health. The theme of "knowing by doing"--that the way to teach 800 million people preventive health measures and health care is to see that they are involved--has meant the broadest involvement of people at every level of society in health care.

The health care system in China emphasizes the provision of services in the rural areas, where 80-85% of the Chinese people live, and the development of services to the masses of 'workers, peasants and soldiers.' The cost of health services in China appears quite low; economies are attained by a combination of low cost local facilities, the use of traditional techniques and medicines, modest salary levels for health workers, and an incentive system increasingly based on social motivation rather than economic rewards. "The greatest lesson that China offers is that a nation can within one generation move from a starving, sickness-riddled, illiterate, elitist semi-feudal society to a vigorous, healthy, productive, highly literate, mass participation society."

In Cuba, the situation prior to 1959 was marked by: an absence of a national health system or of elementary coordination of existing services; insufficient services, with the population being left to its own resources for medical attention, which for many people was unobtainable; predominantly curative services, and a virtual absence of preventive medicine; and a divorce between the teaching of medicine and social needs, as doctors were trained for private curative practice.

Currently, 50% or more of the government budget is allocated to health and education, and the health services system is "accessible and available to practically

100% of the population. Preventive, curative and rehabilitation services are well planned and integrated, and show excellent results in terms of service indicators, mortality and morbidity data." The factors accountable for the success are complete literacy, a high proportion of doctors and other professional staff, good transport facilities, and mass mobilization and full participation of the people.

"A firm national policy of providing health care for the underprivileged of the world will involve a virtual revolution in most health service systems. It will bring about changes in the distribution of power, in the pattern of political decision making, in the attitude and commitment of health professionals and administrators in ministries of health and universities, and in people's awareness of what they are entitled to."

World Bank. World Development Report 1980. New York: Oxford University Press, 1980.

The World Bank has historically based its aid and finance programs on formal models of development economics, emphasizing the rate of capital investment in physical infrastructure--industry, transportation, communications, and agriculture. Investments relied heavily on the capital/output ratio, or the efficiency with which the investment is converted into production output.

"The productivity of investment in people has been shown to be higher than the productivity of investments in physical capital."

World Bank, 1980.

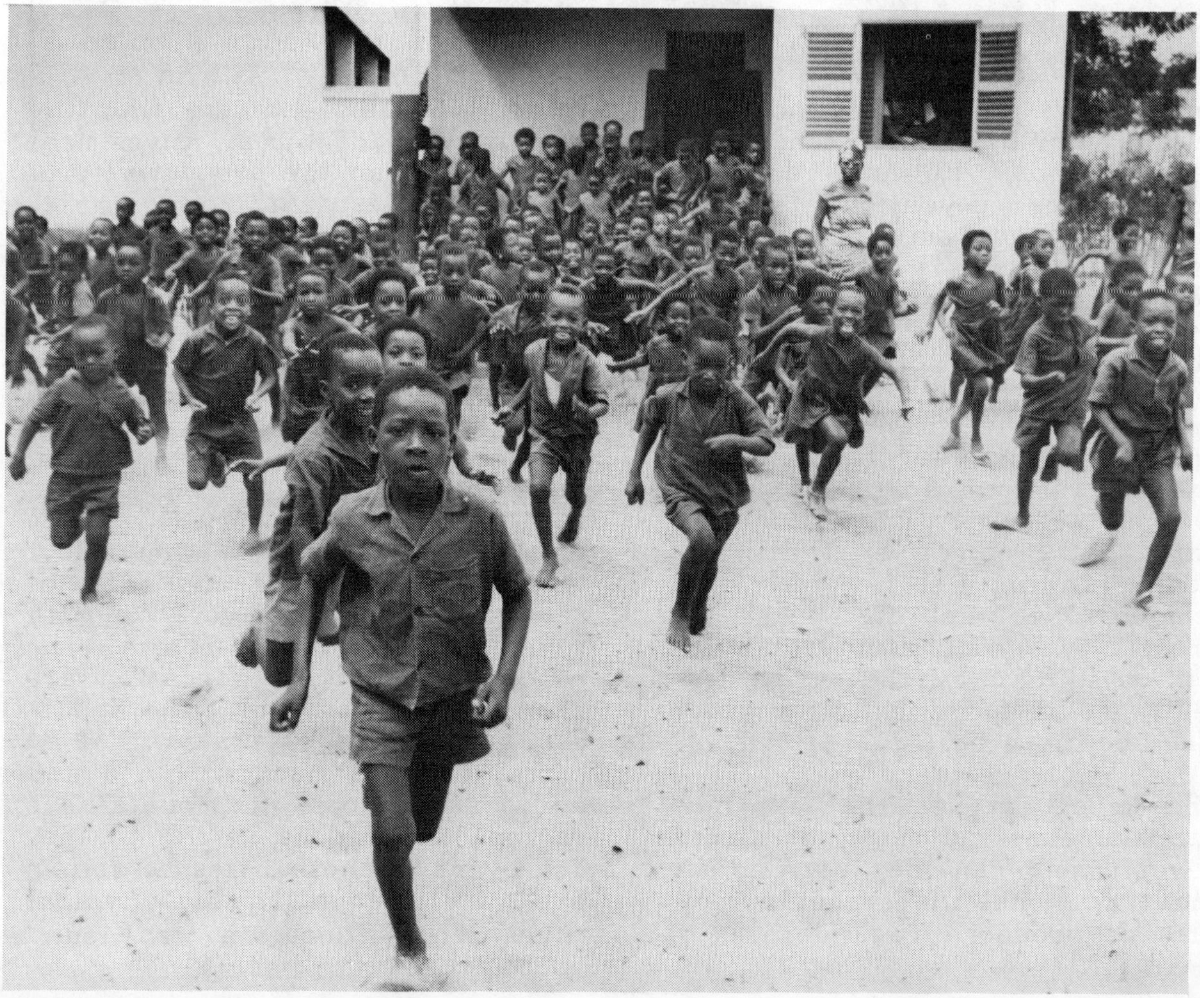

"The medical empire has geared its services, medicines and hardware . . . to such tremendous profits that it has priced itself out of the reach of the majority of the people . . . People are what make health care work."

David Werner, "Health Care and Human Dignity—A Subjective Look at Community-Based Rural Health Programmes in Latin America," Contact,*#57, August 1980.*

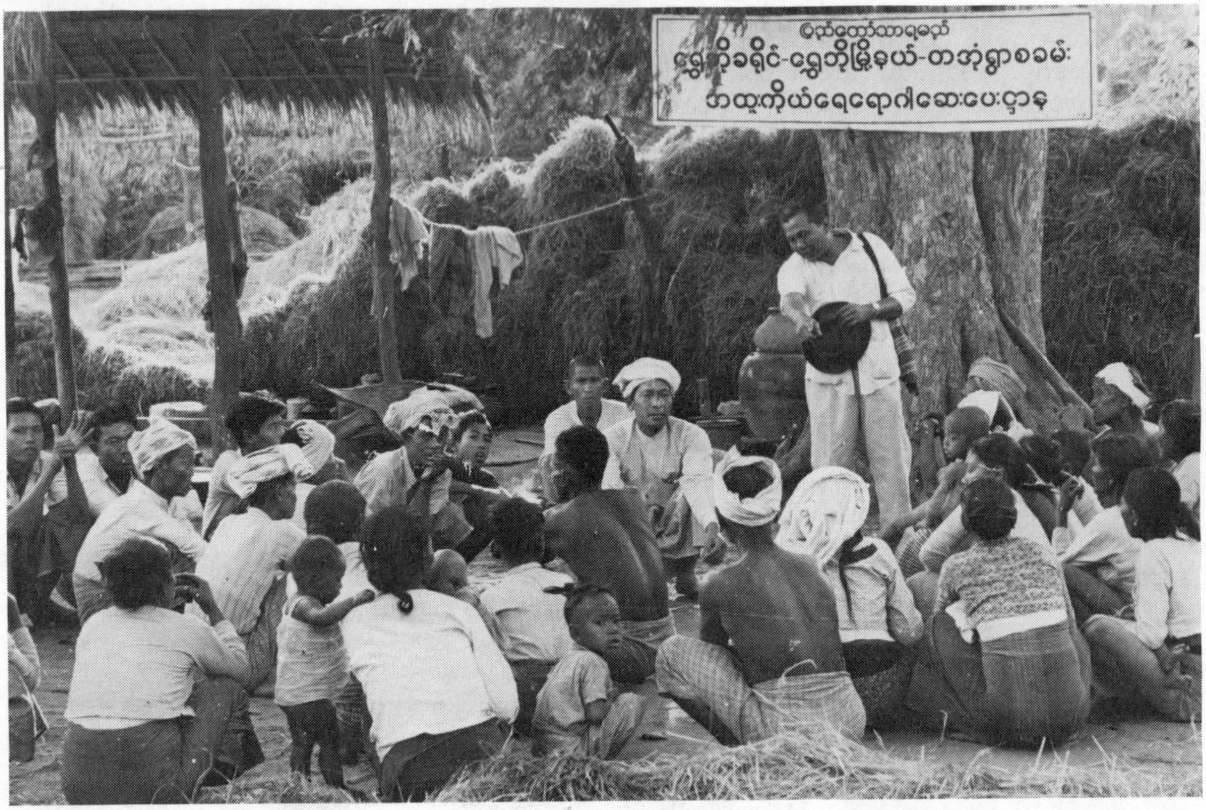

This Report marks a distinct shift in the World Bank's concept of development. Human development--better education, health, nutrition, and family planning at the local level--is seen as promoting economic growth as effectively as capital investment in physical infrastructure. The satisfaction of human needs through increased investment and improved health, education and nutrition are viewed as a means towards economic growth, but also part of the objective of development planning itself. Adam Smith is quoted to the effect that the prosperity of a nation is determined mainly "by the skill, dexterity, and judgement with which its labor is generally applied".

The Report argues that expenditures of time and money on human development can be justified by the traditional investment principles of productivity and rates of return. Studies indicate that the productivity of human investment is higher than the productivity of physical investment. For example, the rates of return on primary education expenditure are as high as 27% for the low income countries and those with low literacy rates, compared with 22% for middle income countries and those with high adult literacy rates. Studies in Korea, Malaysia and Thailand compared the increase in farm productivity resulting from primary education with the cost of the education and found rates of return comparing favorably with investment in other sectors. The rates of return to education are shown to vary though. The Nepalese government estimates that it costs twice as much to build and equip a school in mountainous regions as it does in the plains. Yet overall, these rates of return are rarely equalled by physical investment. Education was found to be the factor consistently linked to the level of human development and to economic growth.

Though the Report does not specifically deal with investments in rehabilitation, it states that "development strategies that bypass large numbers of people may not be the most effective way for developing countries to raise their long-run growth." Regarding investment strategy, the Report points out that the relatively small proportion of people over age 65 in most developing countries considerably reduces the significance of chronic, degenerative diseases, which affect about a third of the elderly in the U.S. The Report concludes that "the most valuable resource any country has is its people, the means and the end of economic advance."

Brown, Joan C. A Hit and Miss Affair: Policies for Disabled People in Canada. Ottawa: Canadian Council on Social Development, 1977.

There is no single definition of "disabled" or agreement on what constitutes disability in Canada. Definitions and standards for eligibility for disability services and programs are often determined by a scarcity of resources available, rather than the level of disability and need. The system might be described as a "gigantic lottery", where under one scheme a person is held too disabled for work, and under another found capable of substantial gainful employment.

While definitions and statistics on the number of disabled persons are crucial to a determination of the needs of disabled people, the level of services required, and the costs of services, this "essential information is often not available to the official and voluntary departments planning services for disabled people, nor to the politicians at the federal, provincial or municipal levels in Canada."

While particular disability programs in Canada are excellent, overall the programs are fragmented and plagued by a lack of coordination in the system. Disability policy is termed a "hit and miss affair". This can be seen in the areas of prevention, vocational and educational rehabilitation, and in the quality of the disability benefits system.

The causes of disability are expanding: mercury, noise, arsenic, and asbestos pollution, nuclear waste spills and other toxic waste contamination have had a profound effect on the incidence of disability. Responsible planning authorities spend 97 percent of their budgets on cure and compensation, and only 3 percent on prevention programs.

There are four systems of medical rehabilitation in Canada--the Worker's Compensation System, the Veterans' System, the Children's System and the General System. These four systems often overlap, and there are considerable provincial differences. There is a lack of adequate facilities, staff and timely access to rehabilitation facilities. Some disabled people receive first class treatment, others little, and responsibility is widely scattered throughout the four systems.

Among the serious problems of the program for integrated education is the inaccessibility of school buildings, inadequate training of teachers, and a poor system for the transition from education to the world of work.

There are two systems for vocational rehabilitation: the Worker's Compensation System, for workers disabled on the job, and the General System for all others. The Worker's Compensation System emphasizes the return to work with the original employer. This provides a familiar environment, maintains seniority, and various benefits. Retraining is given a low priority. A study found that of 95% of job placement cases, 25 percent returned to the employer in lower-paying jobs. The system places priority on the younger age groups both for general admission and training; older workers are encouraged to accept early retirement. The costs of the vocational rehabilitation program are shared between the federal and provincial levels, and these budgetary decisions affect the subsequent caseload possible, screening and referral process, and the general visability of the program. Employment placement policies are also beset by problems such as inaccessible manpower employment centers and low levels of employment in the public sector despite government policy to the contrary.

The disability income system is inadequate. A study revealed that 73 percent of disabled persons had no personal property of value and 93 percent had no real property of value. The current disability income pension rates assume that the disabled, who do not have employment costs such as fares, clothing, lunches and taxes, can live on 75% of prior income. Yet the costs of disability are often higher than pre-disability costs. Eligibility for disability pension benefits is limited to workers who contributed to the pension fund for a sufficient number of years, and thus exclude everyone who never entered the labor force, or who have just joined the work force. A three month mandatory waiting period assumes that other income security programs will provide for basic needs. And the definition of disability and award of benefits differed in each province, often much lower than actual need.

Access to disability income is determined not by the degree of disability, but by the cause or source of the disability. The whole network of administrative and legal systems established to deal with disability adds to the total cost of the disability income system without necessarily improving the standard of living of disabled people. "The categorical systems also involve wasteful duplication of administrative costs and professional services.. Each compensation system has staff spending their time not in paying compensation to the victims of disablement, but in redistributing compensation costs from one system to another." These eligibility decisions also affect access to other rehabilitation programs, medical care, prostheses and orthotics.

Berkowitz, Monroe, W.G. Johnson and Edward H.Murphy. Public Policy Toward Disability. New York: Praeger Publishers, 1976.

Strategies developed by policy makers to deal with disability are influenced by the concept of disability employed in population surveys. In the United States disability is conceived primarily as a medical problem, or a health-related inability to work. This concept "shapes most of the present government policy and societal attitudes towards the disabled."

There are more than 85 separate programs serving disabled people in the United States. Public and private transfer, medical, and survivor payment programs that pay benefits or provide services to disabled persons in the age group 18 to 64 comprise the workers' disability income system. The cornerstone of the system is the Federal/State Vocational Rehabilitation Program, and other pro-

"Every year an estimated 50 million accidents occur in industry throughout the world; about 160,000 each day." *International Labor Organization, 1981.*

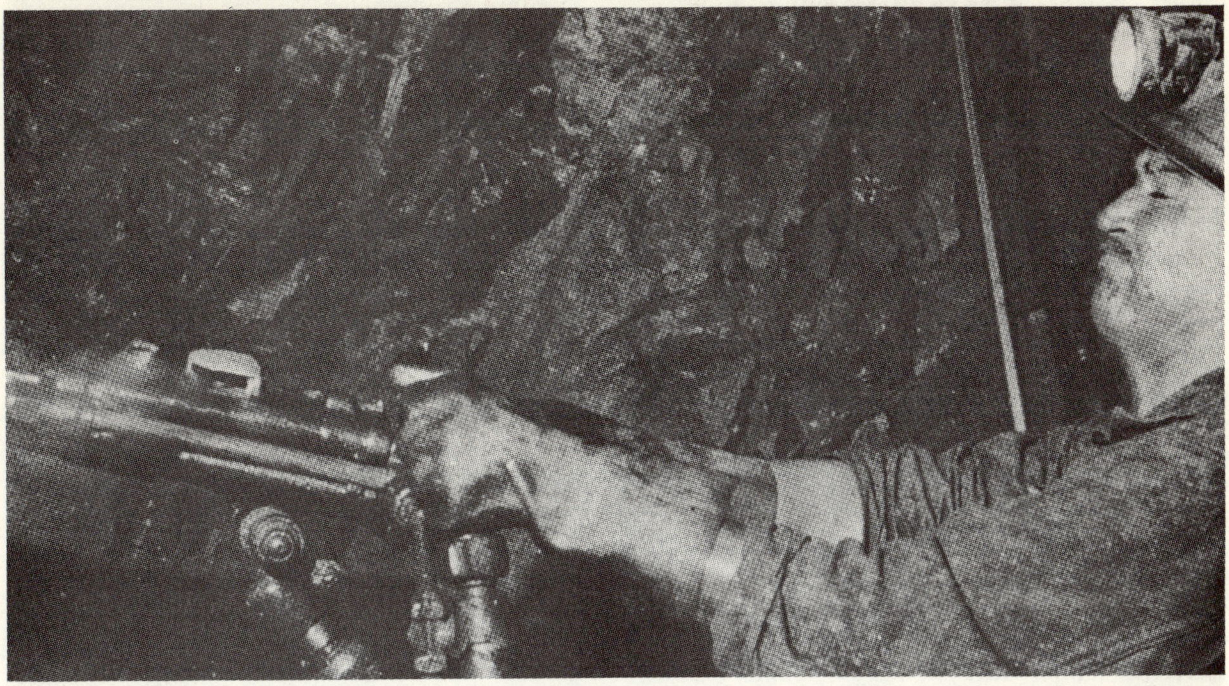

"Economists tell us that if the costs of work-related illness are borne by the firms in which they occur, overall efficiency will be improved because the price of products from each firm will reflect the real costs of producing them—including the cost of damage to human health. Thus one negative result of an inappropriate division of responsibilities among disability programs is diminished overall economic efficiency." *Jonathan H. Sunshine, Disability, 1979.*

grams can be classified into five general categories: risk aversion (private insurance), status (e.g., veteran), social insurance (social security disability insurance), income support (e.g., Aid to Families with Dependent Children or Social Security Income) and indemnity payments (accident liability).

The Social Security Administration has responsibility for making determinations of disability, though disability policy may be modified by the judicial review system. The Congressional definition of disability is "the inability to engage in any substantial gainful activity because of any medically determinable physical or mental impairment." This definition, as well as all of the disability programs, emphasize the medical origins and occupational consequences of disability.

Disability must be conceptualized on the basis of the interactions between health and social and economic influences. The severity of functional limitation is "not the most important influence on differences in the disability status of (noninstitutionalized) impaired persons." Race, age, marital status, education, and access to transfer payments are also important, if not determining factors, in differences in disability status. A labor supply theory of disability, the identification and quantification of these factors that influence individual choices regarding wage employment, nonwage work, or household production, permits policy options to be developed for each variable. Disability programs must move away from a medical concept of disability to one that emphasizes social and economic factors.

II. ECONOMIC AND SOCIAL COSTS OF DISABILITY

Disability is known to have significant effects within all societies. Aside from the more apparent implications of disability for the people directly affected, disability has important consequences for society as a whole. Disability results in a loss of national income. Like other chronic social and medical problems, it may reduce the capacity of the individual to absorb education, to be productive in work, and to function independently. Disability can place heavy burdens upon those who must care for the disabled, sometimes causing a reduction in the economic performance of the care providers. A loss in psychic well-being, while limiting the economic capability of the disabled person, may also affect the economic productivity of his or her family and friends. Economic losses are possible in the future based on the potential effect disability has on the health and well-being of the children of disabled people. Additional indirect effects, such as property losses and marital instability, may be present, but are rarely included within any analysis.

An important category of costs to everyone other than the disabled and their families is that of transfer payments for livelihood support. These costs to the community are offset by the gains to the disabled and therefore do not constitute a net cost to society, although they have other social and political implications associated with the redistribution of national wealth. The analysis of costs is further complicated by the basic differences in social organization which exist between nations.

Relation to the Socio-Political System

Countries vary considerably in their approach to the basic principles of social organization. Some organize their services according to the principles of the "welfare-state", in which the State acknowledges ultimate responsibility for the livelihood of its citizens; others are more allied with the principle of "individualism" whereby ultimate responsibility rests with the individual and the provisions he or she can make for self-help. Societies organized on the basis of socialist systems tend to formalize the responsibility of the State to meet each citizen's basic needs for health care, education and employment. The provisions established by law will be markedly different from those of nations committed to the action and choices of the individual within a broad framework of social institutions. The majority of nations have systems based on the full range of philosophies and policies somewhere between these two polar concepts.

The distinction in philosophical base, and consequent approach to service provision, has an important effect on the economic assessment of rehabilitation activity. It becomes far more difficult to distinguish the costs and benefits of services for the disabled in societies which offer a broad and often centrally controlled range of health, education, counselling and employment services to their general population. It is generally expected that the higher level of universally available

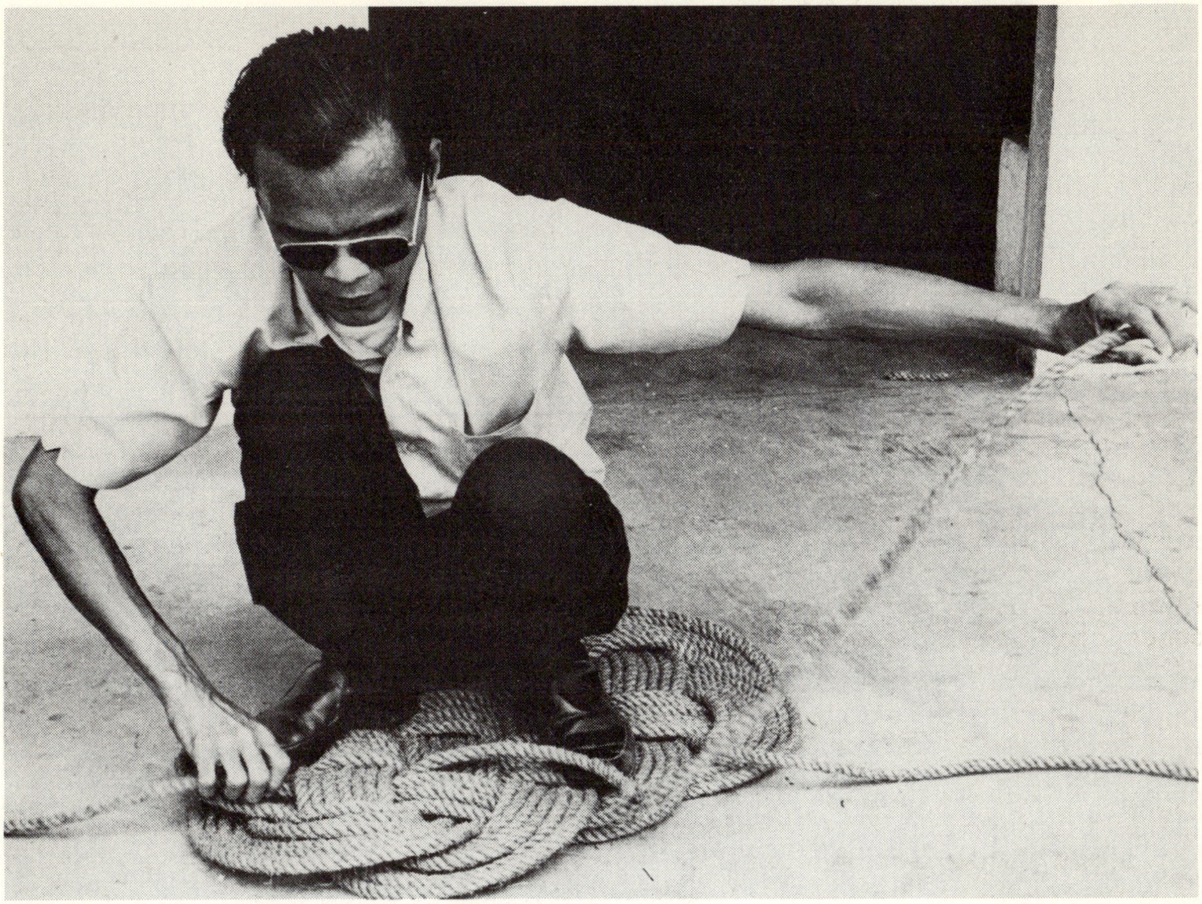

services will reduce the need for specialized services, through the early detection and treatment of disability, through the prevention of certain consequences of untreated disability, and through the integration of the disabled into the existing pattern of service provision.

Thus, for example, in countries which provide comprehensive medical services to their population under state coverage, the identifiable costs of medical services for the disabled will reflect only those highly specialized services such as spinal cord injury units, sheltered workshops, or prosthetic appliance manufacturing units, which are not used by the general population. The physical therapy services, social counselling services, home nursing services, and other such facilities of great importance to the disabled, which are also used by the general public, will not be separately reported as a rehabilitation cost, nor is it possible to estimate their value accurately since the value of services rendered will vary greatly depending upon the number of people making use of the specialized personnel needed.

No society has found the perfect balance between the provision of generally available services and that of specialized services which can accommodate all of the highly individualized needs of the disabled; and no society based in principle on the needs of the individual has found the way to provide all of the necessary services at reasonable cost. Much experience exists in nations which have organized their rehabilitation services on these differing bases; the world's disabled have not yet been the beneficiaries of any systematic international study of the results.

A. REHABILITATION EXPENDITURES

Rehabilitation services, the combined medical, educational, vocational and social services intended to help the disabled person to achieve a social as well as physical adjustment to his or her impairment, can assist the disabled to return to full lives within the community. Several valuable analyses are available of procedures to estimate more accurately the direct and indirect costs of actual service provision. 8/

It is extremely difficult to obtain adequate data on the actual cost of providing rehabilitation services. The International Social Security Association carried out a survey in 1968 on measures and services designed to promote rehabilitation in social security institutions which in part attempted to determine the total cost of the services provided and express this cost as a percentage of the total institutional expenditure. Dr. Charles Berlioz, the consultant for the study, concluded that:

"The information obtained can be used only with difficulty, for very understandable reasons. In many countries the accounting system does not isolate the expenditure devoted to rehabilitation, whether this is provided in special centres, or in other establishments, or for out-patients. Furthermore, even if all the replies had provided information on this point, this would have represented only a fragmentary picture of the real situation since many invalid persons receive rehabilitation outside the specialized rehabilitation services." 9/

Definitive data on the national costs of rehabilitation service provision do not exist for many of the reasons already cited. Likewise, there is little information on the costs of training rehabilitation personnel, one of the major elements of direct cost in rehabilitation, since this training is frequently integrated within larger educational institutions or conducted as a part of research and development activity. It is known that the needs for rehabilitation personnel are enormous, and it is known that the costs to society of rehabilitation service provision are significant. The following examples will illustrate how expenditures for rehabilitation services have been estimated in some countries, in national as well as individual patient terms, and they will demonstrate the magnitude of the costs involved.

The United States of America. A study of 460 severely handicapped patients at a comprehensive rehabilitation center in Chicago, Illinois, carried out in 1968, indicated an average cost per patient of $8,046, with the cost of services ranging from $35 to $55,175 per patient. 10/ It was estimated that in 1970, about $80 million would have been expended by private agencies concerned with rehabilitation in the United States for services and capital outlays. 11/ The Federal Government's Rehabilitation Services Administration expended an average of $2,135 per rehabilitant in 1970. Included in this group were the mildly and the moderately handicapped and a small percentage of the severely handicapped. 12/ In 1975, there were estimated to be more than 10 million people in the United States with severe handicaps. In fiscal year 1973, 85 federal agencies expended approximately $22 billion for services for persons with severe handicaps. These services included, among other things, medical care, services to veterans, income transfer

The global number of people injured on the road each year is now estimated at 10 million, 2-3 million of whom are seriously injured. The costs to society of road accidents include medical care, medicine and transport, administrative efforts by police and judicial processes, social welfare payments to accident victims and their families, reduced tax revenues, and the reduced income for those disabled by accidents. *International Rehabilitation Review, 3, 1978.*

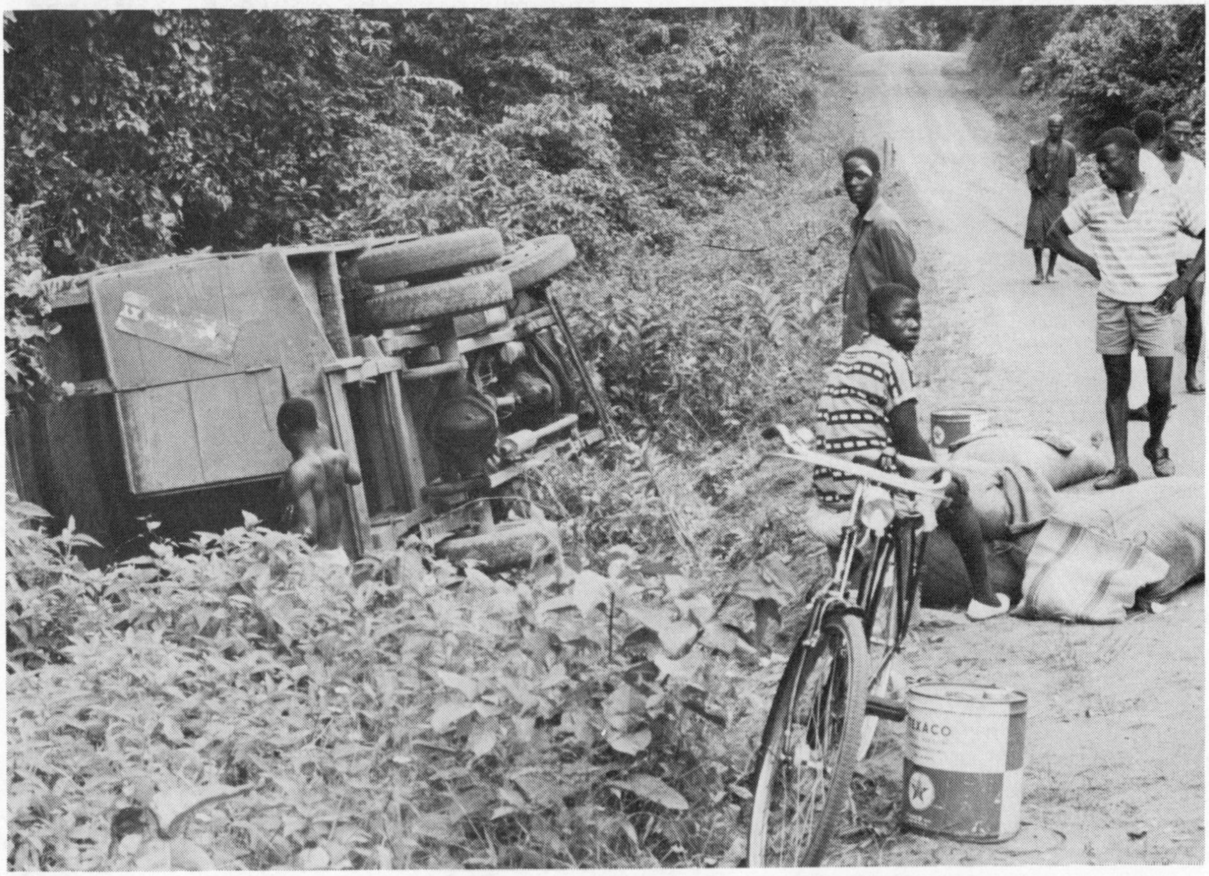

payments, attendant care, social services, and rehabilitation services. Only 2 percent of the total expenditure was provided through the Rehabilitation Services Administration, which has specific responsibility for the rehabilitation and placement of the severely disabled. 13/

Finland. Data from Finland indicates that in 1973 government expenditures for the maintenance of special rehabilitation services totaled: 14/

Fmk 16,612,000	- for institutions for medical rehabilitation;
Fmk 4,426,000	- for institutions for the basic education of disabled children, not including schools for the deaf and blind maintained by the Ministry of Education;
Fmk 798,000	- for disability adjustment training programs;
Fmk 1,160,000	- for work assessment and work training clinics, not including special vocational schools financed by the Ministry of Education;
Total	- Fmk 24,710,000 (approx. U.S.$6,425,000)

In addition, there was during that year an expenditure by the Ministry of Labor for some forms of vocational rehabilitation services -- for example, placement services for the hard-to-employ were allocated more than Fmk 23 million in the Ministry's 1975 budget.

The above data is based on statistics from the National Board of Social Welfare. Studies were also conducted on the number of people in need of rehabilitation services, and the number who could benefit from them if optimum facilities were available. The Finnish National Medical Board estimated in 1971 on the basis of hospital statistics and medical evaluations, that 500,000 people out of a total population of about 4.5 million were in need of medical rehabilitation services. A study by the Research Institute of Social Insurance Institution, using a different methodology based on interviews and evaluations of a sample population, indicated that approximately one half that number of people could benefit from such services if the optimum number of services were available; however, an almost equal number of people could benefit from psycho-social rehabilitation services according to this latter analysis.

<u>Poland</u>. In Poland (1972), the annual average costs and losses attributable to traumatic disability were estimated as follows: <u>15</u>/

992,000,000 zlotys - the value of the social product lost as a result of absenteeism from work due to illness;

64,987,000 zlotys - expenditures for ambulance services, casualty transportation, and medical assistance at first aid stations;

520,829,000 zlotys - costs of treatment at hospitals and sanatoria;

100,132,000 zlotys - costs of treatment at outpatient clinics;

659,977,000 zlotys - total amount of sick benefits paid;

450,800,000 zlotys - indemnities due to accidents and other expenses in compensation for physical suffering;

426,296,000 zlotys - disability pensions;

Total expenditure for traumatically induced disabilities = 3,145,021,000 zlotys. (approx. U.S.$142,000,000)

<u>France</u>. An analysis carried out for the French Institut de la Vie in 1971 based on statistical data from 1967 attempted to calculate the costs to society of disabled people. The calculation was theoretical, and it utilized data from the Sixth Plan of the Social Action Commission, from the National Social Security Administration, and from the French Consumption Research and Documentation Center (CREDOC). <u>16</u>/ The analysis took into account the benefits provided to the families of disabled children, the allotments provided to handicapped adults, and the costs of in-patient treatment in specialized institutions for certain groups of the disabled. In 1967, there were an estimated two to three million disabled persons in France, somewhat less than one million of whom were children and youth under 20 years of age. Their disabilities

included varying degrees of mental retardation, cerebral-motor disability, non-cerebral motor disability, blindness and deafness. The war-disabled and persons injured in work accidents were included within the total figure.

The CREDOC data indicated that a disabled child cost on the average 27 francs a day for daily expenditures including food, housing and education. A normal child cost about 4.5 francs daily. Reducing this amount by the special benefits provided to the families of the disabled, it was estimated that the average disabled child would cost his family on the average five times more than a normal child.

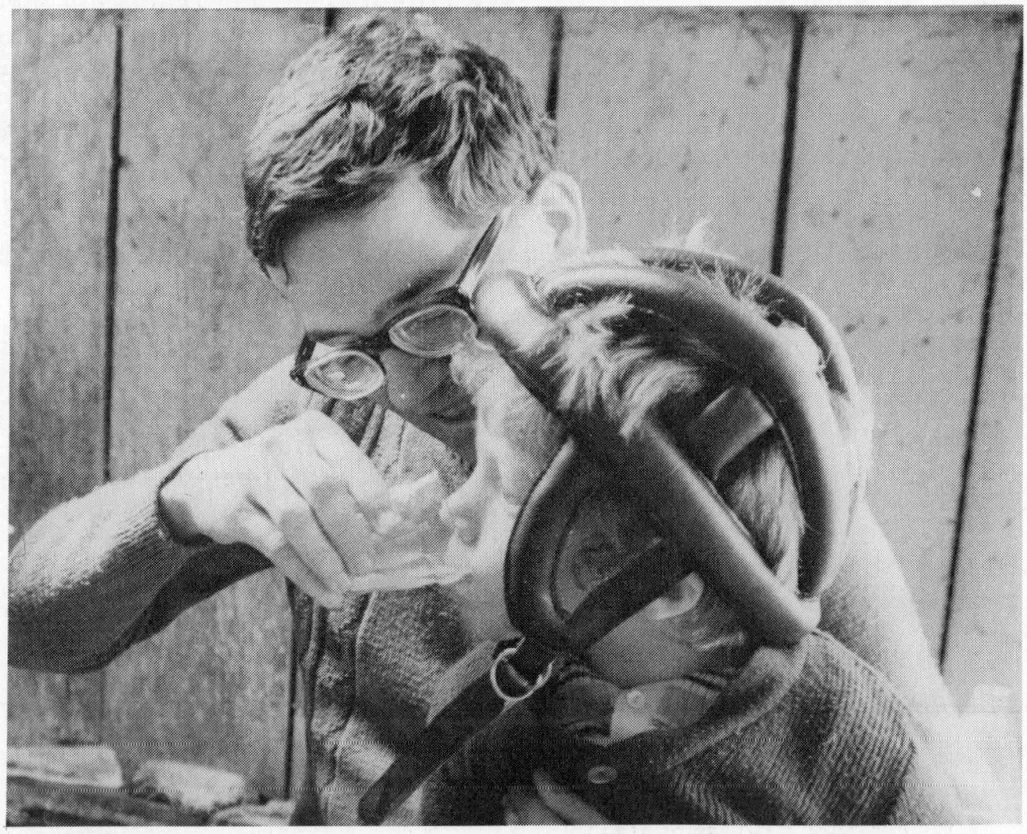

The data from the National Social Security Administration and other institutions which provide lifelong service to the disabled were used to calculate the average lifetime expenses to society. These calculations were based on an average life span of 50 years. Assuming that the average cost of allotments to handicapped minors and specialized in-patient institutional treatment would be 7,000 francs per year per child for 15 years from ages 5-20, an average of 105,000 francs was being spent per child yearly during this period. The cost during adulthood from 20 to 50 years of age, based on an average expenditure of 10,600 francs yearly per person in social assistance allotments and unconditional disability payments, was 318,000 francs. The average cost from ages 5 to 20 and 20 to 50 years were then added to total 423,000 francs per disabled person. Taking into account additional expenditures during the preschool years, and the change in value of the franc between 1967 and 1970 it was concluded that the average cost to society in 1970 of a disabled person having a life span of 50 years would have been at least 500,000 francs, or 10,000 francs per year of life (= U.S. $2,500).

Additional References on Rehabilitation Expenditures:

Berkowitz, Monroe and W.G. Johnson. "Towards an Economics of Disability: The Magnitude and Structure of Transfer and Medical Costs," Journal of Human Resources, Volume 5, #3, 1970, pp. 271-297.

"Possibly one-sixth of the civilian non-institutionalized population of working age is limited in their ability to work because of chronic health conditions or impairments. Nearly one-half of the men not in the labor force were disabled and more than one-third were severely disabled. Disability of the breadwinner is a significant cause of family incomes falling below the poverty line. It is not chronic conditions alone which cause losses; the average currently employed worker loses nearly four days of work per year due to some acute conditions."

It is possible to approximate the economic losses due to disability by estimating disability transfers, which involve no real resource costs, and medical costs, which do involve real resource costs.

Among the major categories of transfer payments in the United States are private disability insurance, social insurance (mandatory government programs), indemnity payments (such as liability insurance contracts), income support to disabled persons, disability payments due to status (such as a veteran), and payments to the survivors of those whose disability leads to "premature" death. The total dollar value of these transfer payments due to disability totaled $14 billion in 1967.

The estimated cost of medical services devoted to the relief or cure of disabling conditions, adjusted for age (18-64) and the elimination of preventive-diagnostic treatment, was $20.5 billion in 1967. The total estimated loss was $43 billion in 1967, or 7 percent of national income.

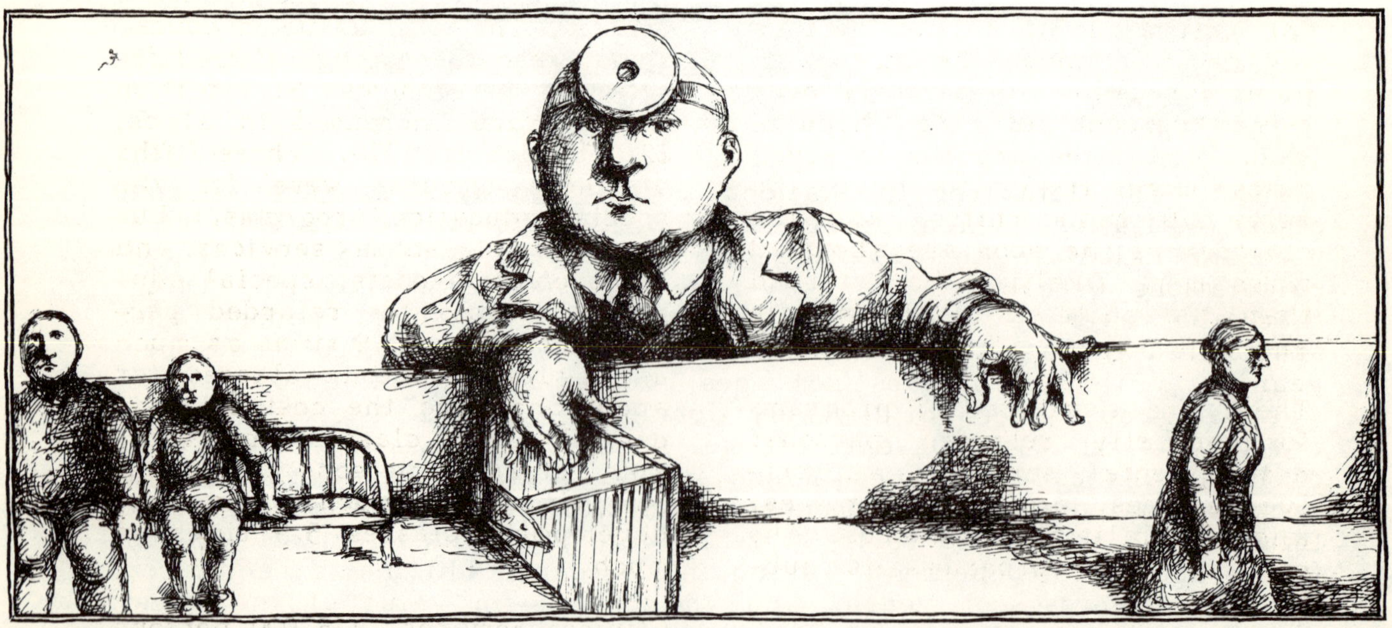

Physician propensities to prescribe costly services are of particular interest from the point of view of total health care spending; it has been estimated that physicians control 70 percent of total health spending.

Alain C. Enthoven, "The Behavior of Health Care Agents: Provider Behavior," 1980.

These statistics reveal that while transfer payments are scrupulously limited in order to avoid disincentive effects to return to work, most medical costs of the same disabling conditions are largely ignored. The effect is to increase the substitution of free medical services for those utilized prior to disability--hiding the costs of disability behind the "general label of poverty."

Conley, Ronald W. The Economics of Mental Retardation. Baltimore: Johns Hopkins University Press, 1973.

"Mental retardation refers to a condition of inadequately developed intelligence which significantly impairs a person's ability to learn and adapt to the demands of society...the effects of mental retardation are, to a greater or lesser extent, borne by all. For example, mental retardation increases the tax burden on the average taxpayer because of the frequent need for publicly provided maintenance and treatment and the reduced tax receipts resulting from lower earnings."

"An estimated 5.6 million persons in the U.S. under the age of 65 have IQs below 70--slightly over three percent of the population...Nonwhites are six to seven times more likely to have IQs below 70 than whites, and the children of the poor are about 13 times more likely to be retarded than the children of the middle and upper classes."

There are a number of programs for mentally retarded persons: developmental services, supportive services, protective services, and rehabilitative services. The cost of these programs is substantial.

Residential Services. In 1968 the cost for 274,852 mentally retarded persons in 24 hour day care was $1 billion and in 1970 the expenditure increased to $1.3 billion

2.1
Expenditures on Selected Programs Serving the Retarded

	1968 (millions)	1970 (millions)
Residential care	$1,284.4	$1,619.5
Special education	1,057.9	1,463.6
Regular academic education	648.0	748.6
Clinical program	26.0	54.4
Employment programs	75.0	124.8
Construction	46.5	41.5
Training of personnel	183.0	235.0
Research	50.0	62.0
Income maintenance	263.5	364.6
Agency operating expenses	7.1	11.8
Total	$3,641.4	$4,725.8

(Adding the value of unpaid volunteer work and the value of land, buildings, etc., the figures increase to $1.3 billion and $1.6 billion). The average per capita costs among adults was $2,300 per year, and for children about $4,400 in 1968.

Education. In 1970, approximately 690,000 retarded children attended special education programs, and 740,000 attended regular academic classes. The total value of educational resources being utilized for retarded persons was $1.7 billion in 1968 and increased to almost $2.2 billion in 1970. (Three-fifths of these amounts were for the special education programs.) Due to extra classroom services and transportation costs, special education classes for retarded persons cost about 1.9 times as much as regular academic classes (or about one-third the cost of residential care); classes for "trainable retarded" persons cost about 3.5 times as much, and day development classes 5.9 times as much.

Clinical Services. 115,000 persons in 1968 were provided clinical services, and 180,000 in 1971. The costs of these services increased sharply from $26 million in 1968 to over $54 million in 1970.

Employment Programs. Approximately $75 million was spent on employment programs in 1968, and 125 million in 1970. These figures include the costs of vocational rehabilitation services and sheltered workshops. The average cost of vocational services for all successfully rehabilitated clients was $2,181 in 1970. Assuming that retarded persons require twice the counselling time of other rehabilitants (almost 30% of rehabilitation funds is used for counselling and placement), then the actual cost per rehabilitated mentally retarded client was $2,830 in 1970.

Income Maintenance. About $365 million was disbursed to 360,000 retarded individuals, primarily "childhood disability beneficiaries" under Social Security and APTD (Aid to the Permanently and Totally Disabled) in 1970.

Though total expenditures on programs for mentally retarded persons totaled $3.6 billion in 1968 and $4.7 billion in 1970, another cost concept is social costs, or excess costs--the value of resources that would be available for other uses if retardation did not exist. These costs are "measured by the difference between what is spent on retarded persons and what would be spent on these individuals if they were in a normal intellectual range." The following adjustments are made from the total expenditure figures to estimate the "excess costs":

a) income maintenance payments and maintenance costs in institutions are subtracted, since these costs would be incurred in any event. Agency operating costs of income maintenance programs are not subtracted, since they represent a use of societal resources that normally would not occur;

b) only the above average expenditures on the education of retarded persons represent excess costs;

c) institutional costs are reduced since this money would be spent on institutionalized school-age retarded persons if they attended normal classes;

d) all other costs are assumed to represent abnormal expenditures.

The estimate of excess costs in 1968 was $1.6 billion, $1.3 billion if research, training and construction costs are not included. In 1970, these figures were $2.1 billion and $1.8 billion.

Apart from the expenditures on programs for mentally retarded persons there are the costs that stem from the effects of mental retardation.

2.2
Total Social Cost of Mental Retardation

	1968	1970
	(in 000,000's)	
Loss of earnings	$3,680	$4,142
Loss of homemaking services	380	424
Loss of other unpaid work	250	276
Excess cost of retardation services (excluding research, construction, and training)	1,319	1,835
Research, construction, and training	280	338
Total social cost of mental retardation	$5,909	$7,015

Loss of Earnings. The earnings loss among retarded persons in institutions was estimated at $676,968,000 in 1968, and $706,553,000 in 1970, based on average earnings and employment rates of others their age and sex. Almost 95% of all retarded persons are not in institutions, and the loss of earnings of non-institutionalized retarded persons in 1968 was estimated at 3 billion, and 3.4 billion in 1970--"four times as great as the loss of earnings among mentally retarded persons in institutions." An estimated 87% of mildly retarded adult males were found to be employed, a rate 4% below the general average. Earnings were estimated at 86% of the average; 33% of retarded females were working at wages that were 87% of average.

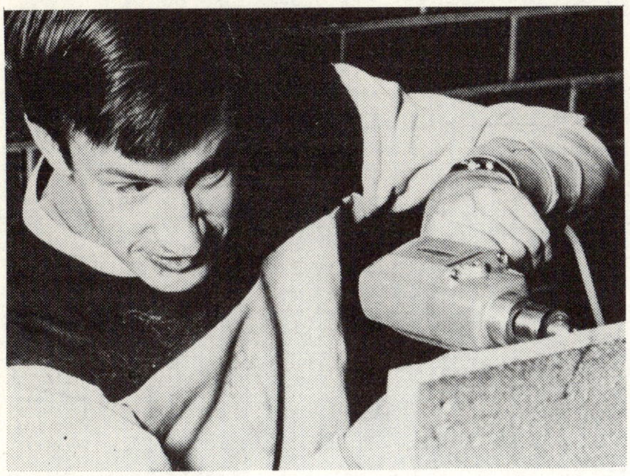

Loss of homemaking and other unpaid work. A housewife's services are valued by what she could earn, if employed, less estimated tax payments; estimates were for female retarded homemakers only. The value of unpaid work, other than normal homemaking services, was estimated at 25 percent of gross earnings. The estimated loss of homemaker's services among retarded females in institutions was less than 150 million in 1968 and 1970, and for non-institutionalized females it was almost $235 million in 1968 and $275 million in 1970; The 25 percent is multiplied times the loss of earnings among male institutionalized retarded persons of all IQs and the non-institutionalized male retarded persons with IQs below 50. Loss of unpaid work is estimated at $250 million and $276 million in 1968 and 1970.

Total Social Cost of Mental Retardation is estimated as the total of excess costs of services, loss of earnings, homemaking services and unpaid work. This figure totaled $5.9 billion in 1968 and $7 billion in 1970.

Commission of the European Communities. Directorate-General for Social Affairs. Comparative Study of the Rehabilitation of Handicapped Persons in the Counties of the Community. Volume I: Belgium, France, Italy, Luxembourg. Luxembourg: C.E.C., 1975.

Belgium: The National Fund for the Social Resettlement of the Disabled (FNRSH), governed by the Ministry of Employment and Labor, is responsible for comprehensive and coordinated programs for social and vocational rehabilitation of disabled persons. In 1972, 133,519 disabled persons were registered for assistance under Social Security legislation, 26,524 of which were for the 1972 financial year.

The total expenditure incurred in 1972, including services provided and subsidies, was over 1,000,000,000 francs.

2.3
National Fund for
the Social Resettlement
of the Disabled
Expenditures, 1972, Belgium

SERVICES PROVIDED (cost in 1000 Belgian Francs	
Preliminary examinations and claims	2,060
Process of rehabilitation	260,200
196,000	Functional rehabilitation
Subtotals 295	Vocational guidance
32,000	School education
33,000	Vocational training
Social aid	42,000
Employment	345,000
Awards	26
TOTAL 72	649,000
TOTAL 71	429,000

Sectors of financial intervention	SUBSIDIES (in 1000 Belgian Francs)		
	Totals	Maintenance	Creation Extension Alteration
Functional rehabilitation	174,000	102,150	71,680
Vocational guidance	4,340	3,520	816
Vocational training	1,360	802	557
Sheltered workshops	180,618	92,200	85,428
TOTALS 72	360,145	158,481	360,145
TOTALS 71	364,866	171,937	192,929

Commission of the European Communities. Directorate-General for Social Affairs. Comparative Study of the Rehabilitation of Handicapped Persons in the Countries of the Community. Volume II: Federal Republic of Germany, Netherlands, Luxembourg: C.E.C., 1975.

Federal Republic of Germany. The costs of rehabilitation are generally borne in full by the insurance funds. In 1973 information was not available on the amounts paid out by the sickness insurance funds, as medical rehabilitation measures were not recorded separately. The following costs were available:

2.4 Accident Insurance Funds 1973 for rehabilitation:	
Out-patient therapeutic treatment	DM 316 484 000
In-patient therapeutic treatment (hospital)	DM 388 134 000
Injury compensation	DM 393 475 000
Occupational assistance	DM 50 641 000
Total	DM1148 734 000

Statutory pension insurance funds (workers', miners, and employees' insurance funds for rehabilitation) 1973:	
Out-patient therapeutic treatment	DM 12 000 000
In-patient therapeutic treatment	DM1920 000 000
Occupational promotion	DM 196 000 000
Transitional cash payments	DM 396 000 000
Follow-up measures	DM 80 000 000
Other promotional measures	DM 567 000 000
	DM3170 000 000

In 1973 the Federal Labor Office spent DM 314 607 000 on the rehabilitation of handicapped persons, primarily for occupational rehabilitation, training, rehabilitation facilities and temporary benefits. The Federal Ministry for Labor and Social Affairs made available an additional sum of DM 40 000 000.

The total expenditure recorded was DM 4 703 341 000 in 1973 (approx. $U.S. 2,025,000,000). In addition, considerable sums were spent by the Lander (states), including social assistance costs. Expenditure on rehabilitation under the war victims' pension and welfare system was also not recorded. Nor does this figure include expenditures by churches and other private organizations.

Berkowitz, Monroe and Jeffrey Rubin. The Costs of Disability: Estimates of Program Expenditures for Disability, 1967-75. New Brunswick, New Jersey: Bureau of Economic Research, 1977.

This study reveals that disability expenditures are increasing at a faster rate than inflation or economic growth without a concomitant rise in the number of disabled persons. From 1970 to 1975, disability transfer payments and medical costs in the public and private sectors almost doubled in current dollars and increased by nearly 40 percent in constant dollars. Total disability expenditures for transfer and medical payments amounted to $38.7 billion in 1967 and comparable estimates for 1975 were over $111 billion. In 1967 these expenditures comprised less than 5 percent of GNP; and by 1975 they totaled 7.6 percent of GNP. Again, no comparable increases in the number of persons who consider themselves limited in the kind and amount of work they can do were found.

Medical payments were responsible for the largest increases, from $21.2 billion to $65.1 billion, while transfer payments rose from $17.5 billion to $46 billion. Factors responsible for growth are the increased number of disabled recipients who have always been eligible for aid, expansion in eligibility considerations that allow other disabled people to qualify for aid, and changes in the amount of aid per recipient (even after correcting for inflation).

Federal payments have grown much faster than state and local government payments, partially because of increases in programs that assumed portions of the disability payments traditionally met by state and local governments or by the private sector, e.g., Medicare, Medicaid, and Black Lung Benefits.

These estimates of programmatic expenditures include transfer payments which are not considered costs in the sense of using up real resources, nor do the estimates include the real costs of lost production and the sacrifice of personal utility. There are only three ways of controlling these expenditures: the prevention of disability, the control of programs by changing eligibility criteria or benefit levels, or rehabilitation to productive activity. Each of these changes will be dependent on the political process.

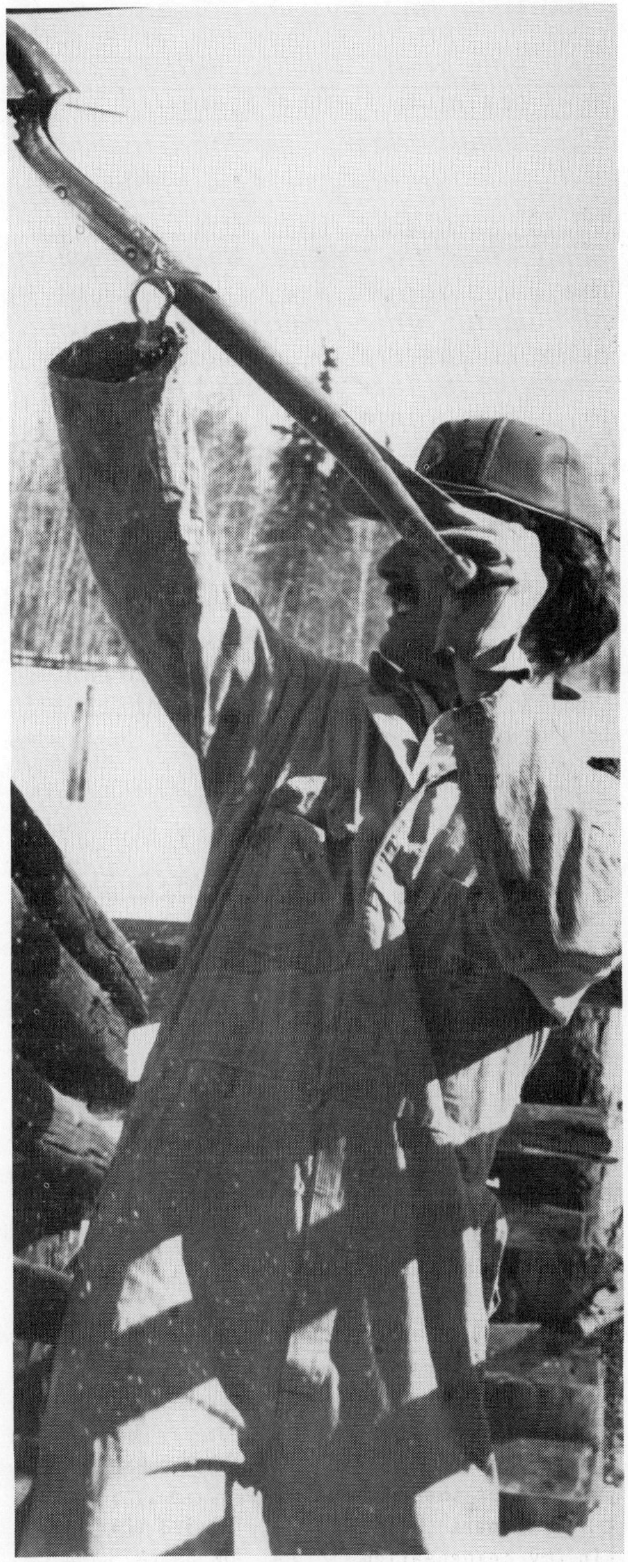

..."rehabilitation to productive activity"

B. SPECIAL EDUCATION

Note: Rehabilitation for the Disabled did not examine the economics of special education; this was done by UNESCO.

United Nations Educational, Scientific and Cultural Organization. Economic Aspects of Special Education: Czechoslovakia, New Zealand, United States of America. Paris: U.N.E.S.C.O., 1978.

It is estimated that 10% of any population is handicapped, yet the handicapped are often left out of account when educational planning is undertaken, sometimes because of a lack of information as to how to adapt educational facilities, or because planners believe that education of handicapped children is more expensive than ordinary education. This work is "designed primarily to demonstrate to policy makers, educational planners and school administrators that special education really pays--that in the long run it is worth while."

Following are the authors and summations of each country study:

Kabele, Frantisek. Czechoslovakia.

The Constitution of the Czechoslovak Socialist Republic guarantees all youth the right to education, and for all citizens the right to work and to social welfare during sickness and old age. The State thus provides medical, educational and social welfare care to all its citizens.

Medical care is basically free. Only when young people stay in an educational, medical or social welfare institution for other than curative purposes do parents contribute to the costs. The size of their contribution is determined according to the social conditions of the child's family. Two factors in particular are taken into account in this context: the income of the parents and the number of children in the family.

Since education interacts closely with medicine and social welfare, the economic aspects of special education cannot be treated adequately without taking these medical and social factors and this interaction into account.

The costs for education and care vary among handicap groups, as is evident from the following figures which represent the annual cost per pupil and which do not include teacher salaries and boarding costs: blind children, 8,200 korunas, mentally retarded children, 7,000 korunas; physically impaired, 51,000 korunas; special apprentice school, 5,600 korunas; and youth with hearing defects, 20,000 korunas.* Hence the costs per pupil at an institute for physically impaired youth is seven times the expense at a special school for mentally retarded pupils.

The reported economic benefits and rates of successful social integration that are the result of special education and care vary according to the type and degree of impairment. Of the graduates of a school for physically handicapped youth in Prague's Jedlicka Institution, about 83% found occupations while only 17% entered social welfare institutions for the unemployable; of the graduates of a special school for the mentally retarded in Prague over a period of 13 years, 95% or 11,300 of 11,900 young people found employment while only 5% became full invalid pensioners.

It was estimated that after nine years the contribution of a rehabilitated and employed person with a handicap amounts to nine times the cost of the special

Though the costs of special education programmes are twice the costs of education for non- disabled children, the contribution of a rehabilitated and employed person with a handicap is many times the cost of the special education. The costs of special education are minor compared to the costs of institutionalization.

UNESCO, 1978.

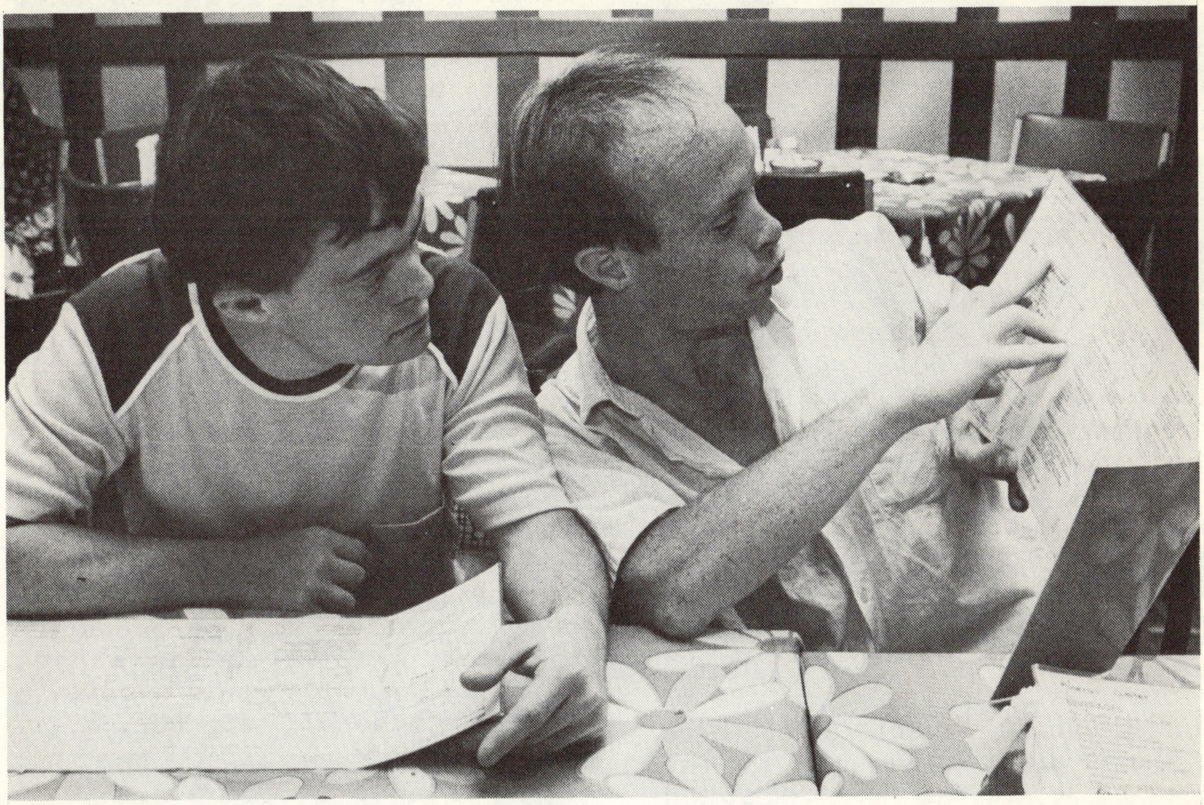

education given. This is an annual contribution of from 30,000 to 50,000 korunas, not counting the decrease in expense for social welfare.

*11.5 Czechoslovak korunas = U.S. $1 (January 1977)

Hyman, Prue. New Zealand.

The effect of handicap which is easiest to assess in a cost benefit analysis* is the loss of potential earnings, but other effects are, in principle, measurable. Inability to manage aspects of life independently requires others to assist, and these costs are either the wages of helpers or the forgone earnings or leisure of other members of the family. The claim that the "economic value of a programme in the education or training field can be assessed by cost benefit analysis with the major benefit calculation being based on increased earnings" should not be made without acknowledgement that the procedure is controversial. Some portion of the increased earnings is probably due to higher ability and more favourable home background, and not all is due to the educational process itself.

The Department of Education of New Zealand estimates an approximate figure of $721 as the average cost for 1974/75 of special education for a child. Education Department estimates for the running costs of education for a "normal" child in the same year average $438. (These figures exclude an allocation for general departmental administration, examinations, land, and buildings.) Therefore the ratio of the average

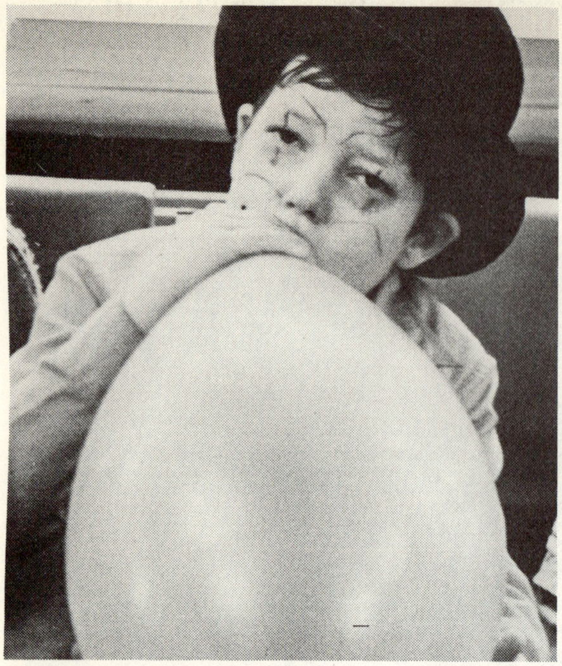

"regular education per child averaged $438"

estimate cost of special education to that in other State schools from these figures is 1.65:1 (primarily because of the lower teacher/pupil ratio in special education).

Concerning placement rates, there is very little difference in the age structure of all completed cases and of clients successfully placed in open employment, and no tendency for the younger age groups to be easier to place. Clients successfully placed earned, on employment, about 70% of the national average wage. Comparison of the present value of benefits and costs show that even with the most pessimistic assumptions for the program, i.e. a ten year working life, no increase in real earnings and the use of a 10% discount rate, together with only 40% of the earnings being attributable to the program, a net present value of $4,657 is obtained. Thus it appears undeniable that quite apart from the social aspects, the program pays in purely monetary terms.

Cost-benefit analysis of education and rehabilitation programs for the visually handicapped found almost all the net present values to be positive. For a person with a full working life, only when the more expensive pattern of education is assumed and not all the earnings are attributed to education does the net present value become negative, and then only with use of the highest discount rate. Yet a rate of return analysis of the education of the intellectually handicapped would probably show that, in terms simply of earnings attributable to their education, it did not pay.

Apart from employment opportunity, the other major benefit from improved education and training of intellectually handicapped people is the increased independence and ability to perform daily tasks. This can yield lower rates of institutionalization. Using a 7% discount rate, the total cost per resident in a New Zealand Society for the Intellectually Handicapped home would be approximately $50/week, but the cost in a psychiatric hospital would certainly be over double this figure.

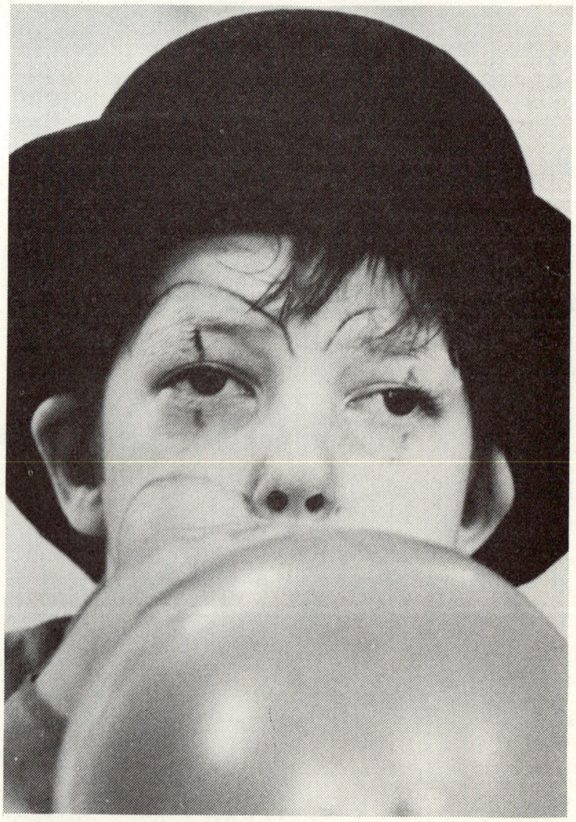

"special education costs averaged $728 per child"

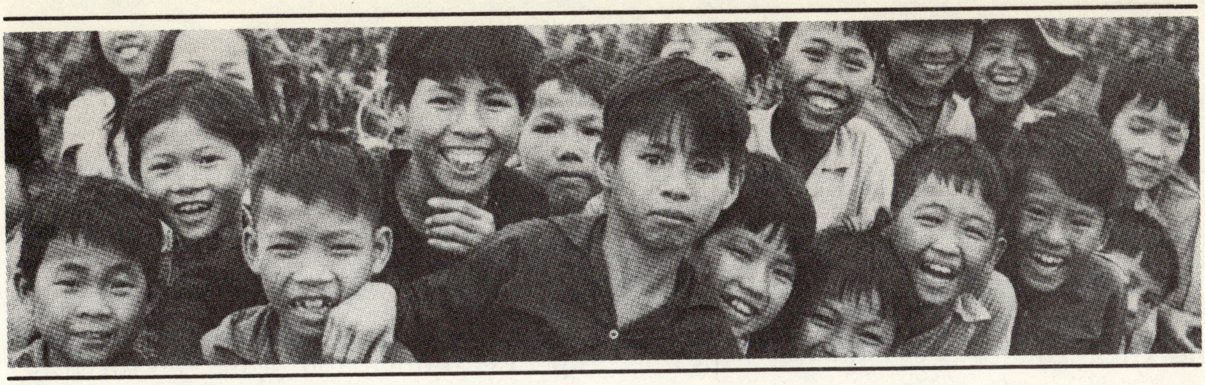

It was estimated that a substantial proportion of mentally retarded patients in psychiatric hospitals in New Zealand could either be cared for in the community or be transferred to homes for the mentally retarded. The majority of those transferred to community units were judged suitable for open or sheltered employment, or for work in occupational workshops.

*See Chapter III on Cost-Benefit Methodology.

Braddock, David. United States of America.

Costs for special education programs in the United States vary a great deal from one group of handicapped persons to another. They also tend to rise or drop in direct accord with the severity of the handicap. Programs for speech handicapped children are less expensive than are programs for the physically handicapped.

The operating and capital outlay costs for special education programs fall into three categories: instruction, public services, facilities. In a recent study, the costs of special education programs were found to range from 1.18 times the cost of educating non-disabled children, to 3.64 for educating a physically handicapped child. The cost index for the entire special education program averaged about twice that spent for regular education. Higher costs for special education were apparent in instructional cost (lower teacher pupil ratios), public service expense (specialized personnel costs and transportation expense), and also in dollars expended for capital equipment investment.

The costs of special education are minor when compared to the costs of institutionalization. "Institutional avoidance costs are a source of long term savings to society." If a disabled individual is institutionalized, the economic consequence of the disability is immediately amplified. Per person maintenance expenditures reported for retardation institutions nationally is $26.02 each day; for mental health institutions, the per diem rate is even higher, $30.86; costs at these levels average about $10,000 per year. Yet 25% of all children admitted to retardation institutions in 1973 were mildly or moderately retarded school age children--children who need not be in an institution in the first place. A recent cost study of long-term care services concluded that substantial savings from deinstitutionalization ($5,000 per year) occur only if the individual is able to live at home. A longitudinal followup study showed substantial net savings to the community after deinstitutionalization: an average ten year net savings--mostly to state government--of $20,800 per person.

Intellectual deficiency, except in the case of relatively severe retardation, was not found to be a major cause of vocational failure. Yet one of the few studies on earnings of severely intellectually deficient people demonstrated adult earnings to be only about one-fifth of the average earnings for adult males. Between 75% and 90% of the subjects followed up in all self sufficiency studies have been found to be totally self-supporting. A small community study found that 87% of mildly retarded adults were employed and their earnings were believed to be between 85% and 90% of the average for the entire United States population. Nearly 60% of the men certified as severely disabled under the United States Social Security program had no earnings at all during a 1966 study. Rehabilitation studies indicate that individuals with orthopaedic handicaps and blindness earn higher wages under sheltered work circumstances and they also pay back their rehabilitation cost in a relatively shorter period of time through regular employment than do mentally handicapped individuals.

An analysis of the ratio of future earnings of retarded workers to costs of their public education, discounted at 7% in 1970 revealed at least three notable findings:

(a) "the lifetime earnings of mildly retarded adults is many times the costs of their education--almost 6:1, adjusted for the percentage employed. Educational services can therefore be justified on the basis of earnings alone.

(b) whatever assumptions are used in the calculation, the benefit- cost ratio exceeds the critical value of 1. The range is between 1:1 and 12:1.

(c) the benefit-cost outlook is much less favourable for the moderately retarded. The range is between 0.1: 1 and 1:1."

In summary, the main sources of social savings as a result of special education and rehabilitation are tax recoupment from earnings, income maintenance cost reduction, and avoidance of the costs of institutionalization.

Another type of cost-benefit analysis is the educational payback period, or the amount of time necessary for an educational program to pay back its costs. Findings vary from a payback period of only 2.3 years for a speech handicapped child to 162.7 years for a severely disabled child. For most categories of disability, the payback period was about 25 years. During the payback period, at prevailing federal government minimum wage

2.5

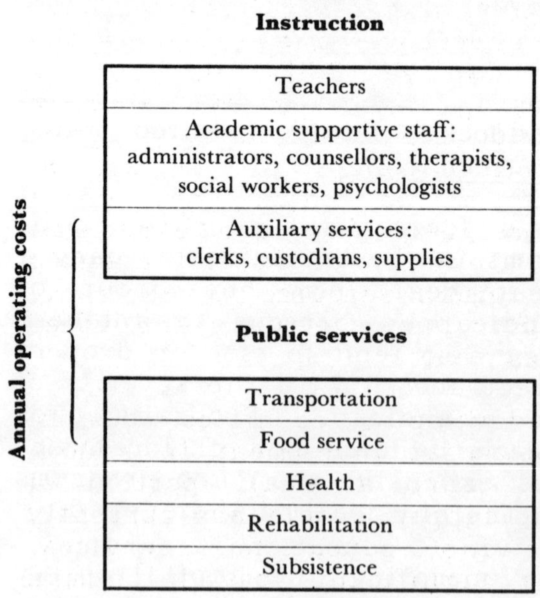

Components of special education costs. (*Source:* W. McClure, 'Alternative Methods of Financing Special Education', *Journal of Educational Finance*, Vol. 1, No. 1, 1975, p. 42).

and tax rates, a non-severely disabled individual will pay $44,840 during a forty year working life in direct taxes. (Education at the highest cost index, 3.64, yields a 12 year special education cost of $52,722. Direct taxes and income maintenance savings amount to $89,680 for a forty year period yielding a net long term savings of $36,958 for this most educationally expensive disability category, even based on a total cost premise.)

Wood, Mary M. et al. "The Economics of Special Education in a Developing Country," International Perspectives on Future Special Education. Reston, Virginia: The Council for Exceptional Children, 1978.

The basic economic problem of most developing nations is not poverty of natural resources, but the underdevelopment of their human capital. Relatively few developing countries are able to provide sufficient funds to offer the full range of educational facilities to which they might aspire. Decisions must be made on the allocation of public revenues for human resource development, industry, agriculture, and other investments.

In developing countries, despite substantial investment in education, only a small portion of handicapped people are currently receiving educational services. This significant loss in human capital could be prevented by investment in an educational program whose benefits to society exceed its costs.

The operation of a special school for handicapped children in Trujillo, Peru--the Manucci School, illustrates this point. This school (80 children) provides an instruc-

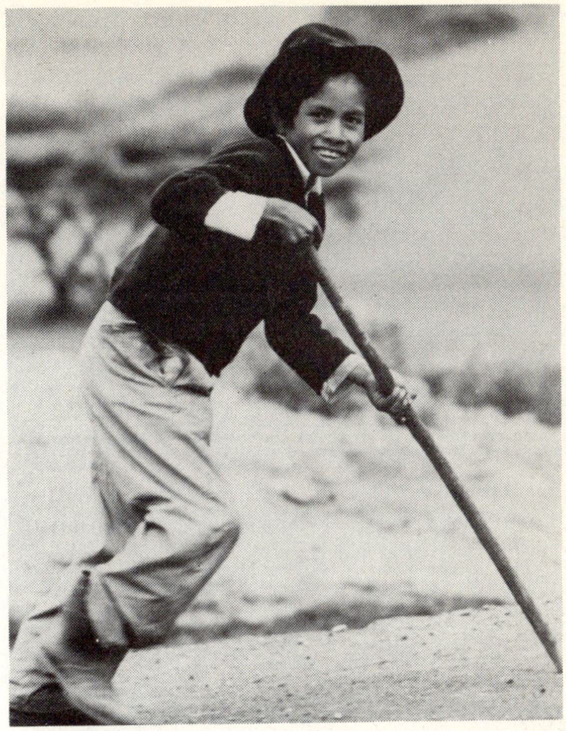

tional program and a sheltered workshop for moderate and severely retarded children, several psychotic and autistic students, and one class for deaf children.

The direct operating costs of $18,000 per year for the Manucci school include: the salaries of teachers and aides, the wages of other service personnel, the cost of instructional material, food, uniforms, and the cost of transporting children. Capital costs of $20,400 include the rent and depreciation charges on the school buildings, and are determined by calculating the value of the buildings and taking 13% (10% rent plus 3% depreciation) of the value of the buildings. The annual cost of school land is also included in the capital costs by taking 10% of its value per year. Total costs are calculated on the basis of an average of 6 years of attendence per student, based on school experience over 10 years. Forgone earnings, a significant cost factor in most educational programs, are estimated as zero, because the handicapped children in the Manucci School would not be capable of work without the special schooling.

The benefits are represented by the estimated increase in income of the student and his or her family resulting from 6 years of special schooling. The school program enables handicapped children to compete for jobs with a portion of the non-handicapped workforce or to perform constructive household tasks in their own home. The estimated monetary value of this work ability for a typical student either within or outside the home is $300 per year, which is equivalent to one-half of the annual income of a non-handicapped maid. There are many other benefits that are not quantifiable in monetary terms.

The rate of return to schooling must be adjusted to reflect the approximately 3% of the students who complete school but are not able to even perform household tasks. Future increases in productivity were projected at 3% per person.

Using these costs and benefits, the adjusted estimated rate of return for the Manucci School investment is 10% per year. All tangible costs and benefits, both public and private, are included in this estimate of net returns, including taxes the students will pay during their working life. This rate of return includes the costs and benefits to society and not just those to the individual students.

These figures compare with the rate of return of 12% (based on C.G. Langoni, "A Study in Economic Growth: The Brazilian Case," Ph.D. dissertation, The University of Chicago, 1970.) to industrial and water development investments in South America, showing that programs for the education of the handicapped are likely to offer relatively attractive investment returns for developing countries.

C. IMPACT OF DISABILITY ON THE FAMILY AND INCOME

The United States Social Security Administration undertook a major national study of disability in 1966 which surveyed a sample population of all disabled adults aged 18-64 living in non-institutional settings 17/ The survey was conducted by mail questionnaire to screen for households with disabled family members, and then in a second phase by personal interview with the adults identified as disabled. The study collected an extensive amount of data on the prevalence, nature and extent of work-limiting disability and on the effects of disability on income, work adjustments and family relationships. Some of the effects of disability on the labor force were as follows:

Disability resulted in a loss of approximately 2 million workers, people who were previously employed, or employed at the onset of disability and no longer employed. About 300,000 men had never been employed; most of these were people who had been disabled in childhood and would otherwise have been expected to enter the labor market.

Relatively few of the men with occupational or secondary work limitations had left the labor force. There was, however, more part-time work and unemployment among the disabled than the non-disabled.

The loss of work and earnings capacity had serious consequences for the economic adequacy of the disabled and their families. Their family income was considerably less than that of the non-disabled.

"In 1971 nearly one-half of severely disabled men and three-quarters of severely disabled women received no benefits from the U.S. disability system...most non-applicants were aware of the programs, but did not apply because of social stigma surrounding beneficiaries...non-beneficiaries often relied on the wages and transfer income of other members of the household so that the household ended up bearing the total costs of disability."

William G. Johnson "Disability, Income Support, and Social Insurance," 1979.

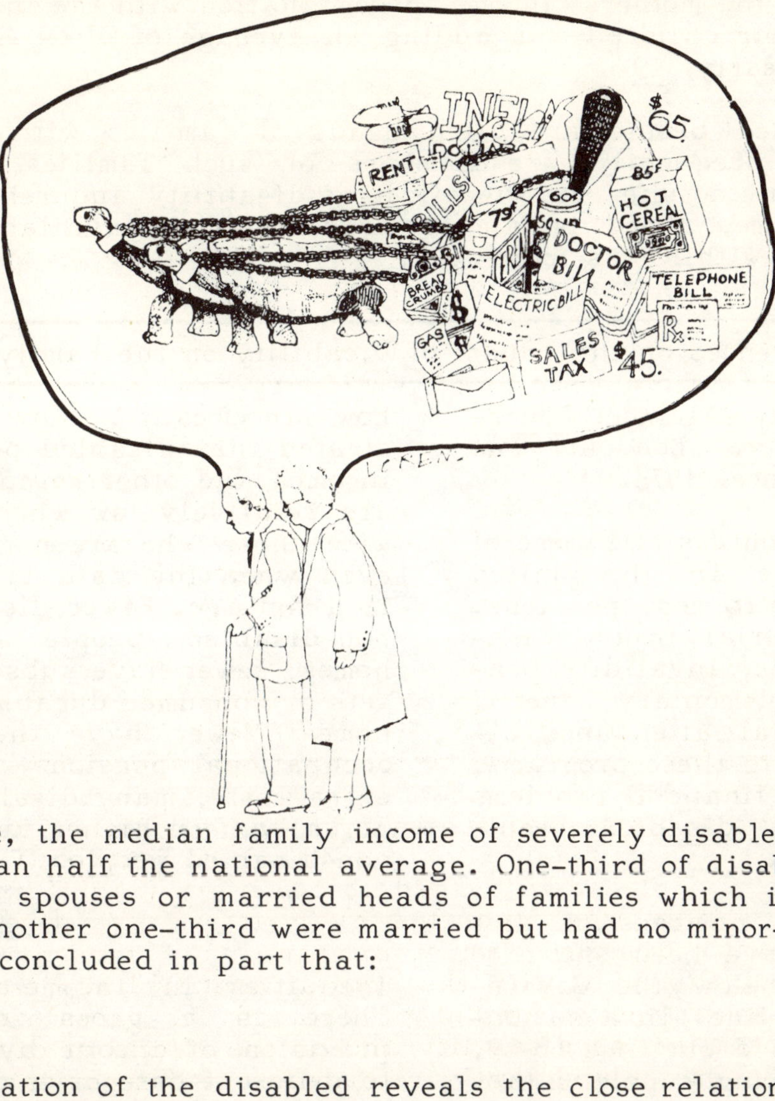

For example, the median family income of severely disabled married men was less than half the national average. One-third of disabled men and women were spouses or married heads of families which included minor children. Another one-third were married but had no minor-age children. They study concluded in part that:

> "Examination of the disabled reveals the close relationship, and at times, dominating influence of disability on such commonly accepted and seriously regarded problems as early retirement, unemployment, underemployment, and non-participation in the labor market; problems of poverty, public welfare, health care and social services are closely correlated with disability prevalence." 18/

Whereas most developing countries do not have social benefit or social insurance schemes which cover the whole or the majority of their populations, the trend is towards expanding the scope of existing schemes. Factors relating to the active work force, and its changing nature thus become relevant as factors to be taken into account through long-range planning.

A recent study in the German Democratic Republic documented the increase in family income which can result from the availability of a rehabilitation service. Using a study group of 586 mentally retarded adolescents, most of whom had some additional physical disability, U.P. Katzenstein of the Rehabilitation Workshop of Berlin was able to analyze the effect employment of the young disabled in a sheltered workshop had upon the yearly earnings of their whole family. Within the client group under 18 years of age, composed of 126 young people, 110 had mothers who returned to work after their children began participation in the program. Eighty-seven of the mothers had not worked previously. It was calculated that the mothers' income in combination with the income being produced by their children was adding an average of DDRM 4,798 to the family income yearly. 19/

Disabled people are often heads of families with minor-age children, and frequently are members of such families. With the exception of some studies on the effect of disability and rehabilitation on family income, there is almost no information available on the economic impact within this framework.

Additional References on the Impact of Disability on the Family and Income:

The Disability Alliance. Poverty and Disability. London: The Disability Alliance, 1975.

The principal sources of income of disabled people in the United Kingdom are retirement pensions, war and industrial injury disablement pensions, invalidity pensions and supplementary benefit, and supplemental attendance allowances. Despite these programs, three principle financial problems encountered by disabled people can be outlined.

Poverty. Large numbers of disabled people have been shown to have incomes below the Government's poverty line. In a national survey carried out in 1968-69, 30% were receiving supplementary benefits and another 7% appeared to be entitled to benefits but were not drawing them (250,000 people). One-third of these disabled people had at least one source of extra expense because of disability. An important indicator of poverty is the rate of unemployment, and the unemployment rate among registered disabled people increased from 7.4% in 1965 (compared to a 1.4% unemployment rate among the non-disabled) to 14.9% in 1972 (compared to 4.1% among the non-disabled).

Low Incomes. A survey demonstrated that disabled people have incomes and other resources which are relatively low when compared with those who are non-disabled, even when the data is standardized for age. Fewer disabled than non-disabled people own their homes; fewer have substantial assets or consumer durables in their homes; fewer have the right to occupational pensions. Yet due to extra costs, many disabled people actually need higher incomes than non-disabled people.

Inequities in income provision. There is a gross inequity of provision of income by the State to different categories of disabled people. Those disabled as a result of war or industrial injury receive a set benefit, irrespective of earnings or national insurance entitlement. The amount of invalidity pension often is unrelated to the degree of disablement. A long-term policy objective must be to eliminate poverty, to bring the incomes of disabled people up to the levels of the rest of society and to distribute resources among people with different types of disability in an equitable manner.

"The paraplegic and tetraplegic patients who come to the centre (Dacca, Bangladesh) are usually victims of accidents directly related to their poverty. Many have fallen from trees while trying to gather fruit and others have suffered broken necks from accidents while carrying heavy loads on their heads. Neither of these are occupations of the rich."

Oxfam News August-September 1980.

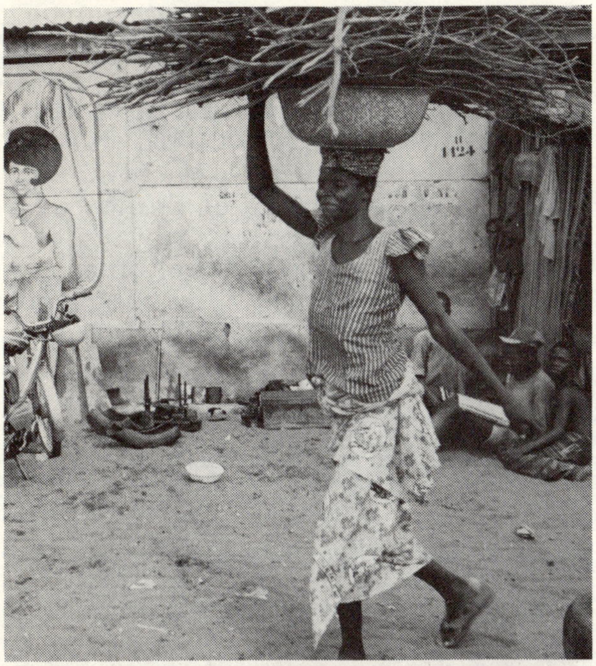

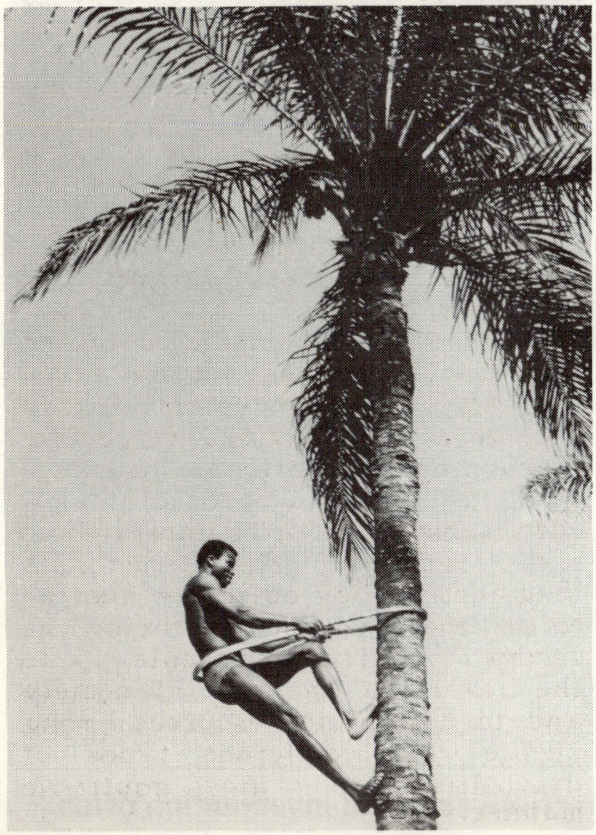

Hyman, Mavis. The Extra Costs of Disabled Living. London: National Fund for Research Into Crippling Diseases, 1977.

This study investigates the extra costs incurred by a sample of 56 wheelchair users in the London Borough of Camden, and the economic consequences of disability for the household. A corollary of the extra costs of disabled living is loss or restriction of income, not only for the disabled person, but for the entire household. "Extra costs and loss of earnings may be separate definable issues but they are closely intertwined for all purposes of living."

The work situations of the people in the sample were as follows: thirteen people were working, and twenty six had given up employment all together. Others were housewives or students looking for work. The problems of the disabled person in employment which emerged from these case studies basically confirmed the findings in another national study: loss of earnings, extra costs related directly to working and restriction of job choice. Personal costs were incurred in the areas of travel, domestic help, wheelchair attendance, work assistants, and working at home. The loss of income was calculated at between L6 and L114 per week. No direct relationship was found between loss of household income and previous earnings. The narrowing or widening of the income gap appeared to be related to severity of dependence in self care ability, other income and sex.

The computation of these extra costs of disabled living examined the bearers of the costs--individuals, families, official organizations, and the characteristics of

"Between 36% and 43% of the agencies felt that their clients were mainly in strained or poor circumstances; the slightly handicapped were less likely to be reduced to poverty because of disability than the severely handicapped; those with a moderate disability, with reduced work opportunitities and the expenses of trying to live independently in the community, were most likely to be brought into severe financial stress because of disability."

Australian Government Commission of Inquiry into Poverty. The Relationship between Poverty and Disability in Australia, 1977.

the expenditures--capital costs, running costs and opportunity costs, and the items on which extra expenditure was incurred.

The author concluded that given the loss of income and relative poverty of the majority of the people in the research sample, income maintenance provisions should not be earnings-related. They should be payable as a matter of right, irrespective of national insurance contribution records, sex, or the cause of incapacity for work. The extra costs component of income maintenance should be paid at a universal flat rate, depending on degree of severity of handicap, and irrespective of sex, age, working status or cause of disability, and that this payment should not be means tested.

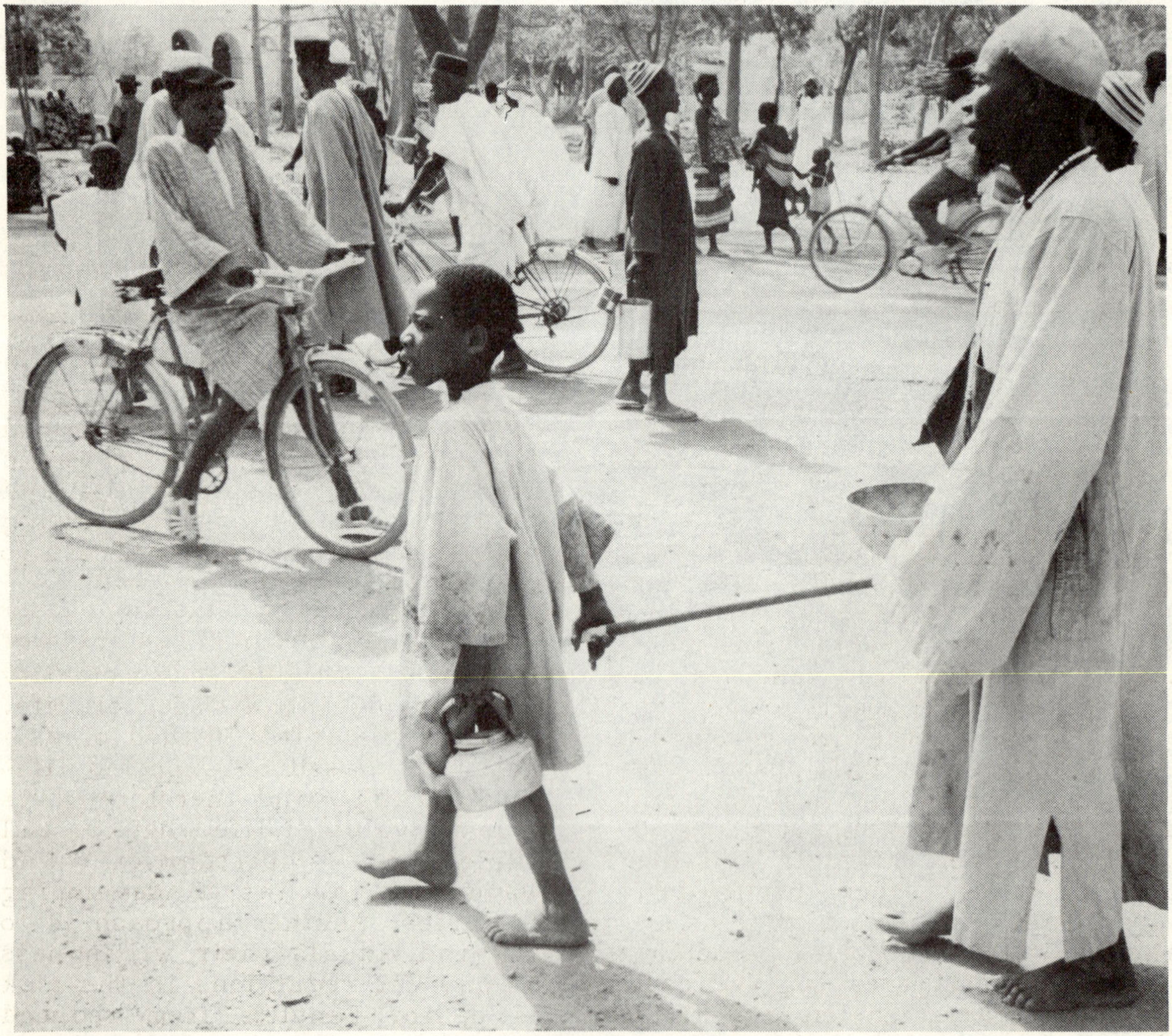

"Calculations of the costs and benefits of various forms of invervention often assume that doing nothing incurs no cost."

Jean Simkins, The Value of Independent Living, 1979

HEALTH CARE EXPENDITURES IN 1972 US
Persons Aged 20 to 64

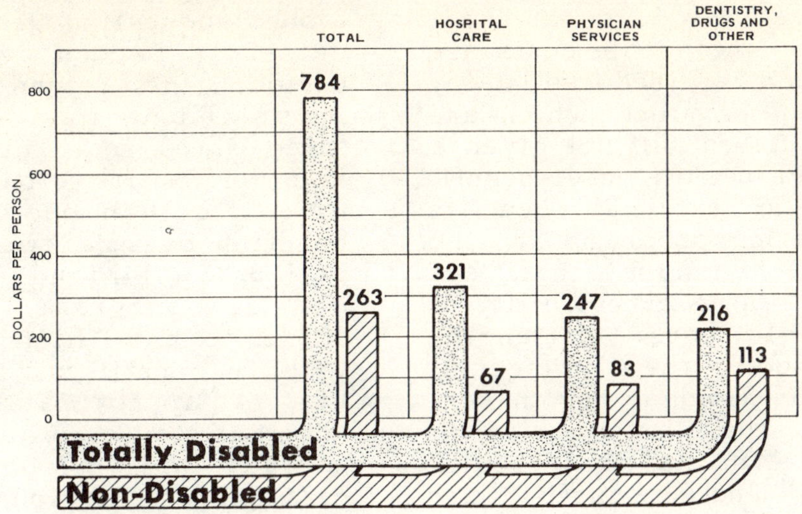

Jonathan H. Sunshine, Disability, 1979.

D. DISABILITY PREVENTION

Note: Rehabilitation for the Disabled did not examine the economics of disability prevention.

Creese, A.L. and R.H. Henderson. "Cost-Benefit Analysis and Immunization Programmes in Developing Countries," Bulletin of the World Health Organization, Volume 58, #3, 1980, pp. 491-497.

This paper applies cost-benefit analysis to health programs in order to analyze investments in universal immunization services. The method is essentially one of comparing the benefits of immunization with the cost of the program.

The principle components of immunization program costs are the wages of the immunizing and supervisory staff, and transport costs. The cost of vaccines in most cases are a small proportion of the total. Studies of immunization costs in the Philippines Expanded Program on Immunization show a range from about US $1.50 to US $6.00 per infant in existing priority areas for infant DPT (diptheria, pertussis and tetanus) and BCG (tuberculosis) vaccinations, and estimates for the cost of measles immunization in Zambia show a range from about US $ 1.30 to over US $12.00 per infant. WHO estimates a global average cost per fully immunized child of approximately US $3.00.

The main categories of benefit from immunization are savings in treatment costs following reduced incidence of disease, reductions in mortality, reductions in morbidity, avoidance of intangible costs, e.g. suffering to children and their families, and external or spill over benefits. Savings in treatment costs take the form of the release of hospital beds and reduction of outpatient waiting time, as well as easier access to care.

Benefits from reduced mortality involves placing a value on life. The human capital method of valuation is based on expected lifetime earnings and therefore gives a lower value of life where formal employment opportunities and wages are low, as in developing countries. Another approach is to ask individuals their willingness to pay for reductions in the risk of death. Benefits from reduced morbidity take the form of reduced incidence of handicaps such as blindness, and the avoidance of subsequent sacrifices by the family in terms of work time and income lost due to disability.

Avoidance of intangible costs are benefits such as reduced pain, anxiety, or discomfort, which are usually described but not given a monetary value in cost-benefit analysis. The "external" benefits of immunization programs are the institutional changes that accompany increased accessibility of effective health care, a strengthening of both the managerial capacities of national health services, and the participation of communities in national health initiatives. These benefits are also difficult to express in monetary terms, so that the net benefits of an immunization program based on cost-benefit analysis are underestimated.

The returns on investments in immunization programs have been substantial. Studies of measles immunization programs in developed countries all show high net benefits. In the USSR, the program was justified economically by part of the treatment savings alone, suggesting very large total gains. In Sweden over a 30-year period, the return on measles immunization was estimated at three times total program costs, and for poliomyelitis, the costs were less than one-sixth of total benefits over a twenty-one year period. In Finland and the USA, measles programs have been shown to have high net benefits, with a benefit-cost ratio in the USA of approximately 10:1. For tuberculosis in Britain, however, a study in 1976 found that immunization was no longer economic, the low risk of infection making the cost of preventing one case very high--about UK L5500 (US $11,000).

In the urban areas of southern Zambia, the benefits exceeded the program costs by factor of four, "based on a conservative assumption that there is no economic value to the saving of infant lives." Attachment of a positive value to each infant life saved would justify (on the narrow grounds of economics) the expansion of the program to the rural population.

Walsh, Julia A. and Kenneth S. Warren. "Selective Primary Health Care: An Interim Strategy for Disease Control in Developing Countries," New England Journal of Medicine, Volume 301, #18, November 1979, pp. 967-974.

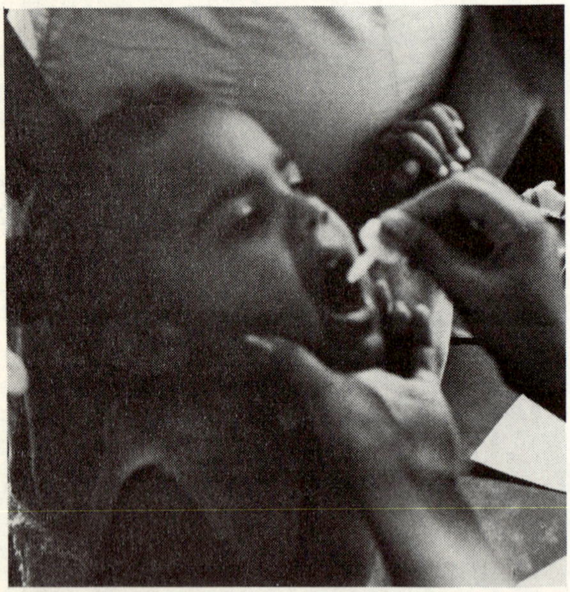

"Although polio vaccine is relatively cheap at about U.S. $0.06 per dose, the costs of storage, transport and delivery normally mean that it costs almost U.S. $0.90 to fully protect a child against the disease."

Nicholas Ward, "Malawi: EEC/NGO Anti-Polio Campaign," Courier, 1981.

"The three billion people of the less developed world suffer from a plethora of infectious diseases. Because these infections tend to flourish at the poverty level, they are important indicators of a vast state of collective ill health. The concomitant disability has an adverse effect on agricultural and industrial development, and the infant and child mortality inhibits attempts to control population growth."

"The World Bank has estimated that the cost of furnishing basic health services to all the poor in developing countries by the year 2000 will be $5.4 to $9.3 billion (in 1975 prices). This investment, which includes only initial capital investment and training costs, would provide one community health worker or auxiliary nurse midwife for every 1400 to 2000 people and one health facility for every 8000 to 12,000 people for every 10 km^2, whichever is greater." The goal is unattainable because of the cost and numbers of trained personnel required.

Therefore, there is a need for selective primary health care directed at preventing or treating the few diseases that are responsible for the greatest mortality and morbidity in less developed areas. "In selecting the health problems that should receive the highest priorities for prevention and treatment, four factors should be assessed for each disease: prevalence, morbidity, mortality and feasibility of control (including efficacy and cost)."

2.7 Priorities for Disease Control in the Developing World, Based on Prevalence Mortality, Morbidity, and Feasibility of Control

Priority Group	Reasons For Assignment to This Category
I. High	High prevalence, high mortality or high morbidity, effective control
Diarrheal diseases	
Measles	
Malaria	
Whooping cough	
Schistosomiasis	
Neonatal tetanus	
II. Medium	
Respiratory infections	High prevalence, high mortality, no effective control
Poliomyelitis	High prevalence, low mortality, effective control
Tuberculosis	High prevalence, high mortality, control difficult
Onchocerciasis	Medium prevalence, high morbidity, low mortality, control difficult
Meningitis	Medium prevalence, high mortality, control difficult
Typhoid	Medium prevalence, high mortality, control difficult
Hookworm	High prevalence, low mortality, control difficult
Malnutrition	High prevalence, high morbidity, control complex
III. Low	
South American trypanosomiasis (Chagas' disease)	Control difficult
African trypanosomiasis	Low prevalence, control difficult
Leprosy	Control difficult
Ascariasis	Low mortality, low morbidity, control difficult
Diphtheria	Low mortality, low morbidity
Amebiasis	Control difficult
Leishmaniasis	Control difficult
Giardiasis	Control difficult
Filariasis	Control difficult
Dengue	Control difficult

Source: J.A. Walsh and K.S. Warren, "Selective Primary Health Care: An Interim Strategy for Disease Control in Developing Countries," 1979.

Barnum, H.N. et al. "Cost-Effectiveness of an Immunization Programme in Indonesia," in Bulletin of the World Health Organization, Volume 58, #3, 1980, pp. 499-503.

An assessment of the cost-effectiveness of a proposed expanded program on immunization (for diphtheria, pertussis, tetanus, and tuberculosis) in Indonesia found it to be highly cost-effective in comparison with treatment (based on hypothetical estimates of program impact). The results remained valid when the costs were increased by 20% and benefits reduced by 50%. A separate analysis was made of the DPT (diphtheria, pertussis and tetanus) tetanus toxoid and BCG (tuberculosis vaccine) components of the program, revealing that although the BCG program may not be justified when operated independently, its inclusion in a joint immunization program is strongly justifiable on economic grounds (assuming a vaccine efficacy of 0.5). The study confirms one of the basic arguments advanced for the WHO programs of expanded immunization and illustrates that other immunizations, such as for poliomyelitis and measles, which may not be cost-efficient by themselves, may be economically justifiable when included as part of a larger immunization program.

2.8
Cost-effectiveness of the Proposed Immunization Program

	Cost per death prevented (Rp)	Cost per case prevented (Rp)	Cost of treating one case[a] (Rp)
Total program	53 963 (US$ 130)	3 942	13 166
BCG program only	188 623 (US$ 455)	42 438	49 000
DPTT program only	55 905 (US$ 135)	3 679	11 459
BCG considered as an added program	42 043 (US$ 101)	9 459	49 000
DPTT considered as an added program	32 027 (US$ 77)	2 107	11 459
Total program in last year of plan (1983-84)	50 750 (US$ 122)	3 620	13 166

[a]This is the weighted average of the costs of treatment of the diseases considered. The weights are the proportions of total prevented cases in each disease category.

Akehurst, R.L. and Sally Holtermann. "Application of Cost-Benefit Analysis to Programmes for the Prevention of Mental Handicap," in Major Mental Handicap: Methods and Costs of Prevention, Ciba Foundation Symposium 59. Amsterdam: Excerpta Medica, 1978.

The medical profession has been known to feel that "when economics comes in the door, good practice goes out the window." Yet there is a common interest in ensuring the effective use of health care monies. Cost-benefit analysis is one important method of evaluating the effectiveness of programs to prevent major mental handicap.

Cost-benefit studies attempt to "estimate all of the consequences, both adverse (costs) and advantageous (benefits), of a proposed course of action, and places a money value on those outcomes."

The stress on non-monetary outcomes in cost-benefit analysis ensures that policy makers review the relative merits of the outcomes--that a net cost must be compared to the non-monetary outcomes gained.

One of the key problems in applying cost-benefit analysis to mental handicap is the lack of information about the relation between service improvements e.g., special care units, and improvements in morbidity and mortality rates. For example, analysis of the changes in infant mortality rates showed that the important variable was change in the number of low birth weight babies, and not the availability of special care facilities or maternity service inputs.

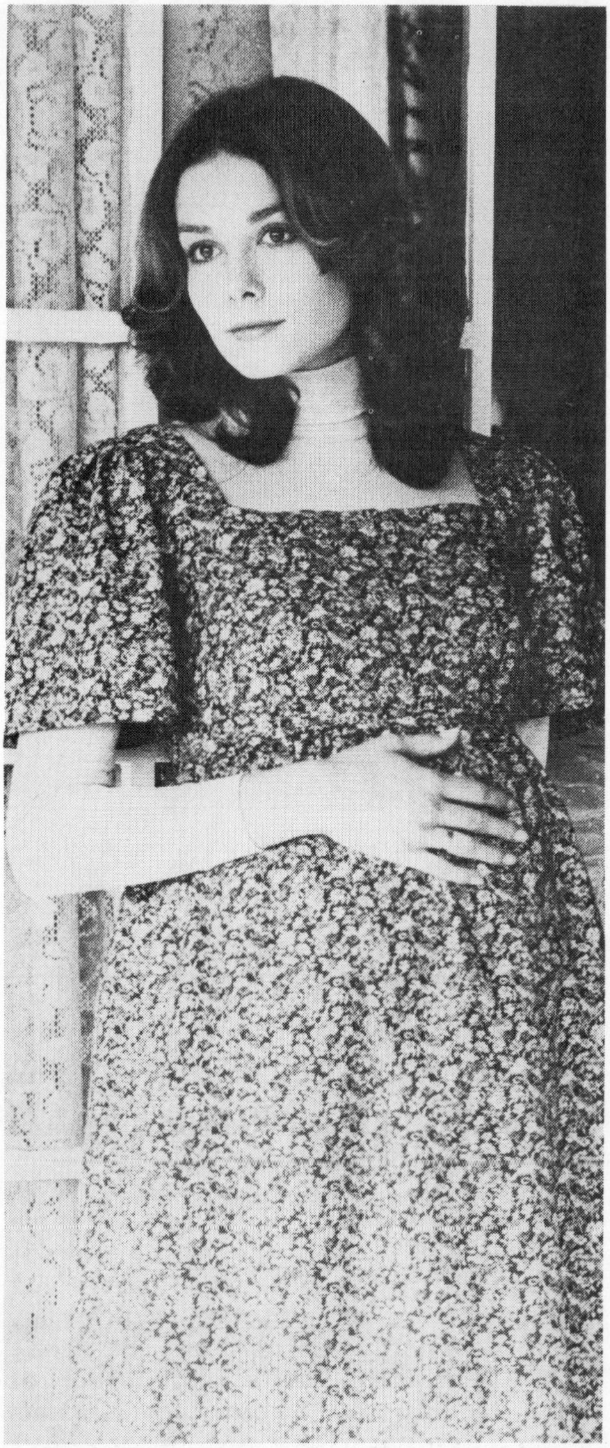

Chaplain, Marie Therese. "Perinatality: French Cost-Benefit Studies and Decisions on Handicap and Prevention," in Major Mental Handicap: Methods and Costs of Prevention, Ciba Foundation Symposium 59. Amsterdam: Excerpta Medica, 1978.

The French Ministry of Health implemented a Perinatal Care Program in 1970-1975 in order to reduce the number of birth-related accidents. A cost-effectiveness evaluation, the ratio (cost over 15 years)/(Number of deaths and number of handicap cases avoided during the same period) was designed to prioritize programs. Among the various policy measures were the training of medical personnel, the development of statistics and research, innoculation against Rubella, intensification of prenatal care, improvement of care during pregnancy and labor, creation of intensive resuscitation units for new borns, and resuscitation in the delivery room.

An evaluation of the proposed measures concluded that in economic terms there would be a return of between 10 francs (optimistic hypothesis) and 5 francs (pessimistic hypothesis) for each franc invested. "If financial advantages alone were considered, the return was 2.5 francs for 1 franc on the pessimistic hypothesis."

"In Sweden, where pre-natal obstetric and paediatric care is amongst the most sophisticated in the world, both infant mortality and the incidence of cerebral palsy in young children are around half the British levels."

Office of Health Economics, 1977.

2.9
Cost-effectiveness of the Programmes

Programme	Cost of programme over 15 years* (million francs)	Number of deaths avoided over 15 years (thousands)	Number of handicap cases avoided over 15 years (thousands)	Cost (francs) over 15 years* / number of lives saved without after-effects over the same period
1 Training	31.9	-	-	-
2 Statistics and research	28.2	-	-	-
3 Inoculation against Rubella	48.0	2.0	1.0	15500
4 Antenatal super-vision	(a) 214.0	18.0	36.0	3800
	(b) 582.0	32.0	60.0	6300
	(c) 1235.0	60.0	110.0	7200
5 Supervision of delivery	29.0	3.7	4.0	3800
6 Resuscitation in labour room	10.6	25.5	25.5	200
7 Intensive neonatal resuscitation centres	173.0	37.5	-5.1	5600

Source: Marie Therese Chaplain

*present value 1970

Mikkelsen, Margareta and Gert Nielson. Cost-Benefit Analyses in Prenatal Diagnosis. Glostrup, Denmark: Danish National Board for Social Welfare, 1974.

This is a short cost/expenditure study of the economic consequences of pre-natal diagnosis for prevention of Down's syndrome, as a cause of mental retardation, in Denmark. Costs consisted of amniocentesis, laboratory exams for interruption of pregnancy; expenditures consisted of care and services for persons surviving with Down's syndrome (institutionalization, special education, pensions, etc., according to life expectancy estimates). The study found substantial savings due to pre-natal diagnosis, and the greatest savings were realized in the "at risk" populations, pregnant women between 35-40 years of age, and families with children having chromosome abnormalities.

Jarvikoski, Aila and Eero Lahelma. Early Rehabilitation at the Work Place. New York: World Rehabilitation Fund, 1980.

Rehabilitation was originally intended to restore "functional capacity to those previously disabled". Morbidity patterns have changed, as chronic degenerative diseases, slow and gradual disabilities, (especially among older age groups) have become more prevalent. Rehabilitation intervention taking place early enough could contribute to the prevention of permanent disabilities, and help to avoid the creation of a permanently disabled population excluded from the labor force. "Rehabilitation research and experience have shown that a disabled or chronically ill individual is as capable of working as a healthy individual, provided the job is adapted to his capabilities." The focus of this project is on persons who are still working and capable of working. Priority is given to preventative measures in the working environment.

The conception of early rehabilitation used in this paper is based on a definition of rehabilitation that consists of comprehensive measures, which

(a) "are directed toward an individual with a chronic or permanent functional limitation or disability, or toward an individual with symptoms indicating a substantial risk of chronic functional limitations or a disability;
(b) are intended to restore an individual's working or functional capacity to its maximum, or to prevent lowering of that capacity, and
(c) aim at developing an individual's own resources or removing obstacles imposed by the environment."

A study conducted in 1973-77 concerned the state of health, working conditions and the need for rehabilitation among 29,000 employees of the city of Helsinki. On the basis of the responses to a questionaire (n=2,324) it was estimated that 10% of all employees were in need of immediate rehabilitative measures(medical rehabilitation, ergonomic or other changes in work conditions, job reassignment) because of chronic disorders. A limited team evaluation of the population found 11-12% of all employees in need of rehabilitation measures, but two years later it was discovered that few of the medical and vocational measures recommended had led to practical measures. It was concluded that only a system of rehabilitation built within the place of employment could guarantee the realization of comprehensive measures.

A model system of early rehabilitation in the work place can be organized in three units: a) contact persons--members in the organization responsible for providing information on rehabilitation activities to other members; b) a rehabilitation team made up of an occupational health nurse, a rehabilitation physician and a rehabilitation counselor; c)a committee for labor protection, consisting of employee and employer representatives to monitor activity.

The rehabilitation measures applied include guidance and counselling, group rehabilitation training, medical treatment, job reassignment (if found necessary), and other measures.

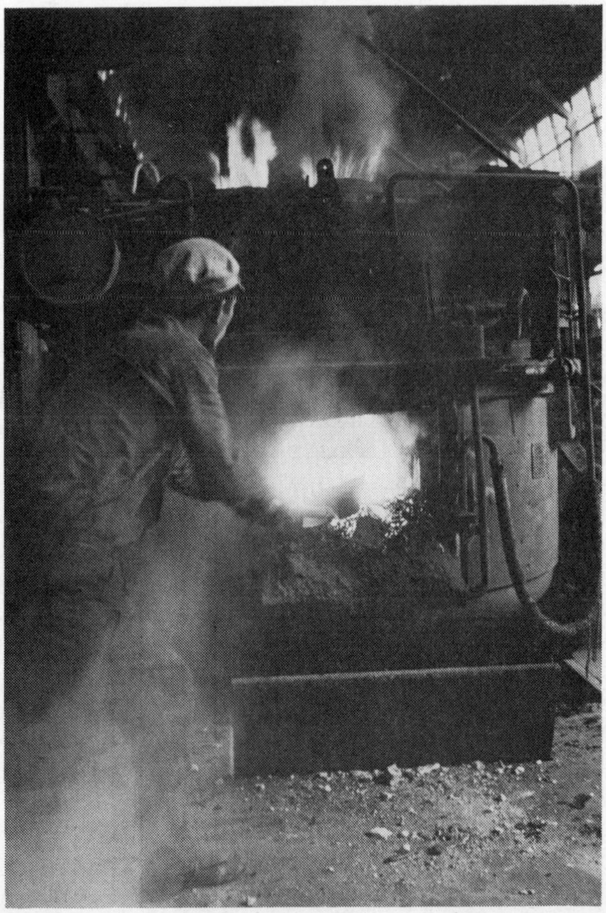

E. THE COSTS OF NOT PROVIDING REHABILITATION SERVICES

The study of economics rewards those with patience enough to cope with its complexities with the possibility of examining each issue from many sides. At times, as in the contemplation of a mirrored image, the most illuminating insights may derive from vision in reverse. The question most frequently asked, "Can we afford to provide rehabilitation services?" may be apparent, while the answer to "Can we afford not to provide rehabilitation services?" is indeed little known. Researchers in some countries have attempted to examine the latter question first and, in fact, their findings indicate that the cost of not providing rehabilitation services is equal to the value of all the economic benefits forgone.

A Comparison of Optimal and Actual Rehabilitation Programs

Researchers in Israel, using patients hospitalized because of cerebro-vascular accidents or heart disease, have attempted to develop a conceptual model for identifying cost factors and analyzing cost structure in relation to non-rehabilitation.20/ They made a comparison of the actual cost of all goods and services provided to such patients in two government hospitals during 1958 and 1959, and the costs of an optimum rehabilitation program which was called the Desirable Program. The medical records of hospitalized patients were reviewed, the patients were interviewed and examined, and contacts were made with the medical and social agencies which had been involved in each patient's program. Both physical and socio-economic functions were examined, and the study classified as non-rehabilitated persons who failed to exploit fully their capacity in either or both of the two functions.

The cost of non-rehabilitation was conceived to be composed of two factors:

(a) Unnecessary services given to the patients under their Actual Therapeutic Program. (The Actual Therapeutic Program included all goods and services actually given to the patient as a consequence of his disability including his hospitalization);

(b) Benefits forgone, which could have been realized under the Desirable Rehabilitation Program and which, for example, might have resulted in increased family income during the rehabilitation period, or might have resulted in greater future productivity of the disabled person. The net cost of non-rehabilitation was obtained by deducting the cost of any additional services needed to provide the Desirable Rehabilitation Program from the net cost of the above two factors. The study was based on the assumption that existing medical and social services in Israel had, at the time of the study, the necessary capacity to provide all resources required for the Desirable Program, but that available resources were not always fully utilized on behalf of the disabled.

While recognizing that many costs of non-rehabilitation are not measurable, the study dealt primarily with the measurable cost factors. Financial outlays for goods and services for non-economic and economic

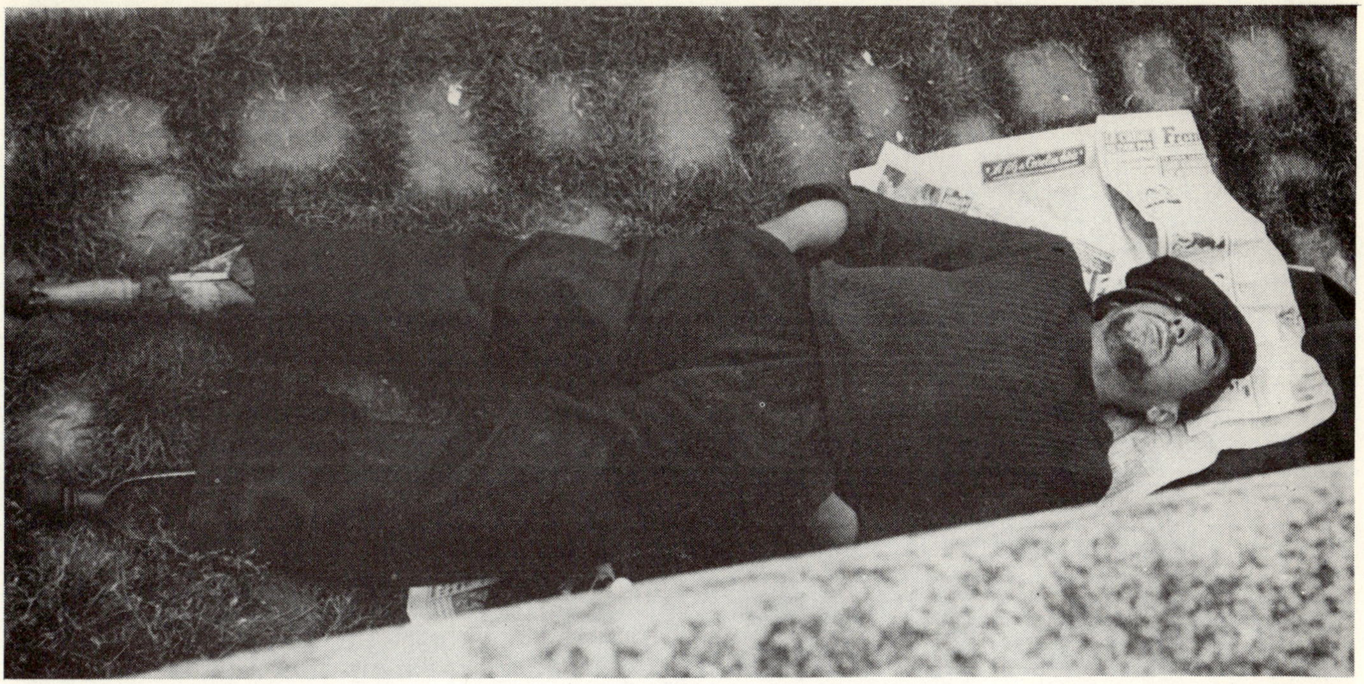

objectives and all expenditures connected with them were estimated. Only those items occurring as a consequence of the patient's disability were included. Patients were divided into groups according to their rehabilitation goals, and cost-benefit balances were made to cover two time spans: the three-year period from discharge until the time of the inquiry, when expenditures for service were anticipated to be relatively high in comparison to benefits forgone, and the fourth and subsequent years when a truer picture of the long-term results of non-rehabilitation was expected to emerge. The cost-benefit balances were performed from the point of view of the family, the public, and the over-all economy.

The study found that:

--Unnecessary costs - primarily expenditures for services which the patient could have dispensed with - ranged from 22 percent to 58 percent of the Actual Program. The largest unnecessary cost was for institutional care.

--Benefits forgone ranged from an annual 33 percent to 89 percent above the income attained under the Actual Program for the first three years, and in the subsequent years benefits lost were greater, ranging from 47 percent to 100 percent above actual income.

--The cost for additional services to attain the Desirable Rehabilitation Program were relatively small in comparison to the benefits forgone. The ratio for the first three years was an annual LI 0.03 to 0.29 spent for every LI 1.00 of benefit, and in the latter years, an even improved ratio of LI 0.04 to LI 0.10 cost for every LI 1.00 of benefit expected. These cost-benefits were not seen to apply to housewives or others who were not engaged in gainful activity outside the home. The primary financial benefit for them was seen to be in the avoidance of costly dependency.

The Israeli study urged further analysis of the concept with other disability groups, particularly for persons receiving institutional care since this was associated in the study with the highest avoidable costs.

A Comparison of Social Security Benefits Provided and Payments Forgone

A study by the Mexican Institute of Social Security, based on pension data obtained in 1967 and presented in 1970, 21/ analyzed the estimation of non-rehabilitation from a somewhat different perspective. Unlike the Israeli study, which developed a model to demonstrate the unnecessary expenditures on services and the benefits forgone by the individual disabled person and his family, the study in Mexico attempted to demonstrate the effect of non-rehabilitation on invalid pension payments, and on the loss of contributions to the social security scheme.

It was first demonstrated that in a follow-up study of 220 people receiving rehabilitation services through the Mexican Institute of Social Security, approximately 60 percent returned to remunerative employment. It was further demonstrated that it costs approximately 7,266,000 pesos annually to maintain a comprehensive rehabilitation center serving 1,000 disabled people annually, exclusive of capital investment costs. (The costs of initial land acquisition, building and equipment were estimated at 17 million pesos.) Based on the number of disability pensions and on the number of pensions provided to workers disabled from work accidents, and assuming that 60 percent of the workers in the productive working age range between 15 and 47 years of age could be returned to work, it was estimated that 17,388,922 pesos in saved pension cost and forgone revenue was lost through non-rehabilitation. In addition, if the disability period for a worker and the expenses associated with it were reduced by only 15 percent, an additional 20,790,000 pesos could have been saved. The total loss through non-rehabilitation of this disabled population group thus became 38,178,922 pesos. Deducting the annual cost of maintaining a comprehensive rehabilitation facility, the annual cost of non-rehabilitation was shown to be 30,912,922 pesos.

The Mexican study further concluded that since the data obtained were for a previous year, the amount of pensioners as well as the annual expenditure of several million pesos has already increased, and will continue to recur year after year without the possibility of reduction until a comprehensive rehabilitation program is introduced. Secondly, the study only dealt with workers insured under the social security scheme. The presence of unremediated disability among the family members of workers would also produce a financial burden for the insured worker, reduce his buying power, and at the same time decrease the income inflow to the social security institution, and to the community. Finally, the study demonstrated that without taking into account the potential reduction in payment subsidies through early pensions saved and incomes received, it is possible to recover within one and one-half years the costs of investments made in the establishment of a comprehensive rehabilitation center.

The Decline in Post-Accident Earnings

A study conducted by the Ontario Workmen's Compensation Board (WCB) in Canada demonstrated that workers disabled on the job experienced an average decline in post-accident income of 18.9 percent in the absence of rehabilitation services as compared to a post-accident income decline of 1.7 percent when rehabilitation services were available. In addition, workers who were provided rehabilitation services had an average increase in lifetime earnings of more than $Can 15,200 when compared to disabled workers for whom rehabilitation was unavailable. These findings were the result of a comparison of two matched groups of workers which differed only in that one had access to rehabilitation services whereas the other had none. The study utilized data on workers injured during during the period from 1965 to 1966 who had available the full range of WCB rehabilitation and retraining facilities, and workers injured during the period 1927 to 1928 prior to the availability of any such services. 22/

Additional References on The Costs of Not Providing Rehabilitation Services:

Bowe, Frank. Rehabilitating America: Toward Independence for Disabled and Elderly People. New York: Harper and Row, 1980.

The crises of inflation, poverty, aging and big government are all directly related to the "problem of disability".

Inflation. Dependency among disabled people now accounts for almost 9% of the U.S. Gross National Product (GNP). Over the past decade, while inflation has grown so fast that the purchasing power of the dollar has been halved, dependency costs attributable to disability have risen much faster, feeding inflation at an alarming rate. Investment on the federal, state, local and private levels in dependency among disabled Americans now accounts for more money than the national defense. Payments to individuals who are dependent on and entitled to government aid is the largest and fastest growing component of the federal budget. These costs are rising at a rate of 11% annually and have quadrupled over the past decade. Benefits for dependent disabled persons account for one out of every thirteen dollars in the federal budget.

Poverty. Disability is a major cause of poverty, and poverty of disability. Of all families on welfare rolls, 20% are there because the head of the household is disabled. More than 60% of all poor families having at least a husband and wife at home include a disabled adult. Almost half of the adult disabled population is at or near the poverty level.

Of the 15 million disabled people in the U.S. between the ages of sixteen and sixty-four, not institutionalized, more than 7.7 million are either out of the labor force or unemployed. Among the severely disabled the proportion not working is nine out of ten.

Keeping disabled people in dependency is costing many times more than would helping them to independence. To do nothing now on the basis that our ability to respond to the problem is constrained by inflation is to feed that inflation and further reduce our capacity to solve the problem of disability. The costs of not eliminating the dependency will vastly exceed the costs of spending to make the disabled independent.

Frank Bowe, 1980

About 25% of all persons not in the labor force are disabled.

Disability is also caused in part by poverty. The rate of disability among black people, for example, is double that of other racial groups; and of the seven million disabled children in school today, almost half are believed to come from poor families living in inner-city areas. Blindness also occurs much more frequently among poor people than among the upper and middle classes. For families with incomes under $2,000 annually, the rate of blindness is 12.3 per 1000 persons, compared to 1.59 per 1000 for families with incomes over $7,000. Malnutrition and poor medical care are two important factors.

Aging. With the changing age structure of the U.S. population, spending on the elderly now accounts for 25% of the entire federal budget. If present trends continue, spending on elderly citizens may triple within the next thirty years.

Big Government. The U.S. spends ten dollars on dependence programs among the disabled for every dollar it spends on programs helping them become independent. In 1967 federal, state, local and private spending on dependence-oriented programs totaled $38.7 billion, while independence-oriented expenditures were less than $.7 billion. The $39.4 billion total was 5% of the GNP for the year. In 1975 the spending on dependence had grown to $111 billion, that of direct services to $3 billion; the total of $114 billion was 7.9% of GNP. These dependence-oriented expenses grew at a rate much greater than inflation, increasing by 40% in constant dollars. Thus enormous sums are spent on income and medical support programs for disabled people, but little on direct, independence-oriented services.

The soaring costs of dependency programs cannot be attributed to increases in the disabled population or a general decline in the national health, but are the result of the perception of disabled people that characterizes U.S. society: the disabled are seen as people who are more disabled than able; the difference between independence and dependence-oriented expenditures is a reflection of this perception.

Independence. Five key programs are required to rectify the problem of disability: expand research, development, and technology-transfer efforts to prevent, cure, and ameliorate the effects of age and disability; remove architectural, transportation, and communication barriers facing disabled and elderly people; increase efforts to train disabled and elderly people; reform the dependence-oriented programing; and make communities "open" to and usable by disabled and elderly people. All of these programs will require billions of dollars, yet the costs of not spending this money--the negative costs--will exceed this sum by enormous multiples.

For example, the startling costs of renovating mass transit systems to provide access for disabled people are minuscule compared with segregation costs. "Dial a ride" (a small van transportation system) would cost $1.75 billion per year. In ten years, it would cost six times as much as would mainstreaming; in twenty years, almost thirteen times as much. Designing for access involves one time cost for renovation and design; thereafter, no appreciable additional expenses are involved. A 1969 Civil Service Commission study of severely disabled federal employees found that 95% of the employees required neither extensive accessibility nor modification of their jobsites, while 3.75% needed only accessibility changes, and 1.25% required jobsite modifications.

Recent civil rights legislation for the disabled is founded in a conviction that "separate-but-equal" is inherently unequal. The statutes proclaim the goal to be one of offering disabled people full access to the programs and activities supported by federal funds.

Keeping disabled people in dependency is costing the U.S. many times more than would helping them to independence. "To do nothing now on the basis that our ability to respond to the problem is constrained by inflation is to feed that inflation and further reduce our capacity to solve the problem of disability. The costs of not eliminating the dependency spending will vastly exceed the costs of spending to make the disabled independent."

"25% of the unemployed handicapped would be able to work if transportation was physically and financially available."

Mayor's Task Force Report, 1973.

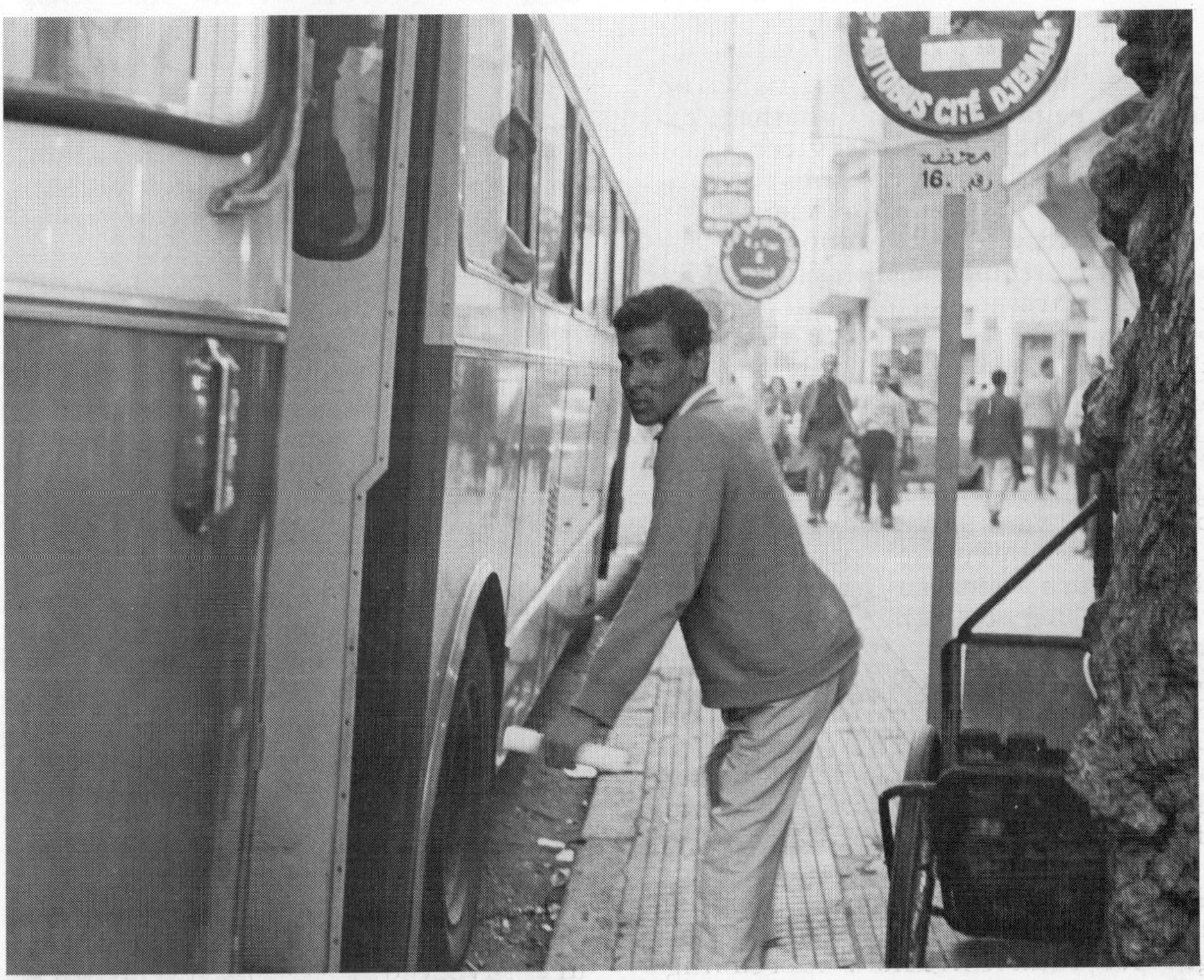

"If time and effort and money are spent on medical and vocational rehabilitation and on measures to make public buildings accessible, and society still continues to deny the handicapped the right of equal access to inexpensive public transportation . . the rehabilitation process is a waste."

Alberta Committee of Action Groups for the Disabled #4, 1974.

Simkins, Jean. The Value of Independent Living: Looking at Cost Effectiveness in the U.K. New York: World Rehabilitation Fund, 1979.

This study examines cost-benefit aspects of independent living in the U.K., where the overall cost of supportive and rehabilitative care for handicapped people is about $5.4 billion, of which two-thirds represents social security benefits. This sum does not include retirement pensions to people with handicaps, estimated at $1.8 billion. Many authorities fear that social welfare sums of such proportion create the danger of transferring the "crippling" effect of disability from the individual to the economy.

Since "the costs of disability accrue regardless of whether or not rehabilitation services are available", many of these costs are the costs of dependence -- both personal and economic. Dependency is not only expensive, but is a status often not desired by those on the receiving end.

A great proportion of the costs involved in cost-benefit studies, such as medical, nursing and custodial costs, will be incurred in some form in any civilized society whatever the conclusions about cost-benefit ratios. One real net benefit, therefore, is the difference between the costs of not doing all that could be done in the way of rehabilitation, and the cost of what is done.

Calculations of the costs and benefits of various forms of intervention often assume that doing nothing incurs no cost. In a recent study of cash provisions for people with handicaps in the U.K., it was found that this is very far from being the case. From one example of a man refused financial assistance for transportation to work, the annual cost to the Exchequer of not making the payment was at least $4,400 (1975 basis). The payment from government funds towards his travel to work was replaced by a much larger payment from the same funds in the form of benefits, to which must be added the loss of his contribution in tax on earnings and National Insurance payments.

Too often systems are designed for the convenience of the administrators without regard for the data providers. No administrative costs, however, are assigned to the recipient families in analytical perspectives. These costs do not cease to exist merely because they are ignored. The opportunity cost of resources of time and human energy in such households is in reality very high.

While rehabilitation services may yield a net social cost rather than a gain when calculated in conventionally measureable economic terms, the drive towards independent living should be maintained as far as possible. The value of social benefits which do not contribute to return to paid employment in cost-benefit analysis is neglected: psychic

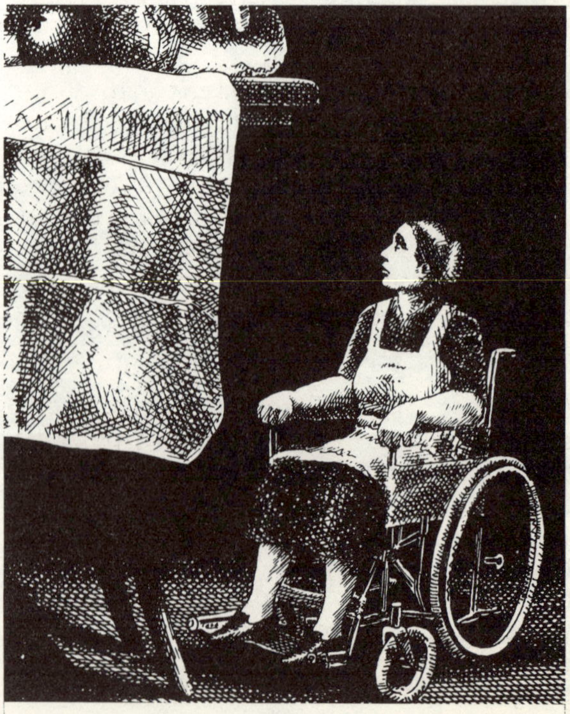

well-being, increased life satisfaction; preservation of the family; reduced medical, nursing and custodial costs; and reduction in delinquency and disturbance of children.

There are substantial differences in the costs of caring for handicapped people in their own homes, with supporting services, as compared with costs in various kinds of institutions. In 1971, the cost per week for care in an acute hospital was $250, in a long stay hospital $100, in a residential home $80, and in a shared accomodation $40.

Shortcomings in service delivery systems have substantial effects on costs. For example, fully qualified nurses should not be engaged in care functions which have essentially no medical content. The Crossroads Care Attendant Scheme, which provides care and services for disabled people in their home, is an example of an economical program, emphasizing "relief at the time and in the way required by the recipient, and with the greatest possible stress on reliability."

The employment and placement services of vocational rehabilitation must be adequate in order to maximize the investment in special education programs. The quality of job placement services for the handicapped is a determining factor in the benefit-cost ratios of such training, and crucial in the effectiveness of the transition from education to employment.

Among specialized employment services for the handicapped in the U.K. there is a quota scheme whereby a percentage (3%) of the jobs in any firm having more than 20 employees must be filled by disabled people. Companies which are below the quotas are not permitted to hire any employee without first obtaining a permit, which will only be granted if no suitable disabled person is available. A strict enforcement campaign in 1975 resulted in only a marginal improvement in meeting quotas. The costs of quota operation in 1977/78 were $4.4 million; 24% of all service office time was spent on the administration of the quota scheme. The conclusion was that "strict enforcement is not justified in terms of the benefits resulting in relation to resources used."

One study which attempted to estimate the costs of housing for disabled people showed the national cost to be only $700–900 for local authority housing, and just over $1700–1900 for owner occupied homes. Yet, "manageable housing can make or break the effort of a family or individual to cope with a handicap. The handicapped mother is particularly relevant, because her housing does not result directly in a return to paid employment."

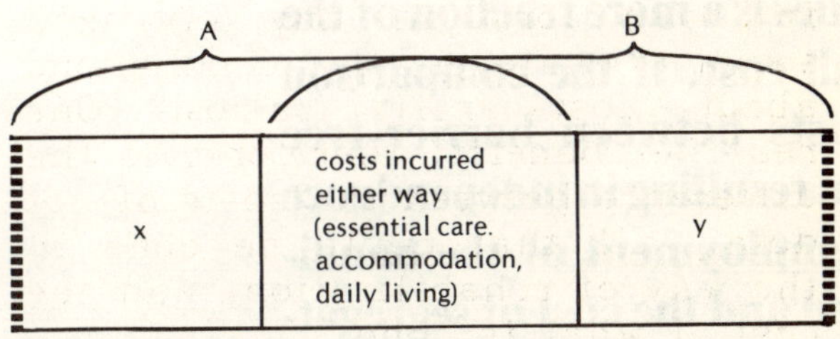

A = "negative" costs i.e. the cost of what is not done
B = costs of what is done
x = the costs of avoidable extra dependence, e.g. more attendants or more active nursing needed as a result of lack of mobility aids; aid in kind because of nil or abnormally low earnings; institutional care because suitable housing not made available; costs in respect of dependents
y = the cost of what *is* done to aid independence: e.g. the cost of self-care training; aids to mobility (physical and financial aids); the provision of suitable housing; help to obtain employment including extra costs for basic education, training and job procurement.

Net benefit arises whenever the amount spent on y leads to a reduction in x which is equal to or greater than y.

The American Society of Landscape Architects Foundation. Barrier Free Site Design. Washington D.C.: United States Department of Housing and Urban Development, 1977.

A section of this study outlines the costs and benefits of barrier-free construction. Concern over the costs of constructing buildings accessible to disabled people, and the costs of renovating buildings already built, is partly due to the lack of research into the cost-benefit aspects of barrier-free site design. Recent studies show previous estimates of these costs to be greatly exaggerrated.

In a study conducted by a firm of architects, it was revealed that the cost to eliminate architectural barriers would not have been an important consideration to authorities undertaking construction projects. Less than ten percent of the architects surveyed felt that a building constructed to be fully accessible would be prohibitively costly.

In a National League of Cities study, of 3 new structures studied, it was estimated that each building could have been constructed in such a way as to provide total accessibility for less than 1/10 of 1% of the total construction costs. And 6 of 7 hypothetical buildings studied could have been constructed barrier-free for less than 1/2 of 1% of the original construction costs.

It is difficult to compare the original construction costs and the costs today of renovating or retrofitting a site or building for access by disabled people. The study suggests that the cost of modifying buildings for accessibility must be carried within maintenance and capital improvement budgets. The costs involved must be compared to the price of not making buildings accessible, and the benefits, in terms of economic gains for the disabled individual, of barrier-free sites.

"The extra cost of barrier-free design in public buildings and facilities is a mere fraction of the overall cost. If the comparison of costs between barrier-free design resulting in independence and employment of the handicapped and the cost of segregating this section of society, forcing them to be dependent of the community were made known, politicians as well as planners would opt for complete integration by means of barrier-free design."

A United Nations Expert Group Report Barrier-Free Design, 1975.

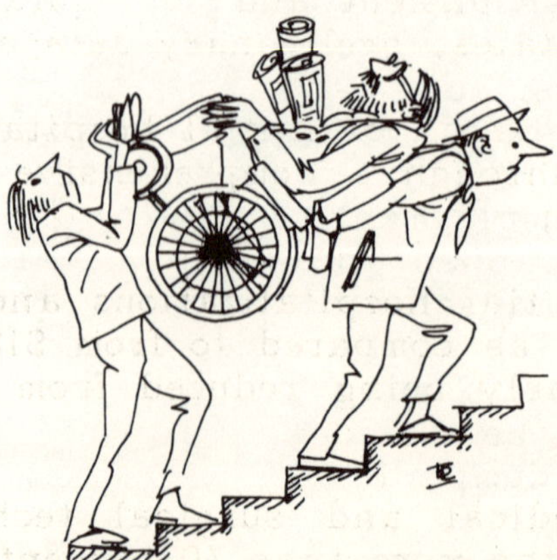

The independent living movement, by challenging what and how services are provided, will continue to have an important impact on the costs of different services. The demand for medical and other professional services will decrease, and the demand for adapted housing and attendant care will increase.

Gerben DeJong, 1979

F. ECONOMIES IN THE PROVISION OF REHABILITATION SERVICES

Health Care Costs

Rehabilitation programs have the potential to reduce expenditures for health service delivery, and the aforementioned study on patients with cardio-vascular and cerebro-vascular disorders in Israel exemplifies some of the possibilities. Reduction in health service consumption can have major economic benefits. It has been estimated, for example, that a reduction in the mean length of stay of patients in a Dublin hospital by only one day each, through the provision of rehabilitation services, could result in an annual savings of L1 million. 23/ Many studies have been made of methods for the more effective delivery of rehabilitation services which may also reduce the cost of service provision and, at the same time, reduce the overall cost of disability. A few of these studies are cited here, to illustrate the range of approaches possible in assessment of this aspect of the rehabilitation process.

In recent years, spinal cord injury mortality has declined markedly during the first five years following injury. In general, the spinal cord injured incur relatively higher medical costs, require greater attendant care, and in only a small proportion of the cases return to gainful employment. The estimated incidence of spinal cord injury in the United States is 35 spinal cord injured persons per million population. There are between 100,000 and 125,000 persons thus disabled in the U.S., and it is estimated that the annual cost of care is $2.4 billion (1975). It has been estimated that the lifetime costs of quadriplegia, based on the costs of initial hospitalization, routine maintenance, attendant care, loss of income and expenditures for environmental modifications, vocational rehabilitation and training, is in the range of $325,000 to $400,000. The lifetime cost of paraplegia has been similarly estimated to be between $180,000 and $225,000. In an effort to reduce the enormous financial burden imposed on both the individual and society by this form of disability, rehabilitation specialists have been attempting to demonstrate that a comprehensive systems approach to the care of the spinal cord injured will not only provide better results for the individual patient but will also reduce medical costs commencing at the onset of injury through discharge from the rehabilitation program and all medical and attendant costs thereafter. 24/

On the basis of patient and cost data collected from selected facilities in the United States, preliminary data appear to confirm that:

--The average length of initial hospitalization and rehabilitation is being reduced through a comprehensive systems approach from 180-240 days to 101 days;

--Costs for initial hospitalizations and rehabilitation are on the average of $11,000, as compared to from $18,000 - $28,000. Annual medical costs are similarly being reduced from $4,000 - $6,000 to less than $1,000;

--Improved medical and surgical techniques are increasing functional recovery for the more than 40 percent of spinal cord injured persons with incomplete lesions. This represents an average savings in care of $150,000 per person.

Similarly, in the German Democratic Republic, a survey of spinal cord injured patients at the Rehabilitation Hospital in Berlin 25/ demonstrated the economic advantages of early and comprehensive intervention, and in the Metropolitan Rehabilitation Center, Konstancin, Poland, 26/ case by case comparisons of the costs of rehabilitation which could have been averted through early intervention were made. In the latter study, savings of from 40,000 to almost 80,000 zlotys per patient were demonstrated.

A study carried out in Finland in 1969 27/ attempted to determine the most effective pattern of treatment for brain-injured patients at the Helsinki University Trauma Clinic. Two hundred and fifty-one patients were divided into groups receiving one of four different patterns of assistance; the treatments ranged from routine medical care to a more comprehensive pattern of medical care coupled with special gymnastics and communication with the patient concerning the nature of his trauma, its prognosis and possible treatment. The patient group receiving the more comprehensive pattern of services demonstrated a significantly shorter period in bed after the onset of injury, and a shorter period absent from work than the group which received only the routine pattern of medical care. Such an approach has important implications for the overall economic effect of the disability sustained.

Institutional Care Costs

Institutionalization may have particularly measurable economic consequences, and it is often possible to demonstrate a marked reduction in this type of cost through the provision of rehabilitation service. The National Fund for Research into Crippling Diseases in the United Kingdom carried out an extensive analysis of the relationship between the cost of institutionalized living for the disabled and accommodation in the community. 28/ The study analyzed the capital and weekly maintenance costs for persons in long-term stay hospitals, in residential homes for the disabled, and in four types of home-care situations which varied according to the need for domiciliary and attendant care. Home care was found to be typically about L10 per week cheaper than the institutional settings due to the lower capital costs and the use of family members for assistance in daily living needs. In addition, home care can delay the onset of institutionalization, particularly in the case of the aged disabled or in forms of disability which are progressive in nature. The postponement of institutionalization represents another form of savings, estimated to be as much as 15 to 20 percent of the cost of one year's institutional care. Furthermore, it was found that while the vast majority of disabled people live at home, many of the most severely disabled living at home were at least as incapacitated as those persons institutionalized in residences or long-term care hospitals. The study also referred to the psychological effect of institutionalized living and compared these to the potentials for interaction which disabled people have with other groups in society through community living.

Professor S. Brattgard, founder of the Swedish Fokus scheme for community living by disabled people, has stated: 29/

> "A disabled person runs the risk of isolation in the community and segregation from other people ... All investigations show the impossibility of improving the individual resources of a person if

he lacks stimulating contacts with other human beings ... Our investigations show that it takes several years of hard work to rehabilitate and resocialize a person who has spent several years in an institution."

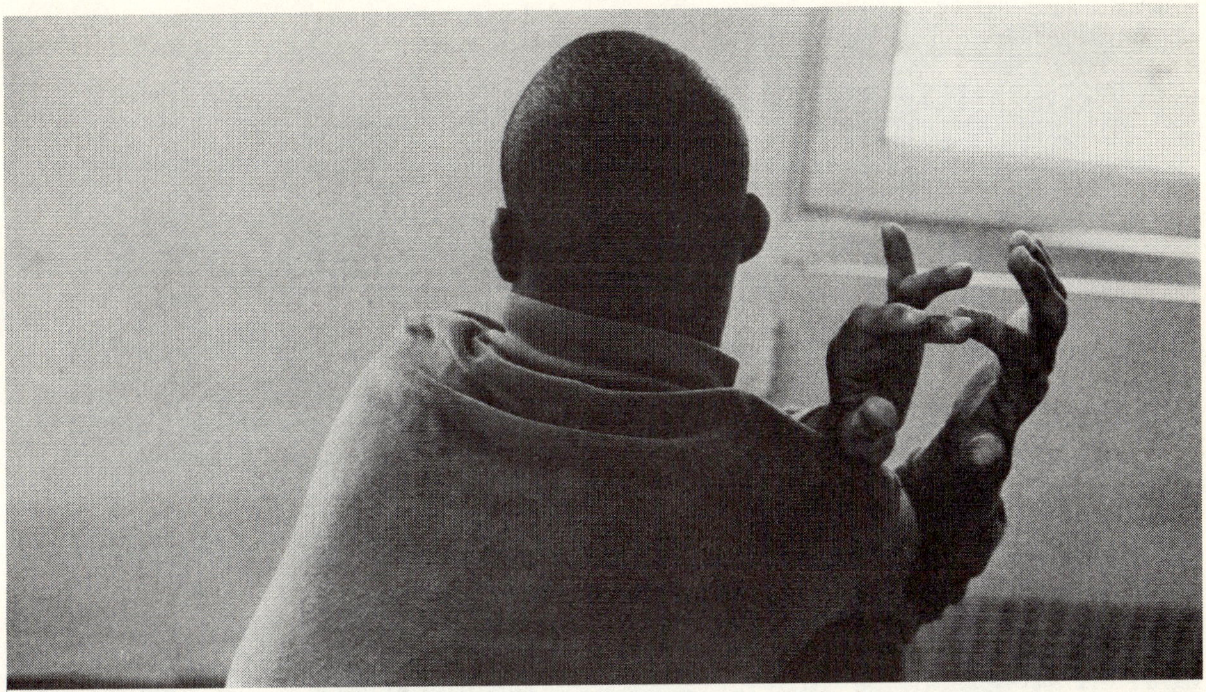

A related study was carried out in the United States to demonstrate the effects of placing mildly and moderately mentally retarded adults in the community to live and work, after an extended period of institutional living. 30/ The subjects of the study had been living in an institution for an average of 15 years, having been either orphaned or abandoned by their families. They were provided comprehensive vocational rehabilitation services including diagnostic evaluation, sheltered workshop experience, vocational training, and half-way-house living when necessary. During the first four years of the project, 128 people were discharged to community living. A follow-up survey of half of this group indicated that 95 percent were employed, and most lived in rented rooms or apartments. Their economic and social adjustment was as good as that of other persons at their social and economic level. The other half of the group placed in employment would not consent to be interviewed although their whereabouts and activities were known to the researchers, and they were believed to be even better adjusted to community living than the study group. After six years, 250 retarded persons had been placed in community living, and the following cost-benefit estimates were made:

--The annual cost of institutionalization for the 250 people would have been $1,800,000 or $18 million over a 10 year period;

--The actual cost of rehabilitating the 250 people was approximately $1 million;

--The total earnings of the 250 persons over a 10-year period will be approximately $10 million, and the group was returning more than $50,000 per year in federal income taxes.

The net gain to both society and the retarded people associated with the project was thus seen to be quite sizable.

Additional References on Economies in the Provision of Rehabilitation Services:

DeJong, Gerben. The Movement for Independent Living: Origins, Ideology, and Implications for Disability Research. East Lansing: University Centers for International Rehabilitation, 1979.

The traditional dominance of "professionals" in disability policy and rehabilitation is being challenged by the rise of consumer groups of disabled people. Disabled persons, not professionals, are argued to be the best judges of their own interests--what services are needed, and of how services are organized on their behalf. Centers of independent living are both an "adjunct to the present human service system and an alternative service provider." The movement for independent living manifests itself at a number of levels.

At the level of vocational rehabilitation, case planning is no longer conducted solely by the case worker, but must consist of an "individualized written rehabilitation plan" to be drawn up jointly by client and counselor.

The movement for demedicalization is based on the argument that individuals can and should take greater responsibility for their own health and medical care. Much of the medical presence and the general management of disability after medical stability has been substantially obtained is seen as unnecessary and counterproductive. "The medical practitioners and disabled patients relationship induces dependency and is therefore in conflict with the goals of rehabilitation and independence."

The movement for independent living rejects the behavioral expectations created by both the sick and impaired roles; "the disabled do not want to be relieved of their familial, occupational, and civic responsibilities in exchange for a child-like dependency." Attendant care--the use of relatively low-skilled individuals to provide personal care in a community setting that would otherwise be provided in an institutional setting by a professional--meets the needs as defined by the disabled person, and also fosters deinstitutionalization.

The independent living movement, by challenging what and how services are traditionally provided, will continue to have an important impact on the cost of different services. The demand for medical and other professional services will decrease, and the

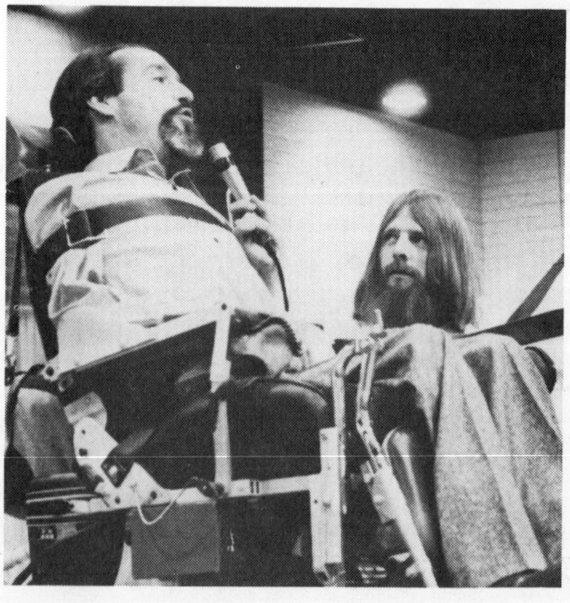

Ed Roberts, one of the founders of the U.S. independent living movement, addresses the 1980 World Congress of Rehabilitation International. Mr. Roberts is Director of Rehabilitation for the state of California.

demand for adapted housing and attendant care will increase.

Independent living is also attempting to develop a new paradigm (the framework and concepts by which problems are identified and solved) in which the problem of disability is defined. The dominant rehabilitation paradigm views the problem as one of the individual--that the individual must be changed. But the independent living movement insists, for example, that the "failure to be gainfully employed does not necessarily rest with the individual but with the market which has been unable to make useful work available or accessible," or with the dependency inducing features of the physician-patient relationship. The independent living paradigm also differs from the rehabilitation paradigm in defining additional outcome variables relevant for research--non-monetary variables such as living arrangement, consumer assertiveness, outdoor mobility, and outdoor activity.

Intagliata, James C., et al. "Cost Comparison of Institutional and Community-Based Alternatives for Mentally Retarded Persons," Mental Retardation, June 1979, pp. 154-156.

An implicit assumption of deinstitutionalization is that community-based residential alternatives are not only more normalized for mentally retarded persons, but are less expensive to operate. This study compares the costs for residential care and professional services in an institution with costs for similar care and services provided in the community.

The costs for residential care included room, board, attendant care and personal items. The comparison of residential care costs was conducted for a variety of living settings, including a large developmental center operated by New York State, group homes, and the home of the natural family.

With respect to the institution, attendant care costs included the salaries of all those staff assigned to resident living units on a full time basis, plus a proportion of institution wide administrative and overhead costs. The costs for residential care in the natural family were based on figures supplied by the Bureau of Labor Statistics Expenditure Survey. The costs of residential care in group and family care homes were based on the combination of federal Supplemental Security Income (SSI) allotments and additional state subsidies which are provided to those persons or agencies operating these homes. Costs for professional services were analyzed separate from residential care costs. The professional ser-

---

2.10
COMPARATIVE COSTS FOR RESIDENTIAL SERVICES

Setting	Cost (Resident/Year)
Institution	$14,630
Group Home	$9,255-$11,000[1]
Family Care	$3,130
Natural Family	$2,108

[1]Variation depends upon residents' levels of disability.

Intagliata, James C.

vices examined in this study included sheltered workshops and physical therapy.

The costs in the institution were found to exceed those of the community settings; costs were also significantly higher in group homes than in either family care or natural family homes. With respect to cost levels for professional services, the institution and community agencies were generally comparable. The variation appeared to depend primarily on the organizational structure of the service agency, the type of service provided, and the type of client served.

Sainsbury, P. and J. Grad de Alarcon. "The Cost of Community Care and the Burden on the Family of Treating the Mentally Ill at Home," in Lees, Dennis and Stella Shaw (eds), Impairment, Disability and Handicap. London: Heinemann Educational Books, 1974.

The problems addressed are whether community-centered services can alleviate the social and clinical impairment of the mentally ill without increasing the burden on the community, which for all practical purposes means the members of the patient's family, and whether community service deployed its personnel and material resources more efficiently than a more traditional hospital-centered one, and in a manner whereby needs were met more effectively.

The study design was to compare all referrals to the community service in Chichester U.K. (population 120,000) with those of a more conservative hospital-centered service in Salisbury U.K. (population 116,000). The following cost-related factors were assessed:

i) referrals: the community service was more efficient in meeting the needs of the mentally ill; referral rates were higher among the "at risk" population--the elderly, single, the poor, thus reducing the likelihood of mental impairment by offering care to more people, but also for those whose needs were greatest.

ii) admission rates: hospital admission rates following referral to a psychiatrist were three times the community rate; though the mean duration of stay in the hospital was significantly shorter, the risk of suffering institutionalization was less in the community service.

iii) outcome: patients treated in the community did not suffer more or less impairment in the two services.

iv) cost to the family of the disabled person: prior to referral the burden on the family was the same: social and leisure activities of a third of the families had been restricted; a quarter had their income reduced by at least 10%; in more than a third, the children were disturbed.

Post referral findings: There was a trend for all aspects of family life to be more adversely affected in the community-based system during the two year follow up, both in terms of financial problems and the effect on the mental health of family members. Families previously categorized as severely burdened were equally relieved in both services. The likely reason for this somewhat paradoxical finding is that more social support was given to patients and their families in the hospital service system. Without efficiently organized collaboration between psychiatric and welfare service, both the patient and those in the community closest to him or her are likely to incur costs--financial, social and emotional.

"It is hard to think of a human being in an institution as a human being, which is one thing that institutions are about—because in institutions, the context is the institution, a context which tries to wall out empathy as it walls in people."

William Roth, "The Uncounted Poor: An Excursion to an Institution," 1977.

Economics Division, South Australia Department of Economic Development. "Community Care and Institutional Care: A Discussion," in National Rehabilitation Digest, Volume 3, # 3/4, 1979, pp. 30-36.

This study explores the "questions of the comparative costs of community care and institutional care of handicapped persons." The question of institutional or community care also concerns the appropriateness of the care delivered, yet the relative costs of each form of care may predetermine the choice in practice.

A 1977 study in South Australia revealed that grants to approved organizations from the government totaled $1200 per handicapped person associated with those organizations. In fact, the vast majority of federal government funds are directed to institutions and not to the handicapped persons themselves. The bias in the direction of funds produces an incentive for persons to remain in institutions. Before clients can live independently, they must find sufficient money to purchase their own equipment. The bias in favor of the institution is also revealed at the work place--those employed in a sheltered workshop received an incentive allowance of $5 per week.

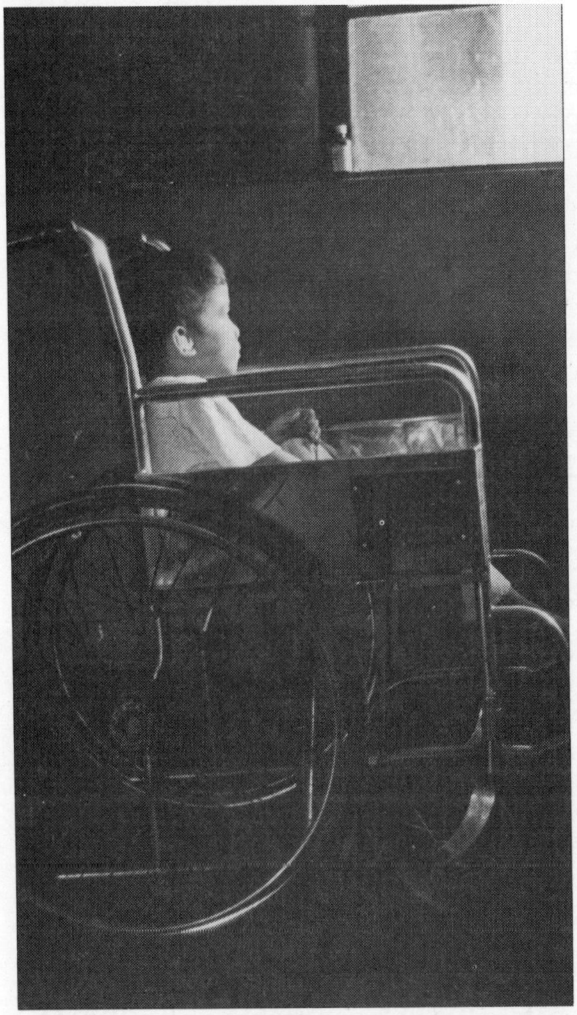

Another study estimated the annual institutional accomodation costs per person at $15,330. By comparison, the costs of living at home would consist of the costs of housing, food and personal ex-

"The U.S. Supplemental Security Income Program, which provides means-tested income support for the elderly, blind, and disabled, reduces by one-third the amount of benefits if the beneficiary lives in or takes up residence in the household of a relative."

John H. Noble Jr., and Ronald W. Conley, "The Search for Fact Amidst Con jecture in the Policy of Deinstitutionalization," Health Policy Quarterly,.1981.

penses, plus appropriate domiciliary care and services. The cost of the last two items may be as little as $5 per week, or $250 per annum. In addition, the costs of modifying a standard ground level dwelling for access by a wheelchair were estimated to be approximately $2,500-3,000. These "threshold" costs of independent living, though substantial, could be covered through "soft" government loans or other subsidies provided directly to the individual.

The study concludes that, given the vast range of individual handicaps, and the various economic and social circumstances that each person faces, the real challenge is to provide optional care systems to meet individual needs at different times.

Creese, A. L. and R. Fielden. "Hospital or Home Care for the Severely Disabled: A Cost Comparison," British Journal of Preventive and Social Medicine, Volume 31, 1977, pp. 116-121.

A case study was conducted of severely disabled patients requiring regular mechanical respiratory assistance (responauts) and a detailed cost comparison of entirely hospital-based care and predominantly home care.

The recurrent costs of hospital care include indirect or shared costs for the building, direct or individual costs attributable specifically to the care of the responauts, and the forgone earnings of the responauts in a hospital. The recurrent costs of home care include inpatient days at the hospital, domiciliary attendance costs of medical, social services, and other personnel, domestic running costs--food, laundry, fuel, power, transport--and forgone earnings.

2.11 Summary of Costs of Home and Hospital Care 1971-72

	Home Care	Hospital Care	Difference
Costs per annum			
Capital	L 737	L 605	+L 132
Recurrent	L5427	L8164	-L2737
Productive time lost			
Men	L1489	L1985	-L 496
Women	L 884	L1041	-L 157
Total			
Men	L7653	L10727	-L3074
Women	L7048	L9810	-L2762

Source: A.L. Creese and R. Fielden, "Hospital or Home Care for the Severely Disabled: A Cost Comparison," 1977.

The capital costs of hospital care include the cost per bed of constructing inpatient facilities, and the cost of specialized equipment. The capital costs of home care include construction cost, medical equipment, non-medical equipment, and alterations to the house. Average costs were used in the study; domestic running costs for home care assumed responauts were single person households, overstating the costs of home care since the marginal cost of an extra adult is less than the average cost of one adult. For capital costs, the use of average costs neglects economies achieved by grouping responauts and equipment in the hospital.

III. COST-BENEFIT ANALYSIS

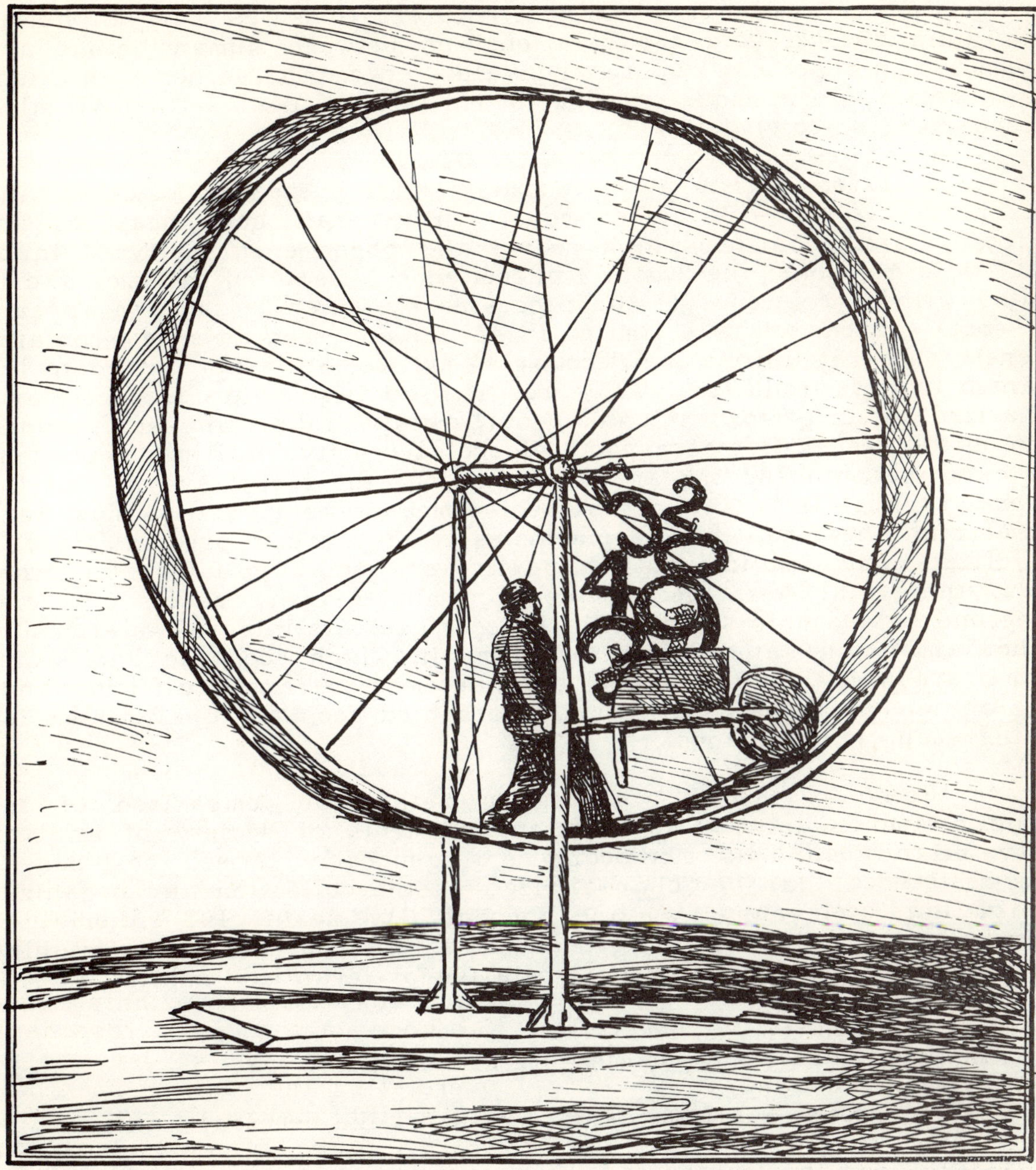

A. CONCEPT, METHODOLOGY, AND LIMITATIONS

Economics has been defined as "the science which studies human behaviour as a relationship between ends and scarce means which have alternative uses". 31/ Traditionally, this study has revolved around the means of production and the organization of productive forces. As governments and public authorities have devoted increasingly greater proportions of national productivity to socially-based programs, an increasing need has developed for social statistics and indicators which can validate the effectiveness of social programming in a manner comparable to the measures applied to assess economic progress. 32/ In traditional terms it may be possible to view such a "social accounts system" as all that is not economic, and thus have it be understood in juxtaposition to an "economic accounts system". In reality, however, social and economic factors are closely linked. Social phenomena, the relationships between human beings, the relationships between human beings and nature, and the relationships between human beings and systems which represent reality and values encompass economic relationships. Social phenomena, in the broad sense, deal with "all that concerns life in society". 33/

Social scientists and economists have succeeded in developing certain indices of social phenomena. In general these measures are limited by methodologies which reduce the phenomenon analyzed in at least two dimensions: the "social" phenomenon is isolated in time, and is studied without reference to the processes by which it came to appear; the "social" phenomenon is limited in space, and seen as a self-contained entity separated from the "economic" sphere; it is not linked to the organization of production. As a result, the indices produce compartmentalized descriptions which do not always take into account the linkages between different aspects of social reality. Multiple dependencies exist between the system of production, the social system and the cultural system. It is known that social measurement systems must take into account these multiple dependencies if they are to predict correctly the effects and implications of particular social policies. In other words, the social must include the economic. As yet, models of social and economic accounts systems which recognize this integral relationship do not exist. The analysis of problems in which economic and social factors are very closely linked thus becomes extremely difficult and, quite obviously, the rehabilitation of disabled people is one problem involving such close linkages.

Economic theory provides a method of comparison of the advantages to society or to different segments of society of a given policy or action. This methodology is generally termed cost-benefit analysis, and it can be "characterized as the collection and organization of data relevant, by some conceptually meaningful criteria, to determining the relative preferredness of alternatives". 34/ Weighing alternatives on the basis of their relative preferability implies several capabilities:

The ability to define and measure criteria;

The ability to collect all or only parts of the necessary data;

The ability to make value judgements on the relative merit of different alternatives, either by the researcher or by the decision maker who uses the research results.

"Traditional cost-benefit models imply that benefits are a result of agency expenditures and efforts. Yet the characteristics of clients and the state of the labor market may have a far greater effect on productivity." R. Treital, 1978.

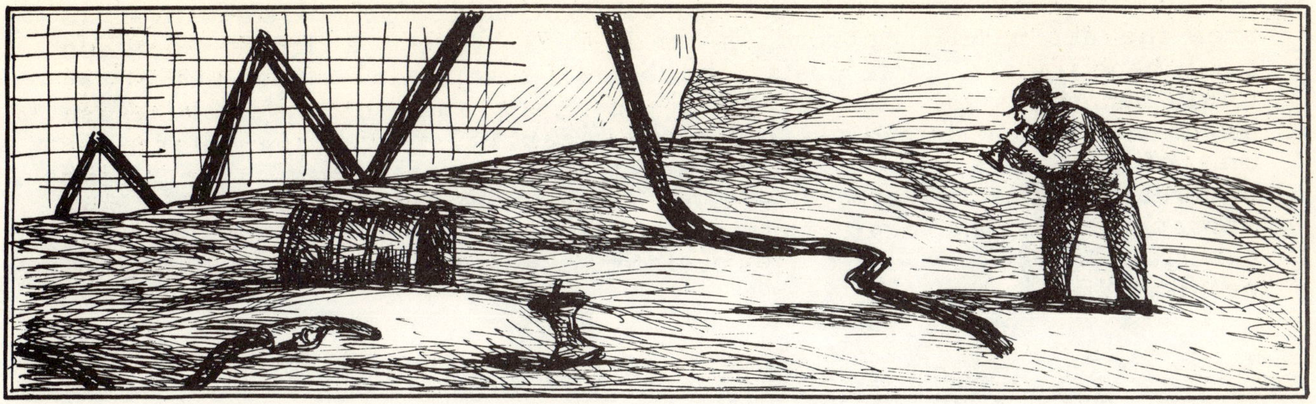

In general, the cost-benefit study will attempt to describe the different alternatives available to achieve a particular purpose. It will describe the side effects of the actions which are relevant, although not necessarily specifically intended. It will describe the "costs" of the different alternatives, and by measuring all effects, side effects and costs in the same units, it will provide a scale of preference for the different alternatives. The method presumes agreement on the value assigned to various effects and costs. Thus, "a cost-benefit analysis should be understood ... as a procedure which to the greatest possible degree:

a. identifies the economic effects, side effects and sacrifices of alternative measures,

b. measures these in terms of economic units, and

c. calculates the net gain or loss of the different alternatives as compared with each other." 35/

Depending on the type of objective being analyzed, it may be necessary to carry out several cost-benefit analyses of the relationship of various alternatives to various population groups or sectors of the economy. Application of the cost-benefit procedure to social programming becomes extremely complex when questions are raised as to:

> "whether additional resources should be used for one programme or for competing needs and demands ... For in addition to the direct and immediate benefits and costs, there will be indirect effects on economic and social conditions that should weigh heavily on any evaluation. Many of these effects will not be subject to precise measurement. Cost-benefit analysis has to steer a difficult course between such near exclusive reliance on quantitative data that the most critical factors in a situation are missed, and a subjective-type evaluation that leads to a biased policy position. Furthermore, the most important policy decisions may involve a choice among values and goals that are incommensurate (e.g., education or health) and can only be resolved through the political process. Research can hope to make that process more informed." 36/

A conclusive cost-benefit analysis requires many capabilities, as indicated above, and at each stage, methodological choices will alter the results possible.

Three alternative approaches for comparing benefits with costs are: the net benefit approach -- this measures the difference between total benefits and total costs; the benefit-cost ratio -- this calculates total benefits over time per unit of cost; and the rate of return approach, which determines the average annual percentage return per unit of cost. The net benefit approach does not take into account the differential size of programs; the rate of return approach is most appropriate to the evaluation of investments in physical assets; the benefit-cost ratio is most appropriate to evaluation of investments in people. 37/

The problem of reducing various benefits and costs to a common scale of measurement is one of the most difficult faced by the cost-benefit analyst. 38/ One major problem is that benefits accrue and costs are incurred at various points in time. Economists adjust such values for purposes of comparison to a common point in time, usually the present, by means of a discount rate. A second problem is that the group to whom benefits may accrue may be different from the group that incurs the costs. If such redistribution or transfer of income is not a concern to the investor, there may not be a question of commensurability. If the redistribution is one of the objectives of the program, however, the analyst must know how the investor, which could well be society as a whole, weighs benefits for the various groups. The weighted values will then affect the outcome of a cost-benefit comparison.

Costs are usually considered to be more easily identifiable and measurable than benefits. This becomes complex in cost-benefit analysis when the analysis includes assessments of forgone opportunities, or opportunity cost. It is frequently impossible to know the full range of opportunities for use of a particular type of capital which has not been utilized in the program under study. Another type of incommensurability may occur when an effect is known to exist but its precise influence cannot be identified. Multiplier effects fall into this category.

The economic benefits of rehabilitation generally can be considered in the following terms:

1. Reduced costs for future care -- for example, independence in self-care, which reduces the need for care-givers, reduced costs services on the basis of improved systems of rehabilitation service delivery, reduced need for medical, social and employment services.

2. Production benefits--the value of added production output or of all future production output. The addition to net production income refers to those products and services which would not otherwise have existed without the economic activity.

3. Reduced administrative costs for transfer payments -- transfer payments such as invalid pensions, sickness and unemployment insurances, income supplement payments, cannot be considered as a rehabilitation cost in terms of the total economy of a country since they only represent a redistribution of the overall wealth, a transfer of income from one sector of the economy to another. If, however, the administrative costs for transfer payments are reduced by reducing the need for such payments through services such as those provided by rehabilitation programs, an actual benefit to the overall economy exists.

(Some studies on the economic value of rehabilitation give attention to the savings in pension and other such payments which result from rehabilitation. It is important to recognize that these savings in transfer payments, while not of overall economic benefit, may have other social and political benefits.)

It is preferable for the cost-benefit analysis to focus upon variables within the ability of the researcher to control, and upon programs which are replicable with respect to both techniques and participants. Economists sometimes argue that the evaluation of effects not measured in monetary terms is not the province of the econometrician, and whereas "cost-benefit analysis allows the economist to identify costs and benefits to different groups, the problem of commensurating them should be left to the political scientist or the sociologist to solve". 39/

Perspective of the Analysis

The cost-benefit analysis may be undertaken from many points of view. Its perspective may be that of society as a whole, or of a specific social or economic institution, or of an individual. The value of each cost and benefit will necessarily be judged differently according to the perspective taken. Thus, for example, a study on the effects of employing a disabled worker may be undertaken from at least four points of view: that of the disabled person, the employer, the state social security or social welfare agency, and the community as a whole. Assuming that some form of pension or income assistance would be available to the disabled person were he or she to remain unemployed, the cost-benefit balances of employment might appear as follows from each of the differing viewpoints: 40/

To the handicapped worker:

Benefit	Costs
Salary	Loss of entire or partial pension, or other such assistance
	Payment of (higher) taxes and social security contributions

To the employer, who may receive a premium from the State for hiring a disabled person but who may have to make special adaptations of the work place:

Benefit	Costs
Value added to production output	Salary of worker
Employment premium from the State	Social security contributions
	Cost of special adaptations

To the state social security or social welfare agency:

Benefits	Costs
Value added to production output	Cost of services or measures to promote employment
Diminution of disability payments and administration costs	Salary of worker
Levying of (higher) taxes and social security contributions from disabled worker	

Assuming that the economic effects of employment of the disabled worker for the community as a whole may be calculated by adding all benefits and deducting all costs, the balance would appear:

Benefits	Costs
Value added to production output	Costs of services or measures to promote employment
Diminution of disability payment administration costs	

There are, of course, areas of overlap between the four groups, and the example is simplified and limited to only one aspect of rehabilitation. The point is that the perspective of the cost-benefit analysis will alter the types of data collected, and the value assigned to the data obtained. The range of possible alternatives will be totally dependent upon the perspective from which the analysis is made.

Limitations

The application of the methods of economic analysis to social phenomena has important potential for social planners, yet it can be seen that major limitations within this process continue to exist. Cross-cultural comparisons offer a similar dilemma: while promising the potential of insights not possible through single-system studies, such comparisons are severely limited by the multiplicity of uncontrollable variables. Rehabilitation specialists have been benefiting from the experiences of their colleagues in service provision in other parts of the world for the past 50 years. Certain difficulties have been consistently evident, however, in attempts to compare statistical data and research findings. The same types of difficulties will naturally apply to the comparison of economic analyses.

In reviewing cost-benefit ratios applied to vocational rehabilitation programs for the disabled in the United States of America, Dr. Ronald Conley found:

> "There has been an amazingly wide variability in published benefit-cost ratios for the Vocational Rehabilitation Program. Most estimates have ranged between 6 and 35 -- all favourable. This annoying variability is largely the consequence of crude and speculative data, especially with regard to mortality, job

retention rates, future earnings, and what would have happened without rehabilitation; the use of different discount rates; and the use of different cost concepts. All computed benefit-cost ratios are based on an incomplete measure of benefits (most measure only the increase in earnings). All benefit-cost studies had methodological deficiencies in the calculation of costs or benefits which seriously distorted the results." 41/

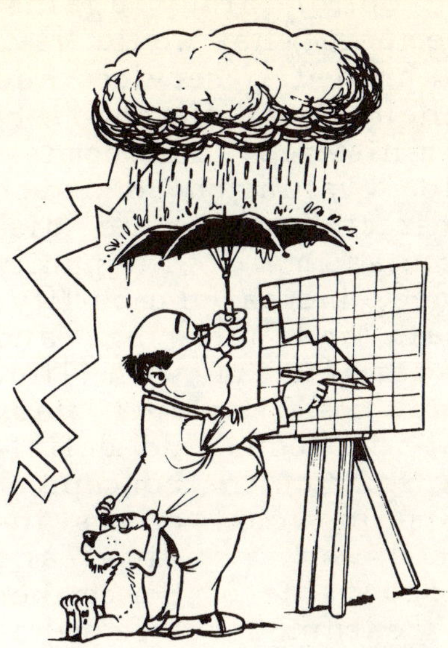

Richard Sterner, who conducted a survey on the social and economic conditions of mentally retarded persons in different parts of the world for the United Nations, concluded that:

> "data both on prevalence rates and on services for the retarded are often not comparable, at least if they are used without taking the conceptual differences into account. In many cases, it seems that there is less difference in substance than in terminology, but in all probability there are differences, too, in real prevalence rates, due to variations in mortality in one direction, and differences in social and economic conditions in the opposite direction. It is seldom if ever possible, however, to measure such real differences. Good epidemiological studies are scarce and it seems that, partly because of institutional differences, it almost never happens that such studies made in different countries are entirely comparable." 42/

Additional References on Concept, Methodology and Limitations:

John H. Noble, Jr. "The Limits of Cost-Benefit Analysis as a Guide to Priority Setting in Rehabilitation," Evaluation Quarterly, Volume 1, #3 August 1977, pp. 347-380.

The serious shortcomings of cost benefit analysis, such as simplistic forecasting of the future earnings of rehabilitants, insufficiencies of data on costs and benefits, and extreme sensitivity of the cost-benefit model to underlying assumptions (e.g. discount rates, rate of earnings before and after rehabilitation), argue against priority setting in rehabilitation investments based on greater rates of return calculated for specific groups of disabled people.

Forecasts of future earnings rely on before-and-after rehabilitation estimates of earnings without benefit of a control group against which to compare what would have actually happened if services had been withheld or different services administered. Economists also avoid evaluation of such possible direct benefits to disabled people as improved capacity for self care, increased mobility, reduced pain and suffering, and increased satisfaction with life. Benefit and cost concepts vary considerably in scope and definition; some restrict the concept of benefit to paid work, others include unpaid work activities and the increased value of homemaker work. The "earnings before rehabilitation" definition varies widely, as earnings are estimated during the week prior to acceptance for services, or for the full year prior to admission to the rehabilitation program. Although all studies discount benefits to their present value in order to take into account the time horizon of future cost and earning streams, the time span and discount rates employed in present value formulas also vary, and have an impact on resultant cost benefit ratios.

$$PV = \sum_{i=1}^{n} \frac{EE_i\ p(S, Em, A, Sx, R, Ed, I, D, G)}{(1+r)^i}$$

The present value of aggregate benefits (PV) is derived by discounting by some rate of interest (r) expected earnings (EE) over time as a probability function of survival (S), employment (Em), age (A), sex (Sx), race (R), education (Ed), type of impairment (I), recurring disability (D), and average growth in the economy (G). n is retirement age minus age at completion of rehabilitation. Σ is the sign for "the sum of."

The sensitivity of cost-benefit models to assumptions is rather great. A 3% increase in assumed productivity can inflate by 50% the resultant benefit-cost ratios; one-half of 1% increase in assumed unemployment among rehabilitants can produce a downward shift of 5%; using a longer instead of a shorter period to define "earnings before rehabilitation" can reduce ratios by 26% to 70%. A discount rate of 13% can yield a benefit-cost ratio 62% less than would a rate of 4%. Given these shortcomings, the political process is the only fair way to prioritize rehabilitation investments.

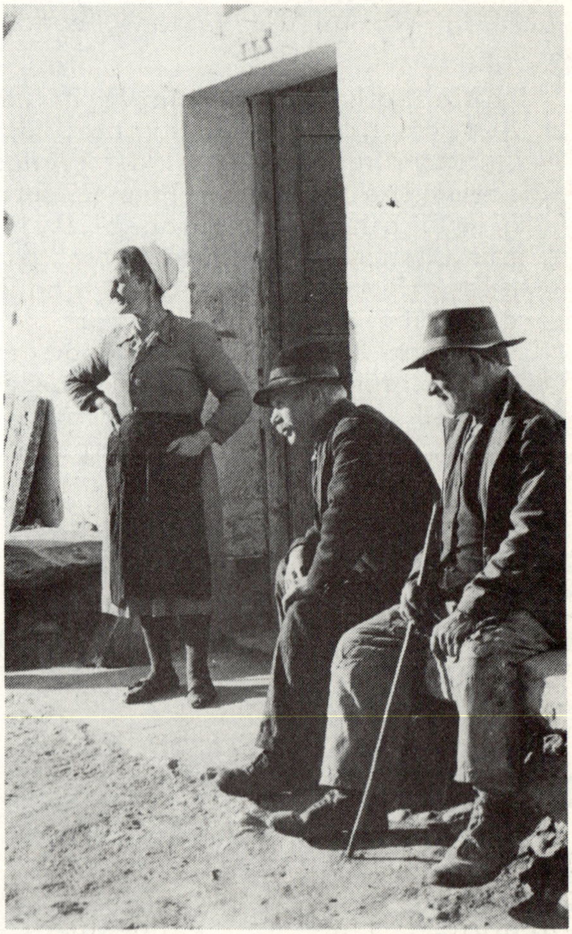

"Cost-benefit models are very sensitive to assumptions. One-half of 1% increase in projected unemployment among those rehabilitated results in a downward shift of 5% in the cost-benefit ratio."

World Health Organization. Cost-Benefit Analysis in Mental Health Services. Report on a Working Group. The Hague, 21-25 June 1976. Copenhagen: World Health Organization, 1976.

Availability of data is a key problem in cost-benefit analysis of rehabilitation services. To illustrate the extent of the problem, seventy percent of WHO member States have no direct information on the health status of their populations. Monitoring and evaluation of mental health services is therefore considered an important tool in the rational planning of health services.

Three main approaches to cost-benefit analysis in the health field can be discerned: pure cost analysis (PCA), which calculates the cost, in monetary terms, to society of a particular disease or disease group; cost-benefit analysis (CBA), has been defined as "the systematic comparison, in monetary terms -- of all the costs and benefits of proposed alternative schemes with a view to determining which scheme or combination of schemes will contribute most to the achievement of predetermined objectives at a fixed investment, or the magnitude of the benefit that can result from schemes requiring the minimum investment"; cost/effectiveness analysis (CEA), which is similar to CBA except that benefit, instead of being expressed in monetary terms, is expressed in results achieved, e.g., number of lives saved or number of days free from absence from work.

The cost of mental health care may depend on three groups of variables. The first and basic group of variables is related to the characteristics of patients themselves. The second group of variables is related to the type of services, and a third group of managerial variables on different administrative levels.

The first group of interacting variables, comprising "estimated care/cure need and demand," contains three groups of parameters: individual characteristics, the microenvironment characteristics (family, etc.), and the macroenvironment characteristics (industrial versus agricultural society, availability of services). The second group of interacting variables, comprising the "care/cure activities provided", contains three groups of parameters: manpower, construction, and tools. The third group of interacting variables comprises "management"--the way to fit the supply to the need. Here planning, programing, and budgeting are crucial variables.

One of the major difficulties in health management is fitting the groups of variables together. Examples of "friction cost", which is the result of poor planning and management, are: construction of tuberculosis sanatoria which became outdated because an efficient outpatient drug treatment program has been developed, or planning at the national level being counteracted by the execution of different plans or policies at local level, etc.

The indirect as well as the direct costs need to be taken into consideration for decision-making purposes. Indirect costs are the costs of dependency; a slightly dependent person (low indirect cost) placed in an inpatient service (high direct cost) is an example of friction cost--supply does not fit the demand/need.

An additional cost at the management level is an "impedance cost--the cost of overcoming inertia, resistance, and friction at each of the different organizational levels.

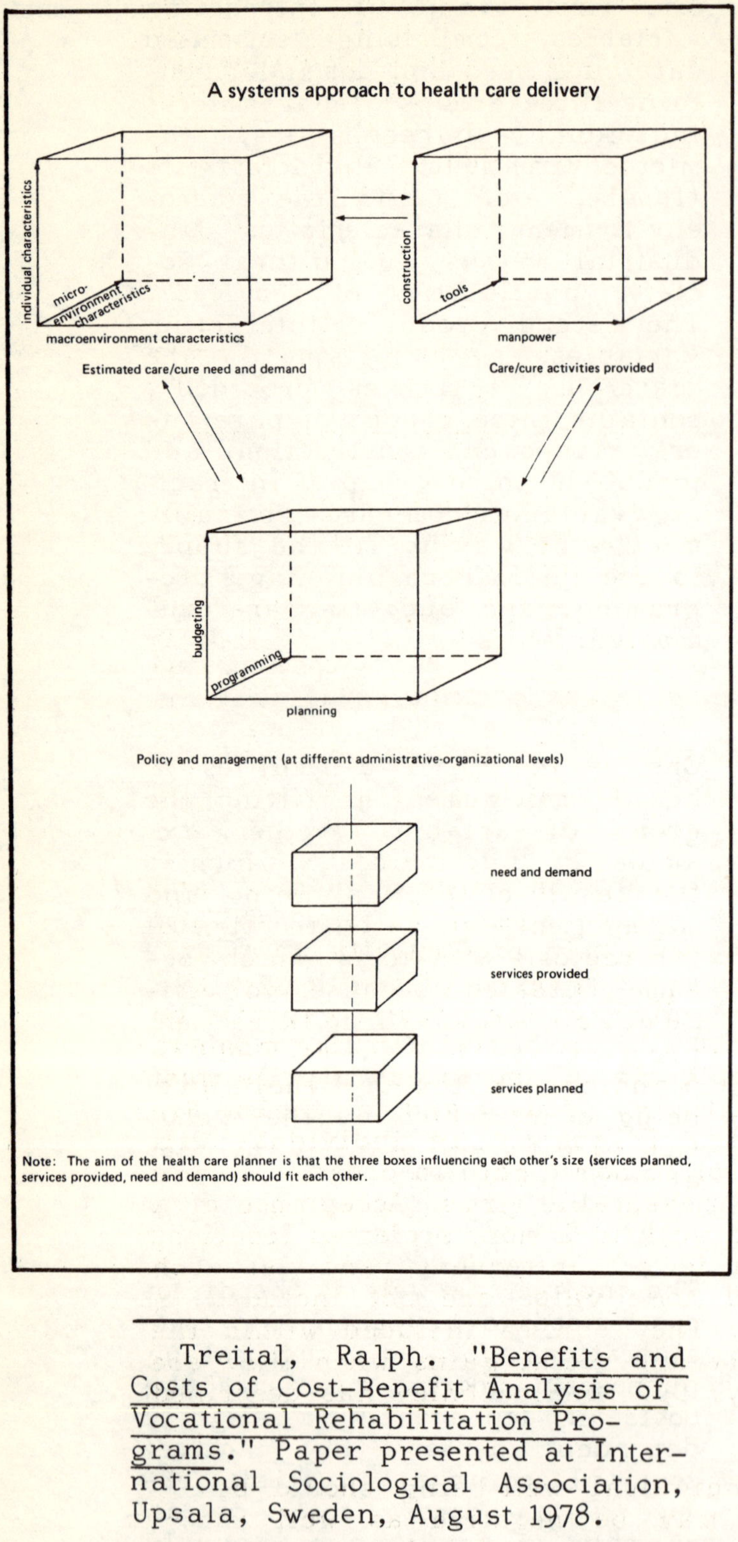

Treital, Ralph. "Benefits and Costs of Cost-Benefit Analysis of Vocational Rehabilitation Programs." Paper presented at International Sociological Association, Upsala, Sweden, August 1978.

This paper reviews the basic limitations in the conventional method of cost-benefit analysis of a single program of services, and suggests improvements in single program assessment, and for comparison of different types of programs.

A common evaluation tool for the assessment of the government programs of vocational rehabilitation services in the U.S. is a comparison of increases in lifetime earnings of successful clients to the costs of the service program. The results of evaluations applying this model have varied widely: Estimates of returns in benefits to costs have ranged from 3 to 1 to 30 to 1; even for the severely disabled, benefits to costs of services have been calculated as 7 to 1 under this model. Some analyses find greater returns in productivity among the most disadvantaged clients in terms of older age, minority and lower income groups, only to be disputed by other studies finding that the disabled with the highest pre-disability income and occupational status realize higher levels of success.

Given these contradictions, major improvements in the method of evaluation would include careful assessment of the functional limitations of clients before and after services and the nature of the services delivered. "Much more important than an artificial ratio of benefits to costs in program evaluation is an assessment of the direction the program is taking--the marginal effects on the cost-benefit ratio of changes in the client population, type of services or level of expenditures." Within this framework, the "definition of costs of services should be broadened to include measures of the dysfunctional effects of large bureaucratic agents of social control in inappropriate labeling of disability and inappropriate socialization of disabled people to work roles that might not be in their own best interest."

Traditional cost-benefit models imply that benefits are a result of agency expenditures and efforts. Yet the physical characteristics of the clients and of the labor market may have a far greater effect on subsequent productivity than the provision of services. The more a rehabilitation agency "creams" through the acceptance of the least disabled and most valued workers, the higher the resultant benefit-cost ratio. A U.S. General Accounting Office study found that a large proportion of clients had returned to working capacity and left the social security disability insurance rolls because of medical improvement unrelated to rehabilitation services.

B. ASSESSMENT OF NON-MONETARY BENEFITS: HUMAN AND SOCIAL GAINS

Within the research based on cost-benefit studies, significant quantities of data have consistently been excluded from analysis due to the existence of non-measurable concepts. Invariably, these non-measurable concepts are seen to be those which relate to the human and societal gains of rehabilitation activity. The process of exclusion does not in and of itself determine that the concepts are of lesser value because of their non-measurable nature, given present economic techniques and assumptions. Nevertheless, the fact that these values have been so rarely examined in economic terms, or included within the overall accounts, has in fact tended to diminish awareness of their importance.

There is, in principal, no distinction between "human" and economic gains. All activities which induce human satisfaction and well-being have implications for the economic productivity they will stimulate. It is widely accepted that improved levels of health care and social service in a nation will be associated with a greater capacity on the part of the citizenry to be economically productive. In like manner, all goods and services for which people are willing to pay a price must satisfy some human need. The capacities to produce and to consume are intrinsically related to human gains. Frequently an individual will choose to forgo some measurable form of economic gain in order to ensure his or her satisfaction in other less measurable terms. Acceptance of a lower-paying job in order to live and work in a more preferred location, or to gain greater job satisfaction is not infrequent, and yet such satisfactions which are certainly of some value are not included in measures of gross national product. They can be included within the term "human gains". Human gains become social gains when they are grouped for all persons in a society. Dr. Ronald Conley has described social gains as follows:

> "All effects of a program on individual well-being should be counted as a benefit (benefits may be negative as well as positive). This includes increases in earnings, home-making services, and other unpaid work, reduction in pain, savings in the costs of care, and psychic benefits. Collectively these effects are termed social benefits. A common misconception is that benefit-cost calculations are limited to variables that can be measured in dollar terms, other variables being described as non-economic. This is untrue. All social benefits are relevant to evaluating a program. If omissions are made, it is because of the difficulty of measurement, not lack of relevance." 43/

Social benefits may thus become the pivotal elements in assessment of the economic value of different types of activity. Just as individuals may decide to forgo certain forms of economic benefit, societies may sometimes determine to forgo certain increases in national income to provide human gains for segments of the citizenry. Actions which offer little or even negative likelihood of measurable economic gain may be chosen as more valuable in societal terms than actions which might engender passivity and feelings of worthlessness.

Another form of social gain is manifest by those gains which are accrued directly by society or by others in society than the disabled and their families. For example, investment in education can provide economic and human gains for the recipients of higher education, through increased income and opportunity, but the widespread availability of higher education can also lead to fundamental changes in the structure of society itself. Greater degrees and depths of communication are possible between all sectors of society; commercial, social and cultural life can be stimulated, and political innovations can take place.

The widespread availability of adequate and comprehensive rehabilitation services for disabled people can also have some such effects on the well-being of people not directly affected by the availability of the services. People who fear the inactivity and dependence which might result from an accident, illness or old age may derive reassurance and satisfaction from the knowledge that alternative possibilities for re-entry into active life exist. Disability recognizes no class or geographical distinctions. It is one of the few universal elements of life to which no person is immune. There are very few people who have not been associated personally, or through their families, with some aspect of disability; there are probably very few people who have not taken cognizance of the possible implications for their own lives. In this sense, the availability of rehabilitation services, like medical services in general, can "not only remove the pains of the sick but also the fears of the healthy". 44/

Application of Economic Analyses to the Rehabilitation Process

It is of great importance to take advantage of the economic tools available for analysis of social phenomena to assess the effects of rehabilitation programs for the disabled. National planners frequently question whether or not rehabilitation programs are affordable and whether or not they should be expanded when other activities of value to a larger segment of the population are in need of funding. Cost-benefit analyses, and other economic assessment methodologies, can be applied to the rehabilitation process to evaluate the relationship of this field of human activity to society as a whole; however, the limitations of the cost benefit tool, and the conceptual deficiencies of economic assessment methodology, cannot be ignored. Economic measures can provide only part of the total analysis which is necessary to fully document the effects of disability and rehabilitation upon society. Nevertheless, much experience exists in countries of greatly differing socio-economic organization in the application of economic assessment techniques to the rehabilitation process.

IV. LABOR MARKET AND MANPOWER POLICIES

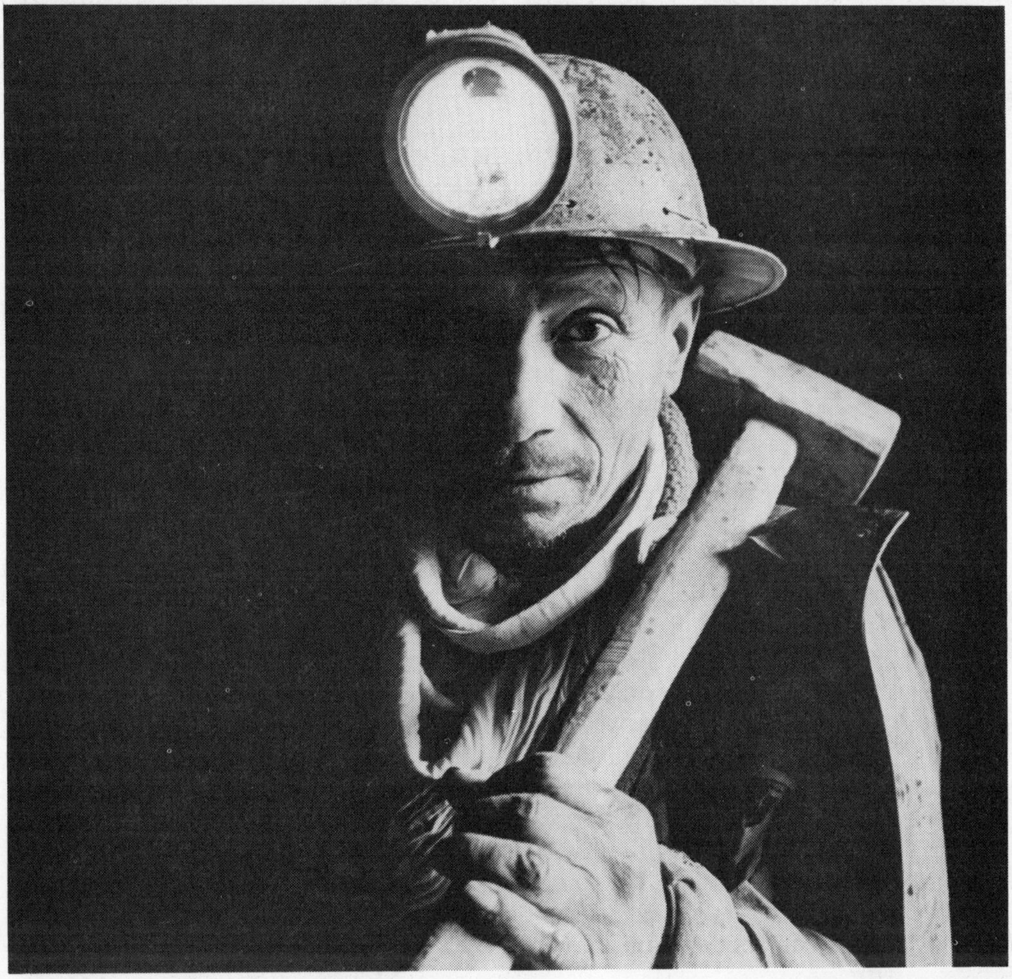

The need for disabled people to "demand from society a fair chance" was the conclusion of a survey on the Social Policy of Industrial Companies in Respect of Handicapped Workers carried out by Anton Heering of the Netherlands. 45/ The survey, conducted by mail questionnaire, dealt with measures employed within industry to facilitate the employment of disabled workers. Responses were received from 54 employers' organization representatives, trade union representatives, government administrators, and social scientists in 17 countries. The results reflected the usual problems of mail questionnaires - only partial agreement between the precoded reply sections, and only partial responses from the various groups surveyed - and as a result, only a rough picture of the situation was obtained. None the less, the author concluded that a significant difference existed between the expressed sentiments of industry in favor of hiring disabled people, and the actual measures taken to facilitate this practice. In situations in which the "economic principle" prevails the disabled worker is less likely to be hired since the employer will tend to take into account the existing state of industrial conditions, and make a determination on the basis of the equipment and arrangements already available in the working environment. There is little likelihood that ergonomic adaptations of the work environment to the needs of the disabled will be considered. A significant proportion of the respondents indicated that the disabled should be given the same chances as the non-disabled, but that special efforts should not be undertaken on their behalf since industries are not, after all, social enterprises. Only in a situation in which a "social principle" prevails, during periods of economic growth or prosperity, is it likely that employers will have more favourable attitudes towards disabled people. Similarly, the majority of respondents believed that disabled workers should have as much participation in decisions about their daily work as other workers, and not more participation.

The survey concluded with an assertion of the importance of giving special attention, under certain circumstances, to disabled people. Disabled workers generally have less flexibility and adaptability than those who are non-disabled, and the risk of failing in a job is therefore greater for them. The working situation for the individual worker has improved greatly since the beginnings of industrialization, particularly through the principle of individualization -- improving the quality of the worker's job placement, improving the quality of his job. As yet, the same benefits have not been extended to disabled people.

A. PRODUCTION BENEFITS OF REHABILITATION

Production benefits refer to the capability of any activity to contribute to the value of the annual production output of a nation, either at the time the activity is undertaken or in future years. Production benefits understandably form the economic basis upon which a nation may develop. It is possible to consider the economic process as being divided into three phases: 46/

1. The creation of values, which generate the gross national product and which are used to satisfy the various claims to income;

2. The distribution of income claims to:

   (a) The active work force;

   (b) The recipients of transfer income;

   (c) Other needs designated by the government;

3. The use of income for the consumption of produced goods, for savings, or for investments.

The three phases are in reality intermeshed and inseparable. They constitute a single dynamic process. All social benefits provided to any group of individuals or to a society as a whole must be derived from within the process, and thus from their relationship to the national product.

Production benefits are of great importance to national planners, and it is not surprising that attempts to demonstrate the economic utility of rehabilitation services have frequently concentrated on this aspect. Activities such as vocational rehabilitation, sheltered employment, and other measures leading to job placement have been analyzed to demonstrate their economic impact. Often the capacity to provide production benefits is seen as the only "economic" aspect, and less easily measured effects are ignored. The possibility also exists that emphasis on demonstration of production benefits has led to a shaping of

"The independent living movement insists that the failure to be gainfully employed does not necessarily rest with the individual, but with the market which has been unable to make useful work available or accessible."

Gerben DeJong, The Movement for Independent Living, 1979.

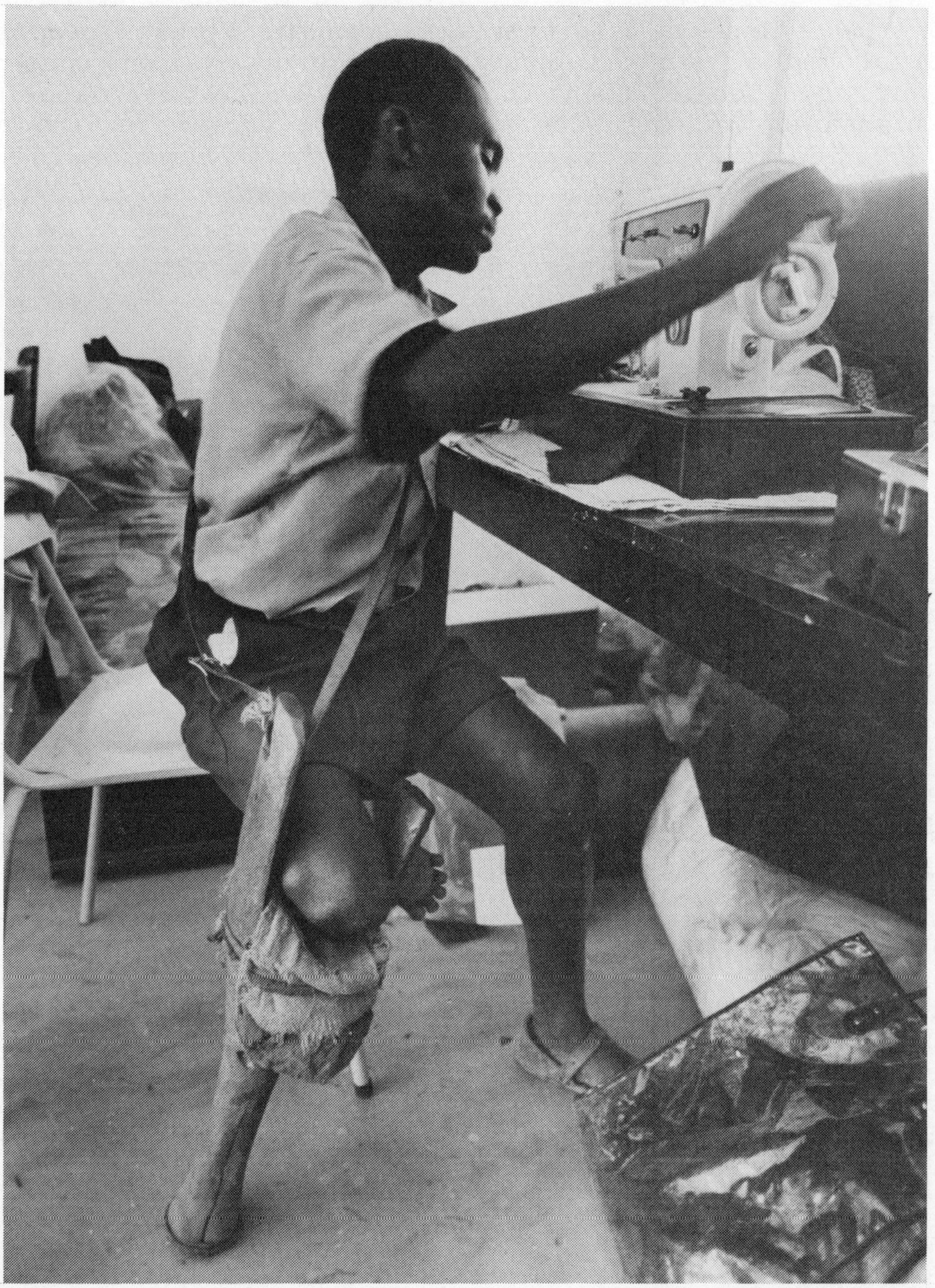

the types of rehabilitation services provided in patterns which do not necessarily correspond to the actual needs of the disabled. This is a problem which requires further analysis in a separate study, although it is only through a more comprehensive understanding of all the economic impacts of rehabilitation activity that such an analysis would have meaning.

Production is dependent upon manpower, and the economic growth of a nation is limited by its available manpower potential. Manpower both assures and creates production by acting both as a consumer and a producer of values. In classical terms, three factors are necessary for the production of commodities: land, capital and labor. Land and capital alone cannot generate an economic yield; they only become useful in conjunction with human labor. As machines have been used to increase the productivity of each worker, human labor has become more and more valuable. Each worker makes use of much higher levels of capital investment. While capital, equipment and technical facilities may be indispensable elements of economic growth, people are the "operational capital" and as such are preeminent. Nations thus make intensive efforts to generate, maintain and preserve the work capacity of their available manpower.

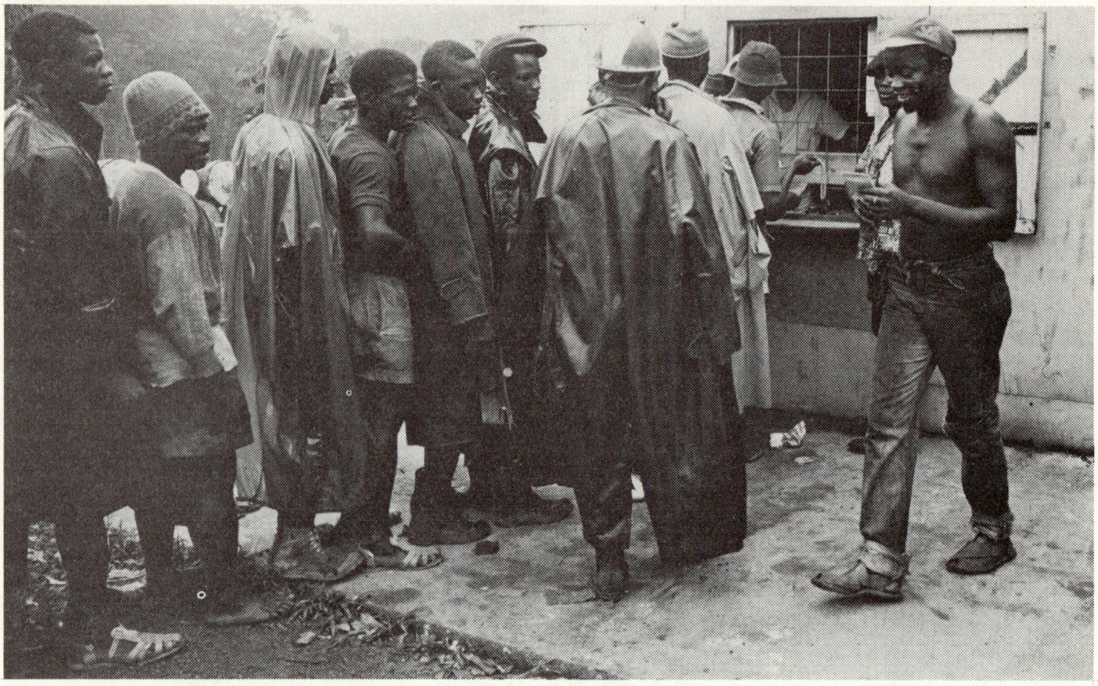

People are not commodities, and their labor is not merchandise. The nature and quality of work produced by each individual is dependent upon many factors related to his or her unique personality. Commodities can be sold, or if not sold, they can be stored, with possible expenses for their storage and depreciation in worth. People cannot be stored. A person, and his or her family, must continue to exist. If because of disability there is a loss in ability to subsist, the costs of "storage" while the disabled person with his or her unique knowledge is recuperating and the costs of "depreciation" from a loss in job knowledge or work capacity will be far greater than they would be for commodities. The greater the costs of educating and training the person, the greater will be the loss caused by his or her removal from the work force because of disability. The effects of disability touch not only those individuals most directly concerned but also their care-providers, spouses, parents, friends and their children, the future producers. Some form of investment is necessary to avert the manpower loss caused by disability, and this is the investment in rehabilitation services. The investment may be directed towards preserving the working capacity of the disabled person or, for persons who have not been a part of the work force, to creating that capacity through training. Disabled people are much more likely to lose work capacity than the able-bodied and require more time and resources to recover from such a loss than do the able-bodied. The earlier that effective intervention measures are established, the more likely it is that there will be success in preserving residual working capability.

The next sections of this chapter analyze research studies on the capacity of rehabilitation services to add to the production output of a nation and on their capacity to alter the available manpower potential. The studies have been selected to demonstrate the variety of methods possible for assessing production benefits in rehabilitation, and to illustrate the assessment process within a range of social, cultural and economic variables.

In addition to the multiplicity of variables within the studies, such as the types of populations sampled, the definitions of disability, the definitions of productivity, the time periods of the studies, the assessment methodologies, and the basic economic system within each nation, the basic organization of social services available within each society constitutes yet another difference of major proportions.

B. SHELTERED EMPLOYMENT

The studies in this section deal with the provision of substitute permanent employment for disabled people in sheltered workshops, workers' cooperatives, and small-scale business enterprises. The studies have been conducted within varying economic structures: the developed market economies of the Organization for Economic Cooperation and Development (OECD) member countries, the centrally planned economy of Poland, and the developing economy of Ethiopia. The comparison is not intended to demonstrate any conclusion regarding the most effective approach towards the organization of substitute employment. It is not intended to reach any conclusions regarding the merits of the substitute employment process. Such conclusions would obviously require greater analysis of a variety of factors than could be covered within the present study. Nor is the intention to advocate any aspect of the service approaches used. Rehabilitation of disabled people is a complex process, requiring the solution of a variety of problems within the social-cultural milieu of each society. Rarely is one approach a panacca.

The studies are presented to demonstrate three approaches to the economic analysis of one aspect of rehabilitation activity under differing economic conditions. Each of the three studies has major limitations which are cited, and each demonstrates some useful conclusions regarding economic implications.

The OECD Analysis

One of the most comprehensive international economic analyses of an aspect of rehabilitation was carried out in 1964 by Bent Andersen for the OECD Manpower and Social Affairs Directorate. 47/ Mr. Andersen conducted the study in conjunction with the Danish National Institute for Social Research. His concern was with persons who are "unplaceable" in normal employment and his study was to determine whether or not the rest of society is economically better off when Measures for Substitute Permanent Employment (MSPE) are taken for such people as an alternative to social cash benefits such as pensions, public assistance, workmen's compensation and unemployment payments. The study examines the economic costs and benefits to the nation, to sectors, and to individual persons, of a system of sheltered employment in six countries.

The basis of the study was a questionnaire sent to 30 sheltered employment facilities in member countries of the OECD. Responses from six countries, Denmark, the Federal Republic of Germany, the Netherlands, Sweden, the United Kingdom and the United States of America are presented, supplemented by information about the general organization of rehabilitation activities and social services in each country. A recapitulation of a segment of this material is illuminating:

> "Germany and the Netherlands are representatives of the continental social security system based upon compulsory disablement and similar insurances for wage earners. In the Netherlands much emphasis is placed on sheltered employment for all kinds of unplaceable persons. In Germany more emphasis is placed on payment of compensation and benefits. A quota scheme provides a high number of jobs reserved for some categories of handicapped persons and a few sheltered workshops exist. ..."
>
> "The social security systems in the United Kingdom, Denmark, and Sweden are characterized by compulsory schemes covering the whole population and--in Denmark and Sweden--to a large extent financed through general taxes. In all these countries there are municipal or private MSPEs with substantial support from the state, but in the United Kingdom there are in addition a number of state owned sheltered factories, organized in a comprehensive system, the Remploy Ltd."
>
> "In the United States of America, social welfare schemes vary from state to state. Voluntary security schemes and charitable organizations play a major role. This is also the case regarding the organization of sheltered employment, but federal support is provided through the Vocational Rehabilitation Administration." 48/

Development of Cost-Benefit Models

The Andersen study was seeking a method of cost-benefit analysis which would be applicable in situations of greatly differing cultural and social organization. The questionnaire methodology was supplemented by direct observation of a small number of facilities, and one of the author's main conclusions was that the latter method of direct comparison would be far more promising than the mail questionnaire which produced responses of limited utility.

Andersen attempted to evaluate two types of data: whether sheltered employment as compared with cash benefits resulted in an increase in the well-being of people unplaceable in ordinary employment, with some indication of the size of the increase and the circumstances under which it took place; and whether there is a net economic gain or sacrifice for the rest of the society connected with measures for substitute permanent employment.

He assumed that society does not neglect the problems of the unplaceable but rather that the responsible powers seek to establish the conditions necessary for providing this group of citizens with what is considered to be a socially acceptable level of living. Possible alternatives to this assumption, as Andersen makes clear, would be:

(a) For the public to neglect the problem;

(b) For various social benefits to be provided;

(c) For measures to be taken to create job opportunities offsetting the inability to compete in normal employment opportunities.

The study excluded programs which aim to restore or improve the working capacity of handicapped persons. A separate extension of the cost-benefit model is provided for facilities which offer training in addition to employment opportunities.

The models developed by the Andersen study may be applied for the cost-benefits of sheltered employment to a society as a whole or for sectoral analyses. Methods are prescribed to assess the addition to net national income provided by MSPE, to assess the value of production, replacement costs, alternative values of the invested capital and normal labor salaries, and the value of input goods and services.

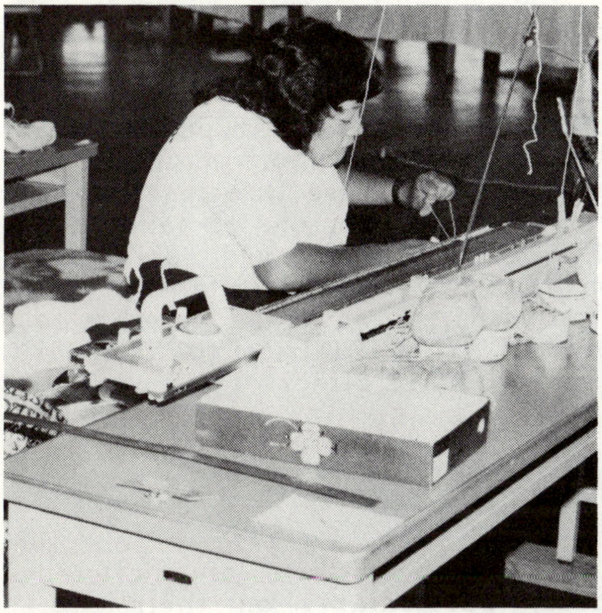

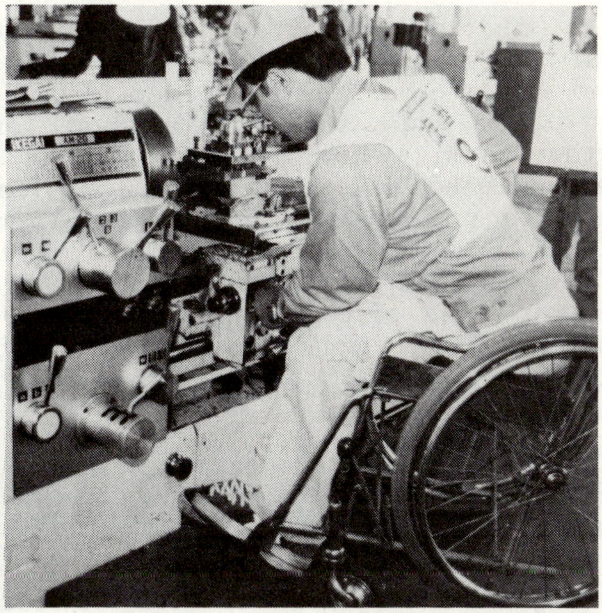

Assessment of Production Output Value

There are certain problems inherent in the assessment of the output of production. Andersen indicates that the actual price obtained for a sheltered workshop product may not always represent its value. If the product is sold to the public on the basis of people's sympathy, the price obtained contains a hidden subsidy from the public which represents their payment for the social value of employing the handicapped. The size of the hidden subsidy cannot be measured directly. It can only be assumed that if the product is not sold in competition, and if the sheltered facility uses its social position in sales promotion or sells a large part of its goods to public authorities, a hidden subsidy is included in the actual price. Such a subsidy will cause the addition to national production to be over-evaluated. In addition, some sheltered employment facilities produce goods and supply services of a kind which otherwise might not be provided. There may be no price for such services, particularly if they are undertaken as a public service to employ the handicapped; and their theoretical value, based on the maximum price which authorities would be willing to pay for the services in themselves, may be completely unknown.

Examples of sheltered employment facilities from the six countries are cited and the cost-benefit models are applied. On this basis, Andersen concluded in part that:

(a) It was not possible on the basis of the study to draw any conclusions regarding the general level of the gains or losses to society of MSPEs. The facilities investigated showed results which varied from substantial additions to net national product to heavy losses;

(b) Those workshops which showed the biggest economic losses to society had either undergone major structural changes during the observation period or employed mentally handicapped persons. The workshops which provided the largest addition to net national product seemed to have relatively more administrative personnel;

(c) It was the general experience of the study that it is extremely difficult to acquire correct information on the consumption of real capital;

(d) In many cases sheltered facilities over-rated the real cost of staff by failing to take into account the costs saved on care-personnel who would otherwise be needed for the most severely handicapped if they were not employed. A workshop for the mentally retarded in the Netherlands, which on the basis of the cost-benefit calculation demonstrated a loss of 319,000 guilders, could reverse this loss if the need were taken into account for approximately 50 persons to take care of the 522 handicapped workers if they were not employed. Using an average wage of 7,500 guilders per year for each caretaker, and reducing the cost of labor by 375,000 guilders, it would be possible to show that the workshop actually provided a net addition to national product of 56,000 guilders. Other such examples are cited.

Effects of Sheltered Employment on other Sectors

The Andersen study also analyzed the effects of sheltered employment on other sectors of society, particularly on their productivity. The study indicated that:

(a) The effects of sheltered employment on other sectors of the economy will be dependent on the general level of employment, the specific sales possibilities of the enterprise, and the production level of the enterprise;

(b) In periods of prosperity, a sheltered employment facility will normally not cause a decrease in the production of other enterprises. If the sheltered enterprise belongs to a sector affected by a general depression, its production may have negative effects on its competitors; however, if the sheltered enterprise is producing specialized products for further production in other firms, there may be a positive connection. The positive and negative direct economic effects may vary within each year, and it is difficult to evaluate fully the direct effects since it is impossible to recreate how the economic development would have taken place without the sheltered enterprise;

(c) It is probable that the total effects of sheltered enterprises on other sectors over long periods will be positive for the following reasons:

(i) The sheltered enterprise helps to maintain the residual working capacity of disabled people and, as such, keeps them in the ranks of reserve workers for the normal labor market. The remaining working capacity of handicapped workers is seen to be more vulnerable than that of the able-bodied and, even though some non-disabled may be kept out of employment during periods of depression while the handicapped are employed, the short-term unemployment for the able-bodied will have a less long-lasting effect;

(ii) The dependants of the disabled person employed in sheltered employment will be positively influenced by the economic and emotional gains of employment. This is particularly important for the children of a disabled individual, who will have a better chance of becoming well-adjusted members of society in the future.

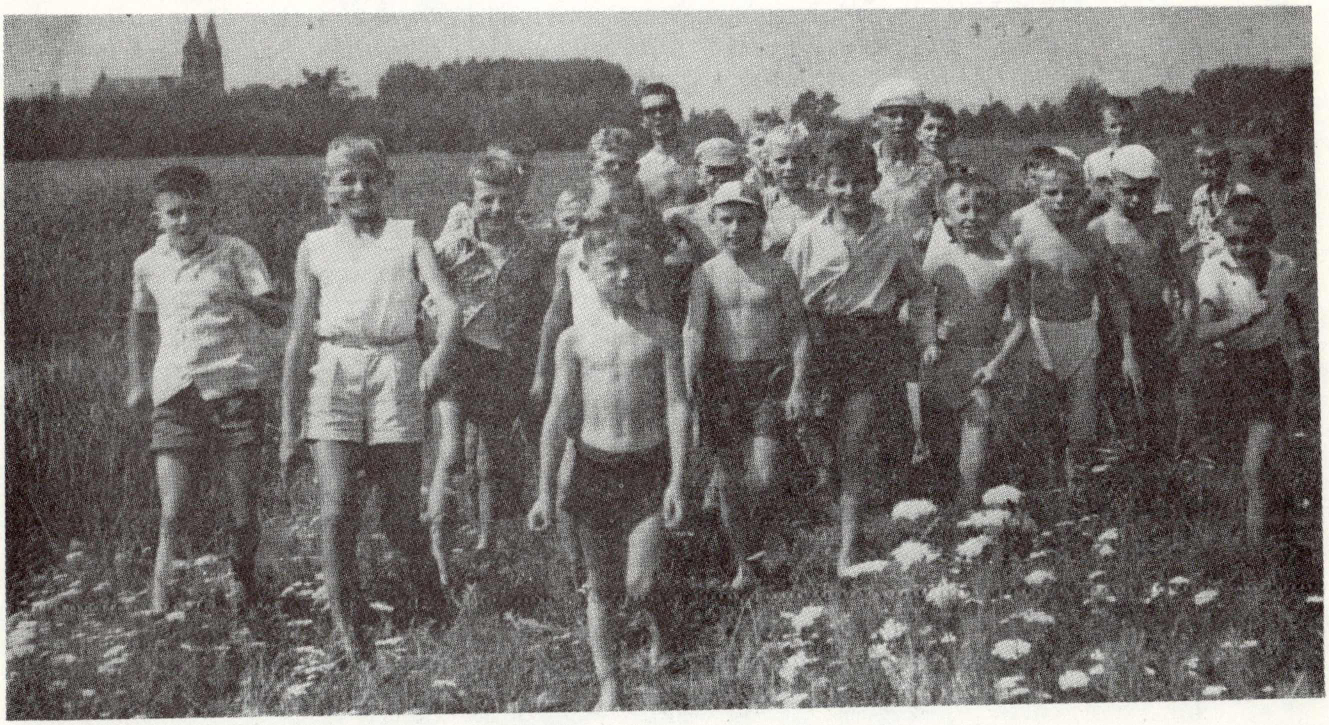

Summer holidays for the children of employees of the Polish Union of Invalid's Cooperative.

The Invalids' Cooperative of Poland

A well developed system of Invalid Cooperatives exists in Poland in accordance with the social, economic and legal structure of that country. They function as an effective Measure for Substitute Permanent Employment, an MSPE according to the Andersen study criteria. The Invalids' Cooperatives have been assessed to be economically self-sufficient in terms of the economy of Poland, as well as providing benefits to disabled people through employment. Membership is open to persons who are disabled or who, not being disabled in terms of pension law, are treated as disabled because of their limited working capacity as defined by the Invalid's Cooperatives Union.

Historical Development and Relationship to the Social Welfare System

The system of Invalids' Co-operatives in Poland 48/ experienced a period of rapid development and expansion in the years following the Second World War. Unions of disabled war veterans, blind people and the deaf were instrumental in this development and, through a cooperative union, they undertook to provide employment and medical, social and educational rehabilitation services for their members. In 1950 the Cooperatives employed 2,000 disabled; by 1960 70,000 disabled workers were employed, and at the end of 1975 240,000 persons, including the more than 180,000 disabled, were employed in Invalids' Cooperatives.

The Polish Cooperatives function within the larger framework of medical, social and vocational rehabilitation services, and they are organized on the legal basis established for cooperatives. Medical and vocational rehabilitation in Poland are administered by the Ministry of Health and Social Welfare, and by the local health and social welfare departments. Disability and Employment Commissions assess the degree of disability of disabled persons and determine their rights to pensions. The disabled are divided into three groups:

Those who are employable, but who require special help;

Those who are unable to work but do not require special rehabilitation help;

Those who can no longer work in their trade or profession or can only work limited hours or within limited circumstances.

Disability and invalid pensions are provided by the Ministry of Labor's Office of Social Security. In 1973 47 billion zlotys (approx. $U.S. 2.4 billion) were spent on pensions in Poland, which had at that time a population of 33.5 million. It was projected that by 1990, 1,200,000 persons would be receiving invalid pensions. In 1973, there were 1.5 million employees with limited working ability in Poland and 600,000 of them were categorized as disabled. In the same year, more than 45,000 disabled people were placed in employment with the help of the health and social welfare departments.

Economic Activity of the Cooperatives

Within the Invalids' Cooperatives, there are approximately 300 sheltered workshops employing a total of 26,000 severely disabled persons. This represents about 27 percent of all disabled people in cooperative production work. The system of sheltered workshops includes those cooperatives regarded wholly as sheltered workshops, special and separate employment sections within cooperatives, and separate sheltered workplaces.

Individuals employed within the homebound workers' scheme represent 30 percent of the total employed in the industrial sector, and in 1973 their work accounted for 20 percent of the overall industrial production of all Invalids' Cooperatives.

The nature and scope of economic activity in Invalids' Cooperatives is determined not only by the type and nature of the industrial and agricultural activity carried out in the town or region where the cooperative is located, but also by the working capacities of the disabled themselves. The main work activity of the cooperatives is concerned with production of articles for the home market and export, i.e., to supply products for workshops and establishments, not for general consumption. The Union of Invalids' Cooperatives organizes production in approximately 16 industrial fields. It is said that there are no television sets, cars or telephone exchanges manufactured in Poland without some component produced by the Invalids' Cooperatives.

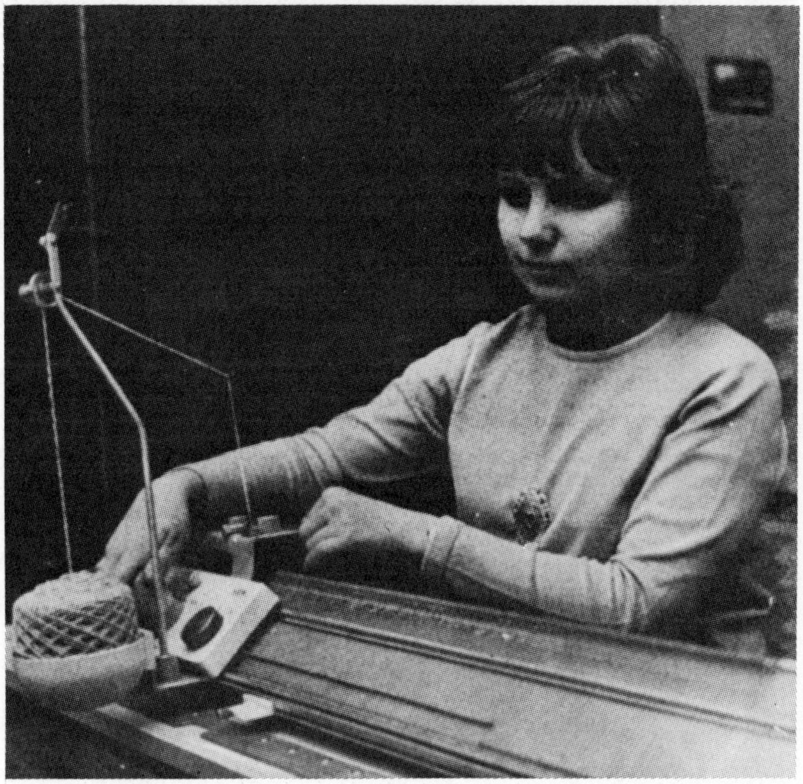

The Invalids' Cooperatives' share of overall national production in 1973 was 1.2 percent. The percentage was far greater in certain sectors: 15.5 percent in the clothing industry, 7.7 percent in the electro-technical industry. Data from 1971 indicated that the value of production for domestic use services and retail trade turnover of the cooperatives that year amounted to 21 billion zlotys, and the value of export goods was 451 billion zlotys. (approx. U.S.$22.6 billion) 50/

In the years following the Second World War, Poland had an excess of manpower resources; however, economic projections indicated that manpower resources would gradually decrease during the mid- and latter-1970s so that the worker reserve capacity provided through the Invalids' Cooperatives will take on new importance to national planners in Poland.

Financial Privileges and Incentives

Employers in Poland are being encouraged to solve the problems of employees with limited working ability within the work place. They are obliged to employ a certain quota of disabled people. Invalids' Cooperatives, in order to qualify for the various benefits accorded this status, must employ disabled people for 70 percent of their labor force. As part of the legislative measures undertaken since the early 1960s, the Invalids' Cooperative movement is provided a system of privileges to ensure its full development. The privileges take the following forms:

(a) Tax reduction in the turnover and income tax -- a 50 percent reduction in taxes is granted to cooperatives provided that they employ the requisite percentage of disabled people. Cooperatives of the blind and those recognized as sheltered workshops may receive a 100 percent reduction;

(b) Exclusive or priority option with regard to the production of certain products and services -- Invalids' Cooperatives have been granted sole production and access rights for some 36 products and services which are reserved for disabled workers. In addition, some 58 articles are produced on a priority basis. In 1973 28 percent of the total Invalids' Cooperative production was produced under exclusive or priority rights;

(c) Facilities in various fields of economic activity -- Invalids' Cooperatives are also given priority in the supply of raw materials when there is a shortage, and they receive guarantees by officials that the production capacity of the cooperative will be fully utilized;

(d) State grants for rehabilitation purposes -- may amount to one third of the sum paid in by cooperatives for the social insurance fund of their personnel, and they are available as a special fund for the construction and modernization of various types of rehabilitation facilities.

The incentives to the cooperatives are viewed as a form of group assistance to the disabled, rather than the individual assistance which is provided through pensions. The incentives are intended to compensate in some degree for the reduced economic capacity of Invalids' Cooperatives in comparison to enterprises employing the able-bodied. They stabilize the rehabilitation and economic activities of the cooperatives while enabling them to grow, increase productivity and provide higher wages. The incentives are regarded as aids to the cooperatives in their efforts to achieve economic self-sufficiency. In addition, the incentives are viewed as a form of compensation to the cooperatives for providing work and vocational rehabilitation for the disabled as well as general social benefits on behalf of the Polish State.

Small-Business Enterprise for Disabled People in Ethiopia

Rehabilitation in Ethiopia had traditionally been the concern of a few voluntary societies, and in recent years the Government of that nation has taken steps to institute a national programme for the disabled. The economy of the country is characterized by unemployment and under-employment of a large percentage of the able-bodied work force. In such a situation the establishment of an economically viable enterprise for employment of the disabled requires considerable planning and skill. An enterprise called United Abilities Company was formed in Ethiopia in 1966 with assistance from the International Labor Organization, and in the past 10 years it has developed into a self-sustaining employment centre for nearly 400 disabled persons. 51/ The Company maintains two factories, one for umbrella production, and one for dry-cell battery production, and it is operated on a commercial basis. Products are sold for profit and workers are paid market-value wages.

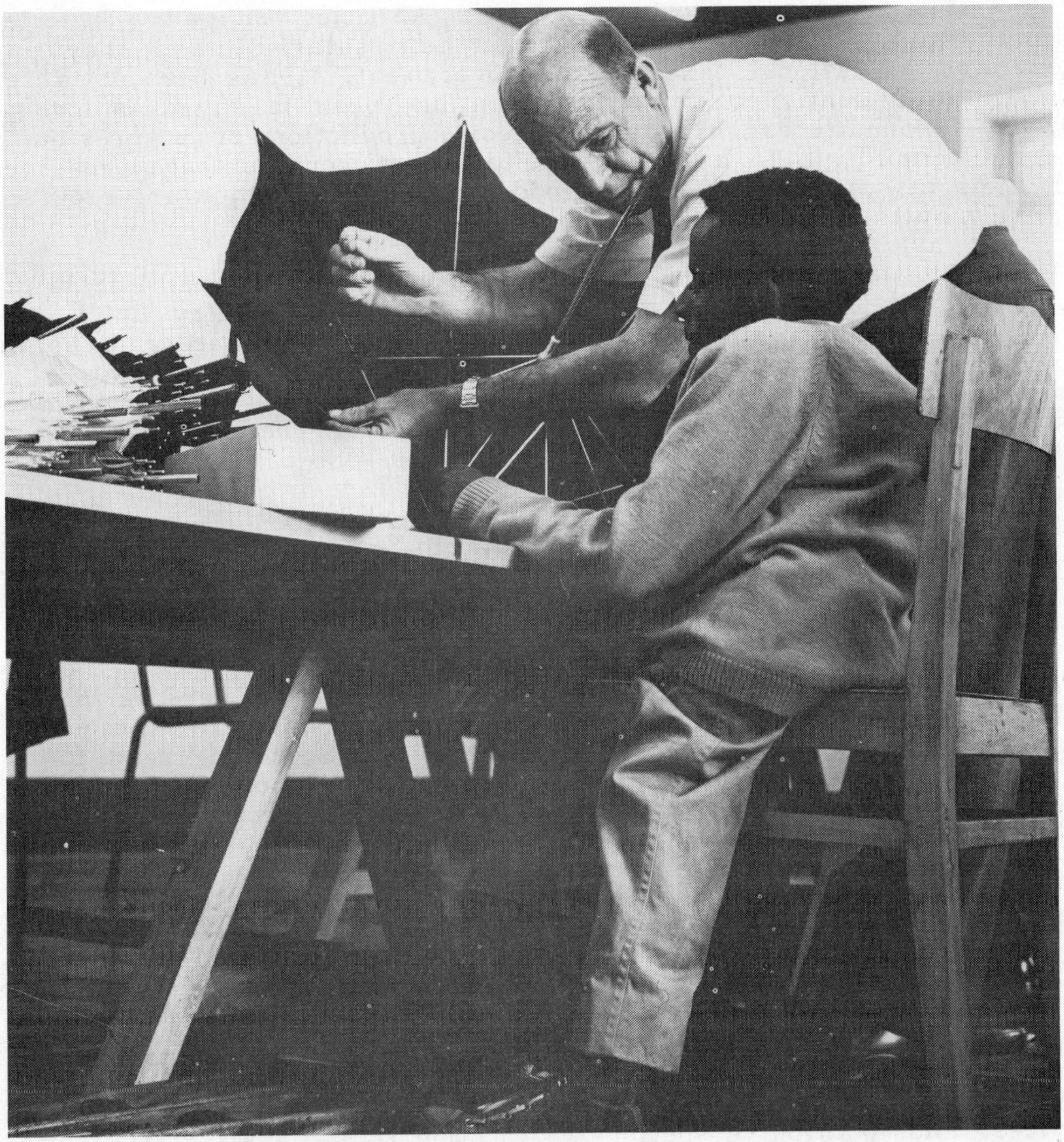

The United Abilities Company was founded with a capital investment from three voluntary agencies for the disabled. It has its own Board of Directors and a manager with full executive authority. The shareholders of the Company can return any profits to further development and expansion.

The Company began its work with a feasibility study to determine the markets available for products of small-scale industry. Considerable attention was given to the selective placement of disabled people in the various phases of production. It was determined that a local market existed for inexpensive umbrellas, and this became the first basis of production. At first the Company, with a labor force of 27, produced umbrellas from imported components; now the unit produces all the accessories and parts which it used to import. Employing 300 disabled workers, the Company produced an average of 2,400 umbrellas per day. Critical to the marketing of the Company's product was the attainment of protection against imported merchandise of the same type but of lesser quality. The dry-cell factory employed 100 severely disabled workers.

The combined workers of the Abilities Company factories support nearly 2,000 dependants with their salaries, and they pay income and educational taxes to the government. It has been estimated that the equivalent of nearly $1 million per year is saved in foreign currency expenditures through the local production of a previously imported commodity. In addition, the disabled workers themselves are, with their new income, consuming goods and services which are provided primarily by their non-handicapped fellow citizens.

The United Abilities Company demonstrates how small-scale industry may be economically viable in a developing country which does not assume a large public expenditure for its disabled citizenry. Certain social elements were necessary for the initiation and development of the effort: the capital investment on a charitable basis and the provision of monopoly production status for the item selected. The economic cost of these items has not been measured.

Additional References on Sheltered Employment:

Greenleigh Associates Inc. The Role of Sheltered Workshops in the Rehabilitation of the Severely Handicapped. New York: Greenleigh Associates Inc., 1975.

This study evaluates the role of sheltered workshops in the U.S., and also provides an International Survey on the role of sheltered workshops abroad, based on the results of research teams visiting the respective countries.

"It is possible to regard the handicapped as clients of a social service system who require a broad range of medical and social services, and to think of sheltered work as an extension of social services, with income subsidized as a form of welfare payment. Conversely, it is possible to consider the existence of large numbers of handicapped persons who want to work as a manpower problem, viewing them as a part of the labor force that is largely unemployed, and for whom integration into the labor force and the economy should be achieved."

The trend in Western Europe emphasizes a view of handicapped people as members (or during the rehabilitation process itself, as potential members) of the labor force. Individuals in workshops abroad are considerably more handicapped than those individuals in workshops in the U.S., though in all cases the number of mentally retarded persons in sheltered workshops is increasing. There is a common trend toward public operation of sheltered workshops. Successful workshop programs usually involve substan-

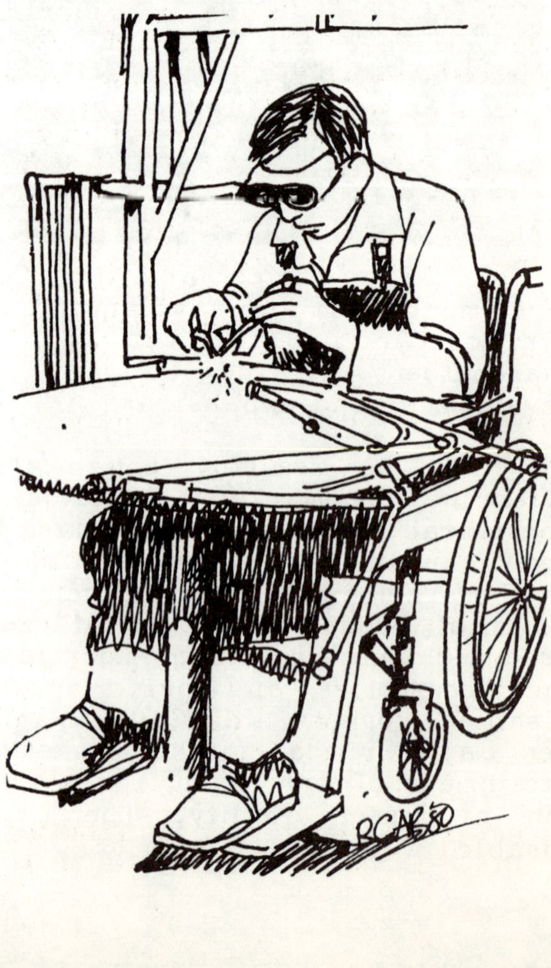

"In 1975, the costs per client in sheltered workshops in Sweden averaged U.S. $5,190 (excluding rent), compared to costs of $1,750 per client in semi-sheltered employment." *National Labour Market Board, Labour Market Policy 1975/76.*

tial direct subsidies in the form of grants, under-writing operating expenses, or tax waivers. Programs to stimulate competitive employment of handicapped people center around quota systems, wage subsidies, or other forms of incentives to employers.

There are two approaches to maintaining income levels for disabled people -- the wage approach and the welfare payment or pension approach. Incomes maintained through the pension approach tend to be lower than those subsidized through the wage system. The level of income maintenance for handicapped people in sheltered workshops in Western Europe tends to be greater than in the United States. The following country surveys provide examples of the operation of sheltered workshops for disabled persons.

Australia: In Australia, rehabilitation is a federal program and sheltered workshop grants go directly from the central government to the sponsers. The federal government subsidizes 80 percent of the capital maintenance, equipment and rent costs of the workshops. Invalid pensions constitute the primary income maintenance system for disabled persons. There were 164 sheltered workshops in 1964, growing at an annual rate of 11 to 20 percent during 1970-74.

Persons eligible for an Invalid's Pension must be certified as 85 percent disabled for work. In 1973, there were 8,393 disabled clients in workshops, 52 percent were mentally retarded and only 15 percent were classified as physically handicapped.

In order to be eligible for federal grants, workshops must have a majority of clients on pension; 71 percent were in fact receiving a pension in 1973.

Due to the heavy reliance on invalidity pensions as income, wages in workshops are low. The average weekly wage for a 31 hour week was $7.86 in 1973, and wages and salaries amounted to about 48 percent of all workshop expenditures. Australia provides incentive payments ($650 US) to workshops that place clients in regular employment for a minimum period of twelve months. Sheltered workshops placed about 10.7 percent of their clients in competitive employment in 1974.

Federal Republic of Germany: Recent legislation in the FRG provides that every employer of 15 or more persons must reserve 6 percent of his jobs for handicapped persons, and workshops have priority in bidding for certain government contracts. The (state) Employment Office operates the workshops, though there are four different agencies that make income maintenance payments to disabled clients in workshops.

The FRG estimates there are 4,000,000 handicapped persons of the population of 62,000,000. In 1971, 3,000 persons were employed in sheltered workshops, and 80 percent of these were mentally retarded. Eligibility for workshop employment requires a 50 percent disability. Movement to competitive employment, though a formal goal, is limited due to the severity of disabilities among workshop employees. The percentage successfully placed in regular employment averages about 5 percent per year.

There is no minimum wage provision for handicapped persons; wages are based on piecework rates and are low. These wages are exempt from social security taxes. Yet many clients receive pensions, disability insurance, and other income support.

Denmark: The rehabilitation and workshop system in Denmark is essentially a social service system, underpinned by the invalidity pension, various supplemental allowances, and daily cash benefits in case of temporary incapacity. Sheltered workshop programs are separate for physically handicapped and mentally handicapped persons. There are two categories of sheltered workshop. Rehabilitation units, the first category, serve workers likely to be capable of earning their own living or supplementing their disability pensions. Sheltered workshops per se, the second category, are for those who "even if in sheltered working conditions, will be able to make only a limited productive contribution." In Denmark, rehabilitation services are provided as part of total social services, which accounted for one third of the national budget in 1974.

Of a total population of 5,000,000 there were 150,000 persons receiving Invalids' Pensions or Benefit in 1972/73. Rehabilitation units served 59,000 persons, of which 23,000 were mentally impaired. This compares with only 700 persons in the sheltered workshops in 1967.

Wages are not regulated by minimum levels, as the invalidity pension is the basic form of support. The pension is adjusted regularly according to the cost of living, or changes in clients' earnings. Officials are convinced that the subsidization system does not constitute a loss in incentive to work.

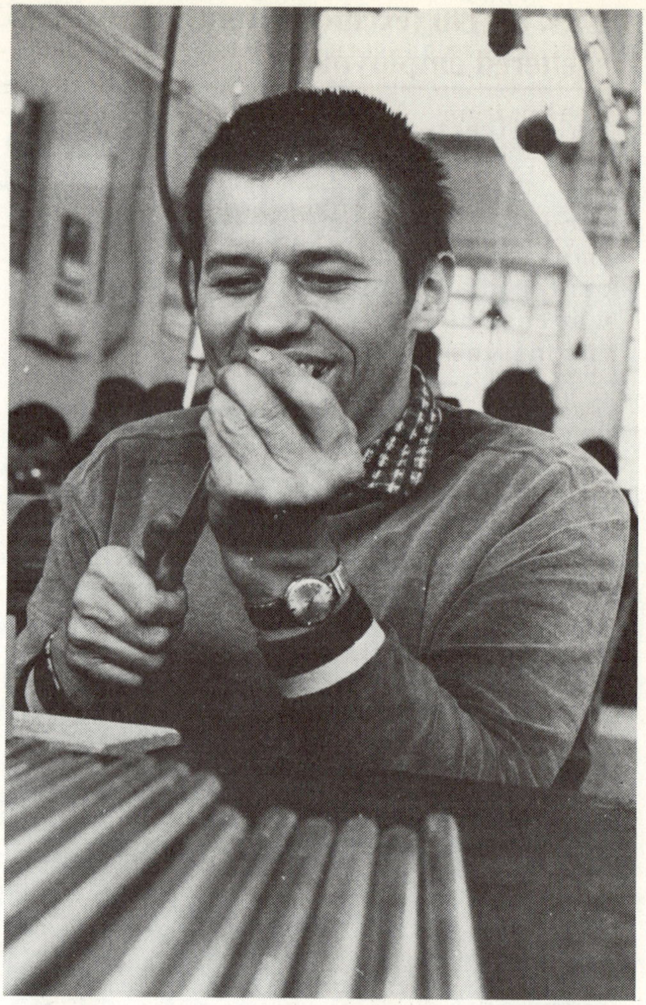

Gennard, John and M. Wright. "A Sheltered Workshop," United Kingdom Department of Employment Gazette, September 1978, pp. 1028-31.

This study compares the income of a sample of individuals in a sheltered workshop with what they would receive if they were getting social security benefits, and examines the contribution they make to the Exchequer from income tax and national insurance contributions paid from the wages they earn in sheltered employment.

The survey was limited to 12 individuals employed in a sheltered workshop. For the majority of interviewees, the sole source of household income was their weekly pay from the sheltered workshop.

The average weekly gain to the exchequer in the form of income tax and national insurance contributions was estimated at approximately L 13.

If sheltered workshops did not exist, the individuals covered would be receiving financial assistance from the State via the supplementary benefits system. A calculation of the estimated supplementary benefit levels for these individuals revealed that employment yielded a private financial gain to the individuals--L 40 average take- home pay versus L 22 in estimated benefits.

The considerable gains to the exchequer would have to be set against the cost of subsidizing sheltered employment. The study concluded that the individuals and the Exchequer were better off financially through the provision of sheltered employment.

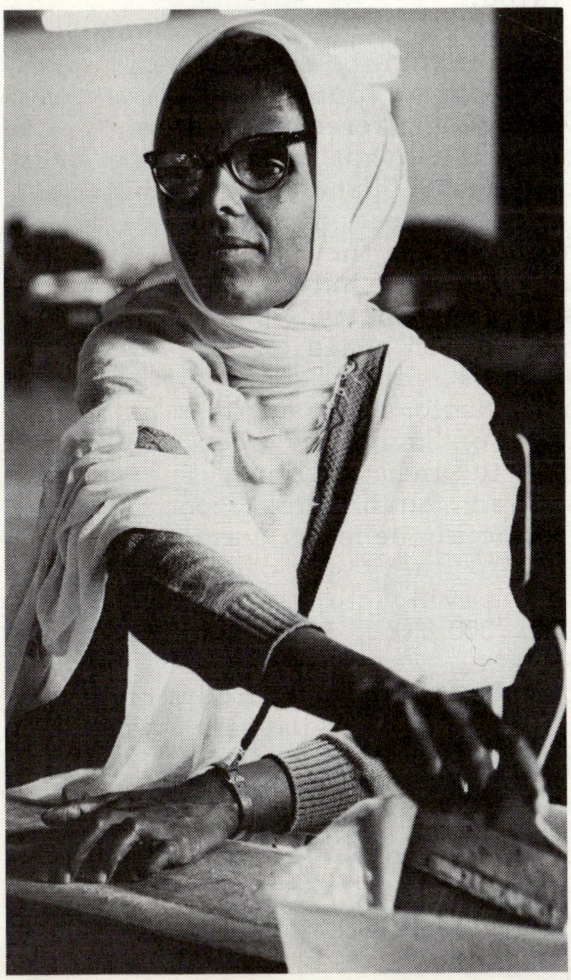

International Labor Organization/Swedish International Development Agency. ILO/SIDA African Regional Seminar on the Organization of Cooperatives for Handicapped Persons. Geneva: International Labor Organization, 1978.

The Seminar reviewed the experience of cooperatives for the disabled in Poland and Iran, and outlined the extent of disability and development of vocational rehabilitation services in Africa. The employment -- creating opportunities for disabled people in Africa were explored and it was argued that: employment is the necessary culmination of an effective vocational rehabilitation program, financial self-sufficiency should be the objective for any type of employment creating scheme, and more emphasis should be given to the development of agricultural projects for disabled people. Included are 12 country papers submitted by participants from Africa, presenting the state of rehabilitation services in Ghana, Kenya, Nigeria, Uganda, Sierra Leone, Tanzania, and several other countries.

Region II Rehabilitation Institute. Rehabilitation, Sheltered Workshops and the Disadvantaged: an Exploration in Manpower Policy. Ithaca: New York: Cornell University, 1970.

The question of economies of scale in sheltered workshop operations is often ignored. Cost-benefit analyses overlook certain production relations affecting costs, e.g., scale of operation. A majority of workshops in five states surveyed were found to operate at highly inefficient, low levels of production. An essay on sheltered workshops, the labor market and unemployment analyzes sheltered workshops as a manpower tool operating within the constraints of price and wage inflation, and full employment policy.

Morgan, P.L., and P. Makeham. Economic and Financial Analysis of Sheltered Employment. Research Paper #5. London: United Kingdom Department of Employment, 1978.

The costs of providing employment for disabled people under sheltered conditions are generally considered in terms of the gross public expenditure costs incurred; this study presents an economic and financial analysis of sheltered employment that goes beyond simply gross costs. It maintains the distinction between economic analysis and financial analysis since they consider essentially different policy questions.

The economic analysis considers sheltered employment from the point of view of resource allocation criteria: the cost of resources used in the provision of sheltered employment is considered in terms of the value of what is foregone in alternative uses. The real resource benefits consist of the market value of the output. Comparison of the real resource costs and benefits indicate the net cost (or benefit) to society of the provision of sheltered employment.

Remploy, a national organization of 87 factories employing 8,000 sighted disabled workers, produced net resource benefits of just over L400,000 in 1974-75 (or L54 per disabled worker). The population of 66 sheltered workshops, separate from the Remploy organization, employing 2,000 disabled people, produced net resource benefits of L374,000 (or L169 per disabled worker). The fact that the population of 52 other workshops, employing 3,000 blind workers, incurred net resource costs of just over L2 million (or L750 per disabled worker) meant that overall net resource costs of about L1.2 million (or L95 per disabled worker) were incurred under conditions of sheltered employment. The study, however, was limited to consideration of those benefits of sheltered employment that were directly quantifiable, that is, the goods that were sold under normal market conditions to consumers. No attempt was made to put a monetary value on either the psychological benefit derived by disabled people from being in employment or the rehabilitative effect of sheltered employment. These are social benefits which do have a real value to the economy but whose value is difficult to estimate in monetary terms; hence the estimates of net resource benefits which were made may be understated and the net resource costs may be considered overstated.

The financial analysis compares the cost to public funds of providing sheltered employment with the costs that would have been incurred if sheltered employment had not been provided. It takes account of the fact that in the absence of sheltered employment, social security benefits would have been paid to the disabled workers, and "contributing tax" and National Insurance payments to the Exchequer would be lost due to unemployment. The results showed that the economic and financial benefits varied according to the type of workshop. A net saving to public funds of L234,000 (or L105 per disabled worker) was contributed by the population of sheltered workshops of non-visually-impaired workers. Remploy's net financial cost to public funds was estimated to be just over L1 million (or L133 per disabled worker) while the population of workshops of blind workers was estimated to have incurred a net financial cost of roughly L2 million (or L716 per disabled worker). From the standpoint of the entire program, the provision of sheltered employment was estimated to have incurred a net cost in public funds of about L2.8 million (or L215 per disabled worker) for 1974-75.

The overall conclusion of this analysis is that the image of sheltered employment as a costly means of providing employment for disabled people is a gross over-simplification; the relative costs and benefits of sheltered workshops vary according to the type of workshop.

4.1 Economic and Financial Benefits (per disabled worker year) £

	Economic benefits/costs		Financial benefits/costs	
	1969-70	1974-75	1969-70	1974-75
Workshops, Blind Workers	-215	-750	-143	-716
Workshops, Sighted Workers	+101	+169	+ 30	+105
Remploy	- 91	+ 54	-203	-133

Note: Minus signs indicate net economic and financial costs.

Source: P.L. Morgan and P. Makeham, Economic and Financial Analysis of Sheltered Employment, 1978.

C. VOCATIONAL REHABILITATION: EMPLOYMENT POLICIES AND PROGRAMS

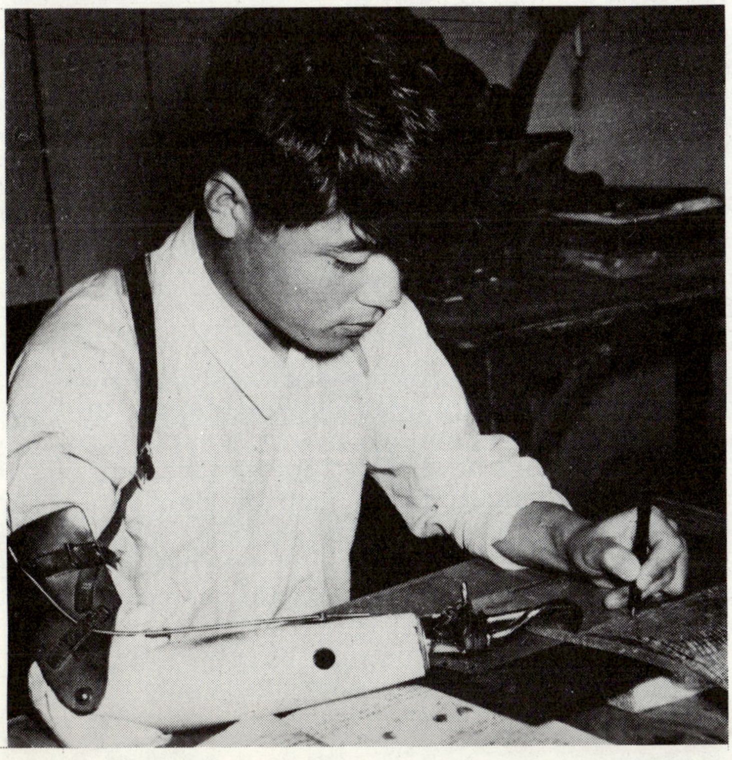

Vocational Rehabilitation and Disabled Client Earnings: A National Analysis in the United States

Rehabilitation services in the United States are provided to disabled people through a variety of governmental and voluntary organizations. Services vary from state to state within the nation; at the national level, major responsibility for the disabled is concentrated within the Rehabilitation Services Administration, Department of Health, Education and Welfare, although many other federal agencies are involved in some form of service provision. One aspect of the overall rehabilitation program, the system of vocational rehabilitation, is based on a state-federal program available to all persons with physical or mental handicaps which prevent their vocational adjustment. The state-federal program provides:

Diagnosis and counselling to help clients choose a suitable rehabilitation goal. Any reasonable vocational goal may be selected, including homemaking and sheltered employment.

Services for physical restoration and vocation training;

Allowances for maintenance, transportation, equipment and occupational licences;

Job placement.

Counselling, diagnosis and job placement are provided without charge. The states have the option of providing the other services without charge or on the basis of a means test to determine whether all or part of the additional costs should be borne by the client.

Economic Evaluation of the Federal Vocational Rehabilitation Program

In order to determine the effect of the vocational rehabilitation program on national output, a study was made of the earnings of rehabilitants during the years 1958-1967 52/ At the inception of the study period, approximately 74,000 people were participating in the vocational rehabilitation program. The number increased gradually over the ensuing years until by fiscal year 1967 more than 170,000 disabled people were involved in the program. The only regularly collected data available for the study were those showing the change in the earnings of rehabilitants between the time of acceptance for vocational rehabilitation services and at the closure of service provision. On the basis of this data, the study attempted to determine the increase in output attributable to the vocational rehabilitation program.

The nature of the data presented certain problems for which compensatory adjustments were necessary:

(a) Earnings of clients vary according to the period of acceptance. Estimates of aggregate annual earnings of rehabilitants based on earnings during the week prior to acceptance are less than one-half of what they would be if based on earnings during the full year prior to acceptance, and about three-fifths of what they would be if based on earnings three months prior to acceptance;

(b) Earnings at closure vary. Follow-up studies indicated that about 80 percent of rehabilitants are working five years after closure, and the decrease in aggregate income is offset by the increase in average real earnings among those who continued to be employed;

(c) The effects of rehabilitation on the earnings of persons, other than the rehabilitants, are omitted. These included the effects of withdrawal of wives from the labor force and eventual increased productivity of children resulting from better care and training. Thus, only a part of increased output was being measured.

Increase in Lifetime Earnings

By comparing the estimated total yearly earnings of rehabilitants at service acceptance and at service closure, and by calculating the average number of years worked by rehabilitants who participated in the vocational rehabilitation program during each year of the study period, it was estimated that the total aggregate lifetime earnings of rehabilitants in 1958 was $2.4 billion and by 1967 this sum had grown to $7.6 billion. (The increase in value was due in part to a gradual price rise of 14 percent during those years.) When discounted at 8 percent, the estimated present values of future earnings was $1 billion and $3.2 billion, respectively, for the initial and final years of the study. Estimated increases in lifetime earnings due to rehabilitation ranged from $1.5 billion to $4.7 billion for the 10-year period, and when discounted at 8 percent, the values of these aggregate increases became $0.7 billion and $2.0 billion, respectively.

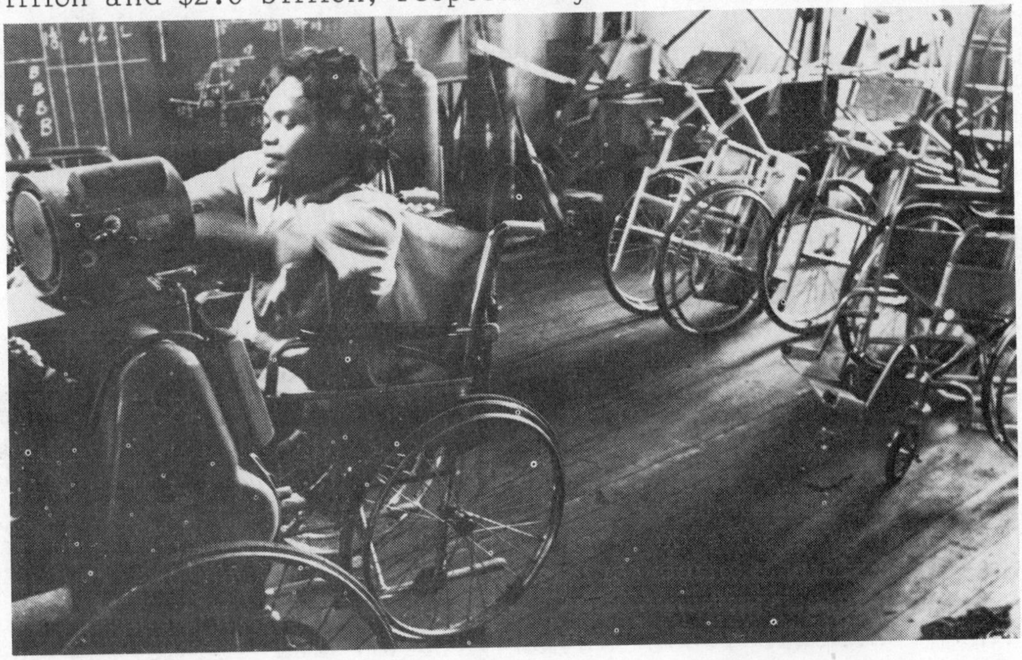

Cost-Benefit Ratio

The increased earnings attributed to rehabilitation were compared to the social costs of rehabilitation services in order to determine the net increases in resources available to society. The social costs of the federal and state programs were calculated on the basis of program costs for the administration and provision of rehabilitation services, from which were deducted and added estimates of many variables: maintenance costs representing transfer payments were deducted; the cost of services provided by agencies and individuals other than the vocational rehabilitation agency were added; the cost of service "repeaters" was added to take into account the one in five clients who return for assistance; and estimated annual earnings forgone during rehabilitation were added.

When the increased lifetime earnings of rehabilitants due to rehabilitation was divided by the social cost of rehabilitation programs, it was found that each dollar spent on rehabilitation set or maintained in motion an output of between $7.90 and $10.90. When discounted at 8 percent, this amount decreased to between $3.30 and $4.70. The study stated:

"Though the costs of rehabilitation in Brazil are high compared to the costs of rehabilitation in the U.S., it was found that after five years a rehabilitated worker returned 2.97 cruzeiros for each cruzeiro invested."

Arlindo Casarin, Avaliacao De Beneficio e de Custo Na Reabilitacao Profissional Do INPS, 1979.

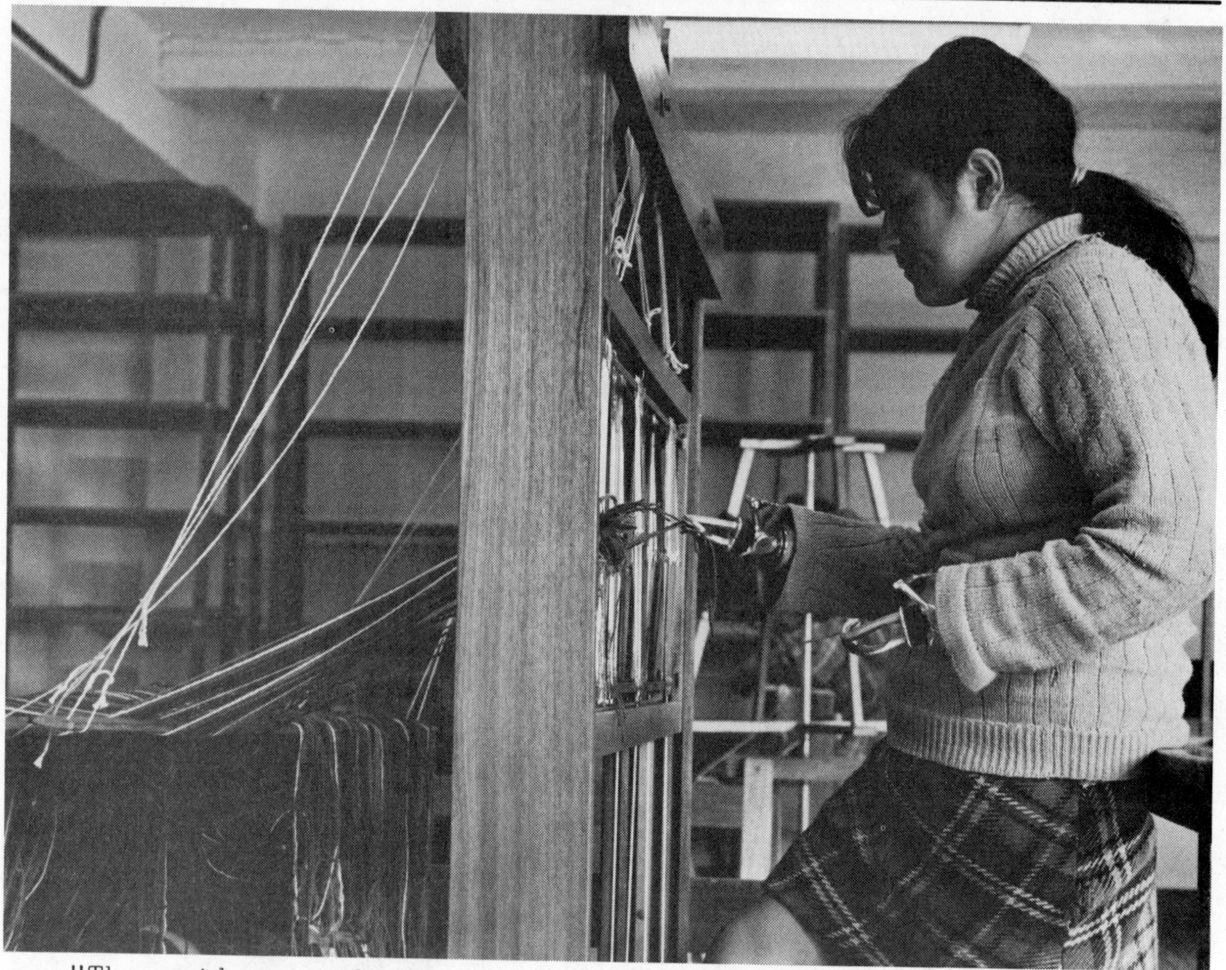

"The evidence indicates that the funds that have been expended on the vocational rehabilitation program are repaid, on the average, many times over in increased output. It must be stressed that the return may be considerably higher than indicated. Not only have we taken a so consistently conservative approach to estimating the future earnings of rehabilitants, but we have also omitted the value of increased homemaking services, other unpaid work, and the important psychic values of becoming a contributing and independent member of society." 53/

Value to Taxpayers

The estimated increase in annual federal income taxes due to rehabilitation in 1967 was $29 million. This too was considered an underestimation since a substantial proportion of future rehabilitant incomes would be taxable whereas the earnings of non-employed rehabilitants are generally not taxable. In addition, federal taxes account for only about one-half of the tax revenues collected by all levels of government in the United States. The number of years required to repay taxpayers their share of the social costs of rehabilitation ranged from 3.1 in 1961 to 5.1 in 1967. The study concluded that:

"Clearly even to non-rehabilitants, rehabilitation is a profitable undertaking, since the average number of years in which most rehabilitants will work is three to four times the number of

> years needed to repay taxpayers ... Moreover, the benefits of rehabilitation are even larger than we have estimated since our approach tends to be basically conservative and we have omitted many benefits, e.g., the value of the assurance to the non-disabled that if they ever come in need of rehabilitation, it will be available; the psychic gains to taxpayers; the value of the better care of the children of the disabled, etc." 54/

Comprehensive Rehabilitation and Disabled Worker Earnings: A Provincial Analysis in Canada

In 1969 the Ontario Workmen's Compensation Board carried out a study to determine the costs and economic benefits of providing a total rehabilitation program. 55/ Rehabilitation services provided to disabled workmen by the Board include physical restoration at the Board's Hospital and Rehabilitation Centre, vocational counselling, vocational evaluation, selective job placement, retraining and follow-up after placement in employment. The Board's Hospital and Rehabilitation Centre can serve 530 in-patients and 60 day patients.

The Ontario Workmen's Compensation system is based on a no-fault system which does not require proof of responsibility for the work accident on the part of the employer or the worker. No limit is placed on the amount of money which can be spent in providing physical and vocational rehabilitation services for occupational injuries, and workers who are unemployed receive 75 percent of their salary up to a maximum figure. In 1969 this was (Can.) $7,000.

Workmen may continue to receive this amount of compensation as long as they are medically judged to be temporarily totally disabled. Monthly pensions for permanent disability are paid of life. Compensation and pension payments are not subject to income tax. They are, however, sufficiently below the total normal earnings of a worker that the Board believes them to still be an incentive to the worker to undertake rehabilitation and return to work.

Ninety-one percent of all disabled workmen provided rehabilitation services by the Ontario Board in 1969 were considered to be successfully rehabilitated. Their estimated initial annual income on return to work was $9,773,601.76. The goal of the Ontario Workmen's Compensation system is to return the injured worker to at least the income level he had reached prior to his or her accident leading to disability.

Comparison of Workers With and Without Rehabilitation Services

The study compared the earnings of workmen who were injured and returned to work before the Board provided physical and vocational rehabilitation services with the earnings of workmen with similar injuries years later who received rehabilitation assistance.

Two work periods, 1927-1928 and 1965-1966, were selected because similar buoyant economic conditions prevailed during both periods. To obtain comparative results, the pre-accident and post-accident earnings of 200 workmen for each period were examined. The selection of workmen was based on similar anatomical disabilities and a matching clinical degree of permanent disability as well as age. All of the individuals had suffered from any of five types of injuries: upper extremity impairment, lower extremity impairment, eye injuries, multiple injuries, and head injuries other than to the eyes. The workers were also matched according to degree of disability, based on a clinical classification of: 10 to 30, 30.1 to 50 and 50 to 100 percent. In the selection of the study data, it was verified that no injury cases in the 1927-28 group received rehabilitation services, that all injury cases in the 1927-1928 sample would have received rehabilitation services had they been offered on the same basis as during the 1960s, and that all injury cases in the 1965-1966 sample did receive rehabilitation services.

The essential difference was that in the 1927-1928 period neither physical nor vocational rehabilitation services were provided, while by 1965, the Board's comprehensive rehabilitation program was fully operational. The study was based on the critical assumption that if no rehabilitation services had been rendered to the workmen in the 1965-1966 sample, they would have had a ratio of post-accident to pre-accident earnings identical to the ratio that prevailed in 1927-1928. For example, it was found that a workman in the 1927-1928 sample who suffered an upper extremity injury which left him with a 10-20 percent disability rating, experienced a 21 percent decline in annual income. It was assumed that an identical disability in the 1965-1966 group would, if no rehabilitation services were provided, result in a corresponding decrease in the disabled worker's income. Calculation of the increase in a disabled worker's earning power, based on the provision of rehabilitation services, was an average of the remaining working lifetime less the costs of providing the rehabilitation services.

The economic cost of providing rehabilitation was based on the direct costs of salary, equipment, travel and overhead costs for program administration. The indirect cost of wages lost by the worker while receiving rehabilitation was excluded since it was believed that the workers would not have been employed during this period and thus no productivity was lost. Payments of temporary total, temporary partial, and permanent disability compensation payments were also excluded from the economic costs because the study was made from the point of view of all citizens of Ontario, and the payments constituted a gain to them equal to the loss to the Board, i.e., transfer payments which were equal. The costs of providing rehabilitation services, which averaged $1,200 per workman, were deducted from their projected earnings to arrive at the net economic benefit.

Increases in Lifetime Earnings

The finding was that rehabilitation services provided to injured workmen yielded an average increase in lifetime earnings of more than $15,200. This amount represents the average difference between the post-accident earnings until retirement of a disabled workman who has received rehabilitation assistance, and one who has not. Calculations were conservatively based on a retirement age of 60. In addition, the average decline in an injured workman's post-accident income in the 1965-1966 period was only 1.7 percent compared with an average decline of 18.9 percent in the 1927-1928 period.

"In 1976 13% of the more than half million people registered as disabled with the U.K. Department of Employment were unemployed, while national average unemployment was 5.4%. Of the 55,000-65,000 employers with a quota obligation, the number fulfilling their quota declined during the period 1960-1975 from nearly 60% to under 40%. Until 1961 the proportion of registered disabled persons in the work force remained at 3% or more, but since that date the figure has steadily declined to 1.86% in 1976."

Report of the Snowdon Working Party, Integrating the Disabled, 1976.

The Workmen's Compensation Board study also indicated that workmen during the 1960s who were disabled showed longer average off-the-job periods than did the workers of the 1920s after their injuries had been treated and they had been medically assessed as being ready for re-employment. This was believed to be in part due to extended periods of partial disability compensation not present during the earlier period, and to the fact that payments could also be made during periods of retraining.

Additional References on Vocational Rehabilitation: Employment Policy and Programs:

Noble, John H. Jr. "Rehabilitating the Severely Disabled: The Foreign Experience," Journal of Health Politics, Policy and Law, #4 (Summer 1979), pp. 221-249.

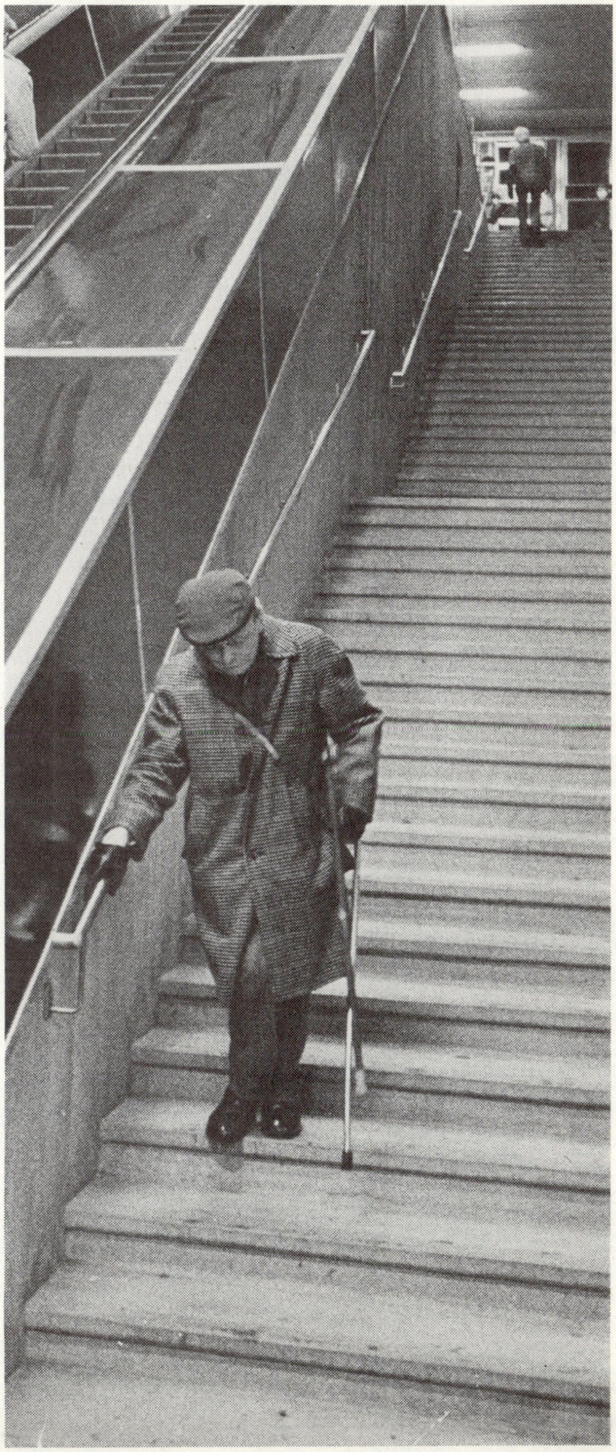

In 1977, the countries of Northwestern Europe were all experiencing rapid growth both in the number of persons receiving transfer payments because of disability and in the amount of expenditures. The "causes of rapid growth in the disability rolls are thought to lie both in the medical advances which prolong life and in the general economic conditions of advanced industrial society, which, through increased automation and rationalization of the processes of production, render obsolete low skilled and physically or mentally impaired workers. Regional poverty and high structural unemployment due to changing labor markets, shifting enterprises, the pressure of imports, and the immediate world economic recession are causing widespread ejection from the labor force of the less able and adaptable workers."

Within this context, the rehabilitation of disabled workers to the status of fully productive members of the labor force is of critical importance. This rehabilitation process takes place with a matrix of disability policies and is only one aspect of a complex process. Thus variations in the structure of the disability policies can influence the outcomes of rehabilitation service technologies. Some combinations of policies and politico-economic conditions may be mutually reinforcing and prove productive; other combinations may simply cancel each other out; still others may be positively harmful to individuals and society.

It is possible to examine the relationships between 14 policy and politico-economic variables and the social benefits and costs of rehabilitation.

1. Wage replacement ratio of benefits: Simon Courant, the Swiss actuary, has documented the fact that the higher the ratio of gross insurance benefits available from long term disability insurance is to previous wages, the greater the incidence of claims. The ratio of actual to expected claims exceeds 100 percent when the ratio of gross insurance benefits to salary reaches 60% to 70%. Therefore restoration to paid work as the result of rehabilitation services is less likely to occur as disability pension benefits exceed 60% of wages. For example, if a worker was earning $200 per week, the likelihood of rehabilitation decreases as disability benefits exceed $120 per week (60% of the prior wage.)

2. A definition of disability as "total work incapacity" is more stringent than a definition which tests incapacity only with respect to occupation. Definitions which relate disability specifically to occupation have a favorable effect on rates of rehabilitation.

3. Community attitudes toward work: a strong work ethic, coupled with stigmatizing or punitive practices in the administration of income transfer programs, may offset the attraction of high benefits.

4. Timing and sequencing of rehabilitation services: delays between the onset of illness, impairment or injury and eligibility for rehabilitation services and benefits may diminish prospects for rehabilitation.

5. Extent of labor market discrimination toward disabled people: employers who hire handicapped people often incur additional production costs by virtue of workplace modification necessary to accommodate disabled persons, and higher absenteeism due to sickness.

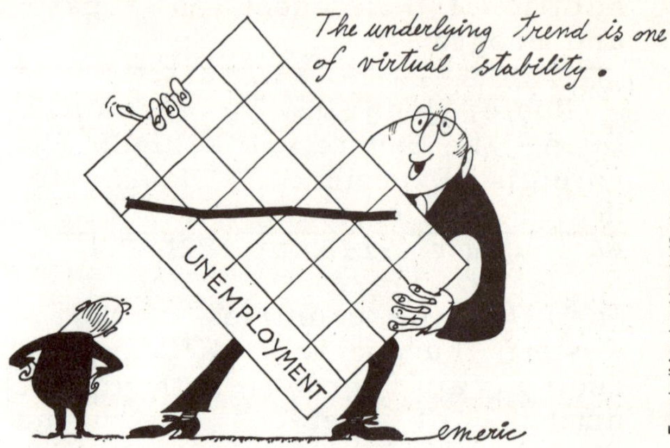
The underlying trend is one of virtual stability.
UNEMPLOYMENT
emeric

Emeric/Morning Herald/Sydney

6. Demand for labor: when economies are expanding and labor markets are tight, disabled people are more employable. But during economic recession, jobs for handicapped people become more difficult to find. Officials in Denmark recognized the near term futility of trying to move people into nonexistent jobs in an economy experiencing very high unemployment, and lowered the retirement age to 55 for persons less able to adapt to changing labor market conditions.

7. Organizational patterns may influence the outcomes of rehabilitation services. For example, in Denmark social services, vocational rehabilitation, and means-tested public assistance are being simultaneously decentralized and integrated.

8. Force of antidiscrimination policies: the efficacy and force of antidiscrimination measures can be expected to influence the outcome of rehabilitation efforts. In the Federal Republic of Germany, where the quota system is enforced by fines for noncompliance, over 400 million Deutchesmarks have been collected

in fines which serve to finance an array of rehabilitation and training centers. In the U.S., the Federal government is required to withhold its contract and grant allocations from employers and service agencies that discriminate against handicapped people.

9. Method of disability benefit disbursal: insurance versus assistance: countries vary in their policy preference for disbursing benefits--social insurance covers certain risks as a matter of legal entitlement on the presumption of need, and social assistance is based on actual need determined by means of a test of income or assets. The stigma attached to social assistance causes some persons with legitimate needs to shun it and do without, and contributes thereby to the reputation of social assistance as "target efficient".

10. Income redistribution ideologies and policies: countries in which income redistribution is viewed as a positive goal may not regard means-tested social assistance as stigmatizing; whereas, in countries in which negative views of social assistance recipients are predominate, pressure may be created for them to seek rehabilitation.

11. Intergovernmental financing arrangements between municipalities, counties, and the central government can provide either incentives or disincentives to rehabilitation efforts. One level of government may label unemployed persons during periods of economic recession "disabled" both to avoid politically embarrassing high unemployment statistics and to shift the burden of unemployment compensation or public assistance onto another level of government.

12. The process of labor force ejection is influenced by the degree of industrialization and is

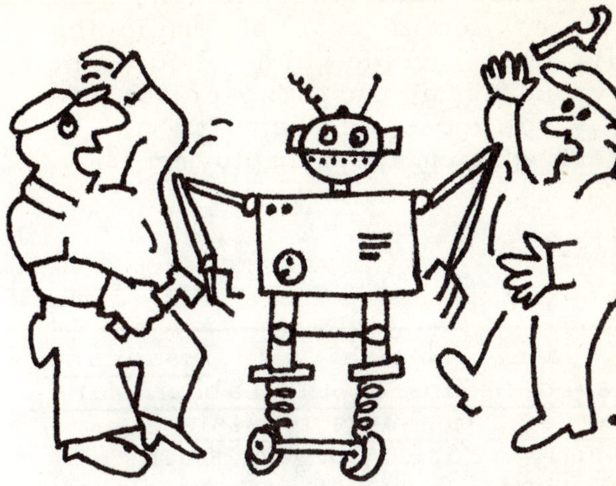

also dependent on the availability of higher technology in the economy, stability of labor force participation, and the age composition of the work force.

13. The age composition of the workforce and of the general population may interact to ease or aggravate the process of labor force ejection and the associated burden of transfer payments for disability. Except in the Netherlands, large scale withdrawal from the labor force of men in the 50-64 age group is the rule in Northwestern Europe and in the U.S. The need to provide transfer payments to persons who give up work and to pay for retraining of those whose attachment to the work force is weak (marked by prolonged periods of unemployment), coupled with reduced male labor force participation, may create a greater cost burden for the economically active portion of the population in some countries.

14. Displacement effects of the employment of disabled people and labor force ejection: In an employment market where available jobs are fewer than the number of unemployed, simply providing preferential access to jobs for some workers may produce a gain for them, but at the expense of others with equal or higher skills. To the extent that the less-able obtain jobs through preferential access and turn out less work than those whom they have displaced, the economy will

suffer a net loss of productivity. This loss must be counted as part of the social cost of employing disabled people and should be evaluated against the entire array of possible benefits to be derived from their employment.

Jain, Harish C. Disadvantaged Groups on the Labour Market and Measures to Assist Them. Paris: Organization for Economic Cooperation and Development, 1979.

There are a variety of approaches, policies and programs to deal with the disadvantaged in the labor market. This study reviews the concept of "disadvantaged worker", and labor market policies for disadvantaged workers in the United States, Canada, the United Kingdom, France, Germany, and Sweden.

Sources of disadvantage in the labor market consist of both internal factors, such as the policies of the enterprise or trade unions, and external or labor market demand and supply factors. Among the internal factors are job barriers and employment discrimination practices--methods used in hiring personnel, such as the use of credentials that are higher than necessary and employment tests often unrelated to actual job performance. Interviews that search out preconceived stereotypes of "good employees", and general hiring practices that bear little relation to the requirements of the job are additional barriers. Handicapped persons are often barred from jobs on the basis of physical appearance even though those physical qualfications are not job related. Restrictive entry requirements and discrimination by unions are also sources of barriers to employment. Within the firm, narrow recruitment practices, post entry level discrimination in promotions and wage increases accentuate the problems of employment discrimination for the disadvantaged.

Policy measures and programs for the disadvantaged in the labor market may also address external factors: the demand side of the labor market--the creation of jobs, or the supply side--human capital improvement measures such as manpower education, vocational rehabilitation and training. The following principles outline the various types of programs employed in the study countries; these measures are not mutually exclusive, and national programs may consist of a mix of different concepts and policies.

The equal employment or equity concept "emphasizes the elimination of discrimination in access to employment and in careers...-which has disproportionate effects on certain groups." This is the approach emphasized in the U.S., the U.K. and Canada.

The income distribution and the poverty approaches are designed to improve the income of people in low income brackets, or to remove poverty. The income distribution approach is more a European policy, and the poverty approach more characteristic of the U.S.

Segmented and dual labor market theories view the labour market as being "segmented in two sectors according to the criteria of wages, employment stability, working conditions, chances of advancement, and equity in the administration of work rules." The primary sector is one with high wages and stable employment, and the secondary sector is one of low wages and instability. The policy measures drawn from this theory emphasize the creation of "good" jobs in either the public or private sector. These are called "demand side measures", since job creation increases the demand for labor.

The disadvantaged or less competitive groups approach emphasizes particular categories of people that are especially prone to unemployment--women, youth, the elderly, and migrants. This approach emphasizes both the supply and demand sides of the labor market. All six countries in the survey are shown to subscribe to this approach in one form or another.

The specific characteristics approach "identifies the physically handicapped, the blind and others with specific handicaps in securing employment," and emphasizes the development of jobs or other remedial action.

"For example, in Sweden, handicapped persons unable to work in the open market may work in semi-sheltered jobs in firms. There is a subsidy for wages and payroll tax accounting to 75 percent in the first year of employment, 50 in the next, and 25 in the third and fourth." Subsidies reduce income maintenance payments, return revenues to the government in the form of taxes paid by workers, reduce hiring costs to the employer, and break the dependency of the unemployed on welfare or other forms of public assistance. In France, Germany, the United Kingdom and Sweden, there is a system of quotas which obliges employers to take on a percentage of people in

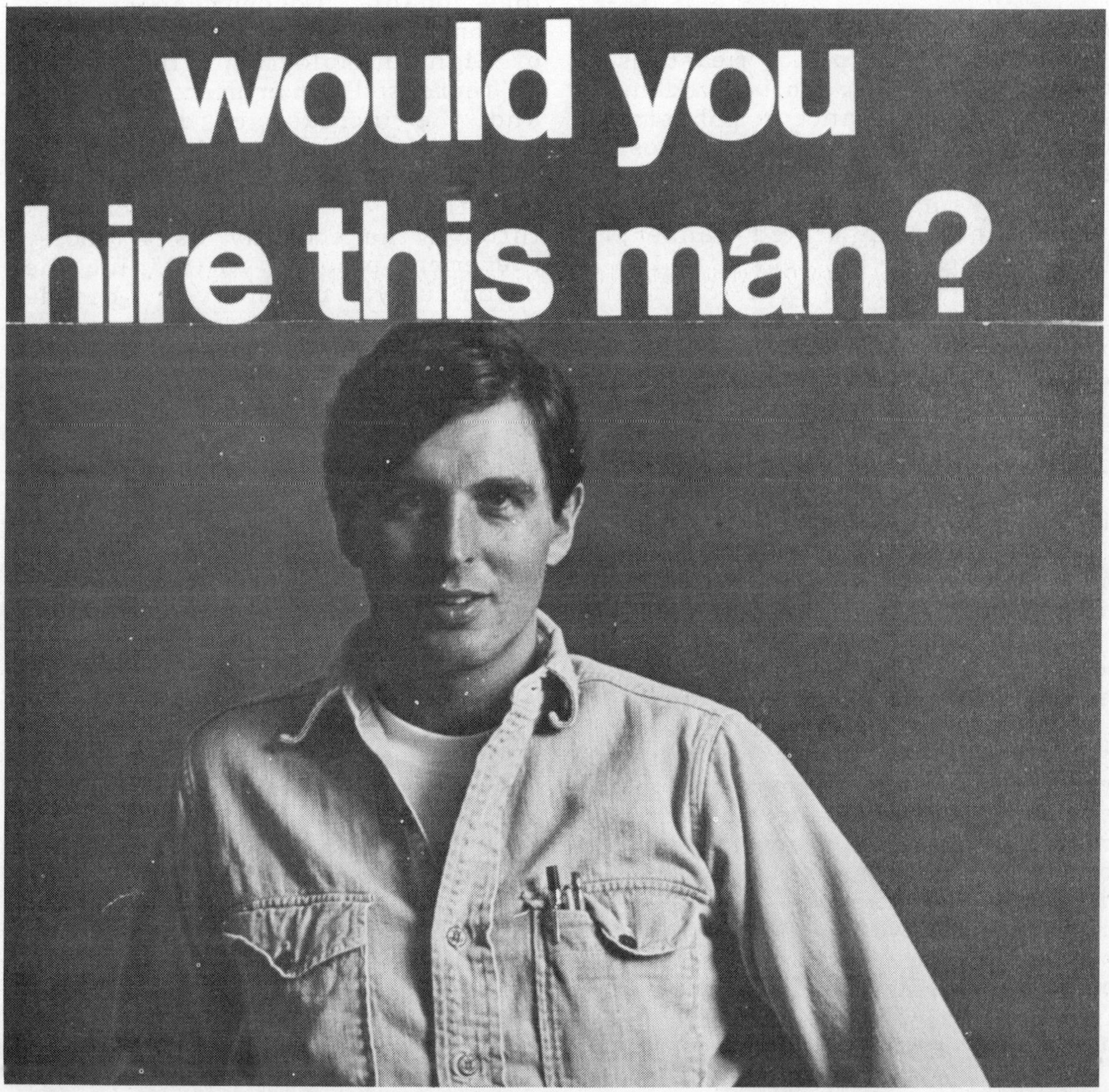

this group (the handicapped). "In the United Kingdom there is also a system of reserved jobs in particular occupational categories; two occupational categories have been so reserved for the handicapped." In the U.S., government contractors are required to hire "qualified handicapped" individuals. At the same time, "reverse discrimination"--the awarding of employment positions to less competitive groups--may result in inefficient workers and increased costs passed on to consumers. Sheltered workshops, for those who cannot work in the competitive sector, exist in most countries; in the U.S. and Canada they provide permanent employment for seriously handicapped people.

The U.S., Canada and Britain seem to emphasize policy measures on the supply side, while Sweden, Germany and France emphasize the demand side. Yet in "most cases public policies to deal with the disadvantaged are being formulated in a fragmented manner, often dealing exclusively with the supply or demand side of the labor market." Systematic handling of the problems of the disadvantaged workers requires coordinated and mutually supportive action on both the demand and supply sides of the labor market.

The current economic environment of stagflation--high levels of unemployment accompanied by high rates of inflation--makes government planners reluctant to use expansionary fiscal policies, such as job creation programs, to alleviate unemployment for fear of increasing the rate of inflation. Yet "selective countercyclical job creation programs, and subsidies to employers to employ the less competitive groups, will avoid the inflationary impact of these programs and avoid the cost of income support programs... Efforts concentrated on less competitive groups during periods of high unemployment generate little inflation...though countercyclical programs must be able to phase in and out swiftly."

The introduction of minimum wage legislation where it does not exist would be inflationary if the earning increase were not offset by higher productivity. It might have the effect of reducing employment opportunities--those who were earning slightly below the minimum wage may have their wages increased to the minimum, but those less productive workers with wages far below the minimum wage level may become unemployed.

The effectiveness of manpower training programs in reducing the inflation/unemployment tradeoff is questionable. Government misallocation of resources during periods of high unemployment, the impact of increased government spending and the increase in demand for goods that results from higher levels of employment, could create inflationary cost increases through the economy as a whole. Placement priority on training the chronically unemployed disadvantaged, rather than unemployed workers with an established attachment to the labor market, could be a questionable policy. Manpower training may also be of little use to the disadvantaged who are locked into a secondary labor market of low wages and persistant unemployment.

Haveman, Robert H. *A Benefit-Cost And Policy Analysis of the Netherlands' Social Employment Program*. A Report Submitted to the Ministry of Social Affairs of the Netherlands. Madison, Wisconsin: Institute for Research on Poverty, 1977.

This study is an economic analysis of the Netherlands Social Em-

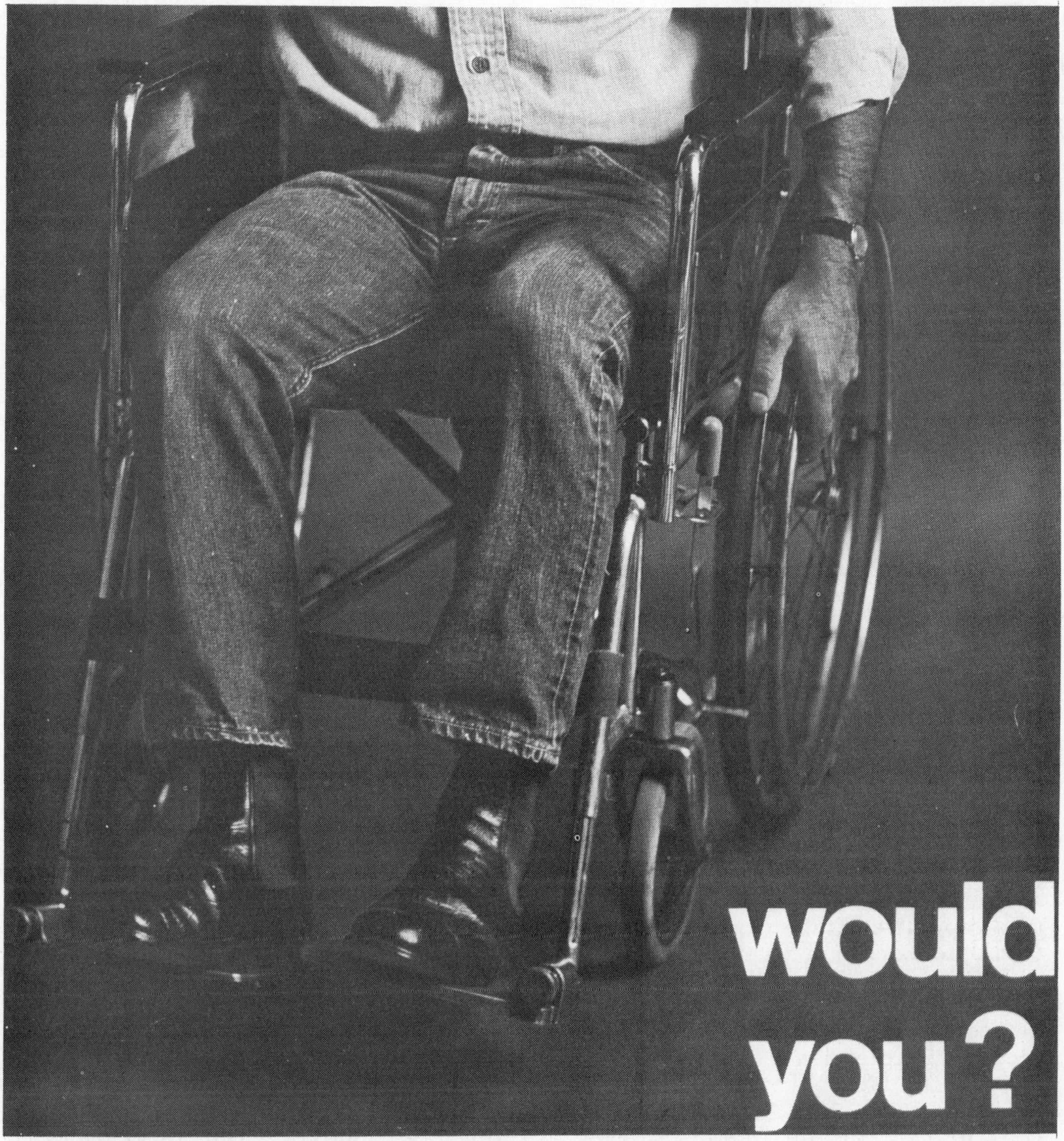

ployment Program; in 1976, 64,000 workers or 1.5% of the total work force in Holland was employed in the Program. Since 1969 the national government's Ministry of Social Affairs has accepted responsibility for providing employment for handicapped and other workers who cannot find work in the private or regular public sectors. The program has two primary components: an industrial centers program and an open-air and administrative activities program. The industrial centers produce revenue, while the latter activities involve maintenance and clerical work.

From 1955 to 1976 the number of workers employed in the Social Employment Program grew from 8,800 to over 64,000; in the period 1970 - 1976, the Program gained 20,000 additional workers,

4.2
Outflow of Social Employment Workers to Open Industry Employment

Year	Number of Persons	Percent of W.S.W. Employment
1967	1938	5.4
1968	3151	7.7
1969	3426	8.4
1970	2092	4.8
1971	1900	4.1
1972	1899	4.0
1973	1946	3.9
1974	1413	2.6
1975	1000	1.6

Source: Social Employment Report of the Joint Ministry of Social Affairs and Finance Commission, Ministry of Social Affairs, March, 1973. Netherlands.

primarily due to the recession and high unemployment rates. The bulk of this growth was in the open-air and administrative projects, increasing from 13,000 in 1970, or 30% of the total, to 24,000 workers in 1975, or 42% of the total program employment. It was estimated that in 1975, 40-50% of incoming Social Employment Program workers in administrative activities had a "NEC"--non-medically diagnosable handicap. This pattern is largely due to subsidy arrangements which tend to give municipalities incentive to relax admission criteria to the program.

During the past decade, the number of workers moving from the Social Employment program to open industry declined precipitously. In 1969, 3,400 workers (8.4 percent of the total) left the Social Employment program for employment in private industry. By 1976 this number had fallen to 1,000 (1.6 percent of the total). As a result, the program has substantially reduced its function as a transitional program to move handicapped workers into private sector or normal public sector employment through training.

Growth of Revenue (Costs). Using estimates of total program revenue to estimate total costs, total costs increased from 660 million guilders (U.S. $264 million) in 1970 to over 1,700 million guilders (U.S. $680 million) in 1975--an average of 20% per year. The subsidy provided by the national government also grew rapidly over the period: from 460 million guilders ($184 million) in 1970 to 1,270 million guilders ($508 million) in 1975.

Sales revenue as a proportion of the total revenue fell continuously during the period; in 1970, sales revenue was one third of total revenue of the industrial centers, while the national government provided 65% of the subsidy and the municipal level 2%. In 1975 sales output accounted for only 27% of total revenue, a and the national share of the subsidy increased to 70%, while the municipal level remained constant. This marked a significant increase in the national government's cost burden.

The pattern in the open-air and administrative projects component of the program was different. Sales revenue as a percentage of the total increased from 4% in 1970, and remained constant at 8% through 1974. The contribution of the municipalities to program costs fell from 8% to 5%, while the national government subsidy remained relatively constant.

As a result of the growth of revenues (costs) exceeding the growth of employment in the industrial centers, the total revenue (costs) per worker has risen rapidly over the period. In 1970 total revenues (costs) per industrial center workers were 16,000 guilders ($6,400); in 1975, per worker costs had more than doubled to 36,000 guilders ($14,000).

For the industrial centers component of the program, the national government subsidy increased from 10,000 guilders per worker ($4,000) in 1970 to 26,000 guilders ($10,400) in 1975. This was an increase of almost 20% per year. In the open-air and administrative component of the program, the national government subsidy to the program increased from 11,000 guilders in 1970 to 19,000 guilders in 1975--a 12% increase per year. Yet this growth was significantly less than that of the industrial centers. The growth rate of the total subsidy to the program was significantly in excess of the growth in the economy of the Netherlands during the period 1970-75.

These substantial increases in the taxpayer subsidy per worker can be linked to the following multiple causes:

- significant increase in the minimum wage over the period
- the increase in social premiums which must be covered by the Social Employment Centers over the period
- the failure of sales revenue to grow as rapidly as program costs
- the increase in raw material and supervisory personnel costs due to inflation over the period.

4.3
Number of Recipients of Disability Benefits in the Netherlands, 1968-77

Year	Number of recipients
1968	164,000
1969	194,000
1970	215,000
1971	237,000
1972	261,000
1973	287,000
1974	313,000
1975	345,000
1976-77	530,000[a]

Sources: Centraal Bureau voor de Statistiek, Statistisch Zekboek, 1977, and preceding issues; and for 1976-77, author's estimates. Figures are rounded.

a. Average for 1976 and 1977. Includes 70,000 self-employed workers and about 30,000 early-handicapped workers who came under the law in October 1976.

A comparison of the growth in employment and revenue between the industrial and open-air and administrative projects reveals

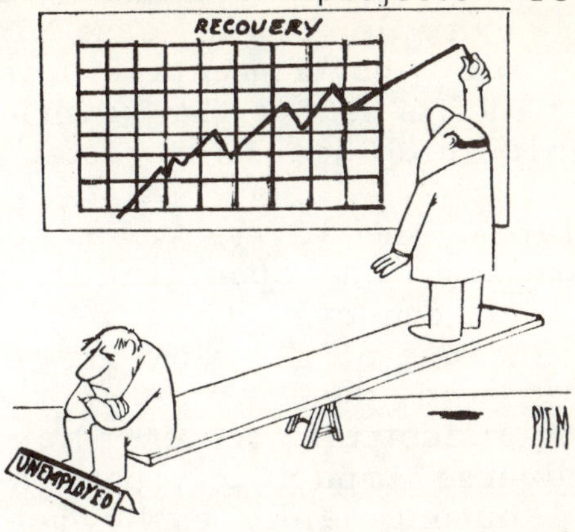

Piem/Le Point/Paris

that during 1970-75, employment in the industrial centers grew by only 4% over the period; in the open-air and administrative projects, employment increased 90% during 1970-75. This huge disparity in increased employment compares with a relatively small disparity in increased costs: 315% in the open-air and administrative component, versus 242% for the industrial center.

Following are several of the key conclusions of the study:

The subsidy arrangements in the program give municipalities enormous incentive to hire Social Employment workers to perform municipal functions. These functions have likely been filled in the past by regular municipal employees. By substituting Social Employment workers for regular employees, the municipal function becomes performed, but with the national government paying 98 percent of the cost. Evidence of the prevalence of this practice is seen in the very rapid growth of the Social Employment workers in open-air and administrative activities, relative to industrial activities. Decision-makers in the program have no more than token incentives to reduce the real social costs of the program.

"The national government has few instruments for imposing fiscal and efficiency controls on the performance of the program. On the other hand, the national government budget covers 75 percent of the total costs of the Social Employment program. This is a classic example of a case in which the governmental unit which benefits is not the government unit which bears the costs."

On balance, the adverse effect of the program on open industry sales and employment is negligible. Because of the slow growth of sales and the nature of the output, industrial centers have less adverse impact on open industry output and employment than in prior years. Moreover, because of the reduced (and low) level of flexibility of Dutch enterprises in altering their labor force in response to changed economic conditions, the existence of Social Employment industrial centers has, in some cases, been of benefit to private industry.

The economic performance of the Social Employment program is related to--and in recent years has been adversely affected by--the structure and growth of the Disability Program. In recent years, the Disability program has been characterized by: 1) high and rapidly rising benefit levels, 2) rapid growth in the number of benefit recipients (See chart), 3) an apparent decrease in the ability of medical and psychological personnel to control eligibility to the program, and 4) the likely abuse of some program recipients in receiving but not reporting income from work done in the home.

A benefit-cost analysis of the public employment program shows that the net social cost of generating social-psychological benefits to handicapped workers is high and rising rapidly. In 1970 the cost to society of providing each industrial center worker with whatever social-psychological benefit the program provides was about 1,500-2,000 guilders. By 1973 this social cost had risen to 5,500-7,500 guilders, and was estimated at 7,500 - 10,000 guilders per worker in 1976. If this same social cost estimate applies to Social Employment workers in the open-air and administrative component of the program, the total social cost of the program in 1976 was at least 500 million guilders (approx. $U.S. 200 million).

Bernhardsson, Gote and Anne-Marie Qvarfort. Employment for Handicapped Persons. A Report to the O.E.C.D. on the Work of the Swedish Government Commission on Long- Term Employment. Paris: Organization for Economic Cooperation and Development, 1980.

This study suggests that there is an international trend whereby less efficient labor, principally elderly and handicapped persons, are channelled out of the labor market and thereby rendered increasingly dependent on transfer payment funds.

Part of the increase is due to a relaxation of statutory provisions. In 1969 the Swedish Confederation of Trade Unions requested that elderly workers in declining industries be awarded premature pensions. According to present law a Swedish citizen between the ages of 16 and 64 is eligible for an early retirement (disability) pension if his or her work capacity is reduced by at least half (or 5/6 to get a full pension). The increase in the number of early retirement pensioners, however, has also been considerable in the age groups below 60. Therefore, in addition to legislative and medical factors, labor market considerations are responsible for the increases.

The level of disability pensions in Sweden varies among different municipalities within the country. There are municipalities where up to 15.6% of the male population between the ages of 25-64 receive disability pensions, as against a mere 1.3% in other municipalities. The main factor in the difference is the level of unemployment in the municipality. In municipalities with heavy unemployment, the workers least competitive in work, the elderly, disabled, and others, are the first to be eliminated from the work force. Additional factors are the proportion of unmarried persons in the adult population, the proportion of low-educated persons, and the general level of illness in the municipality. Higher employment rates among women were not found to be responsible for men being ejected from the work force and rendered unemployed or pensioned off early.

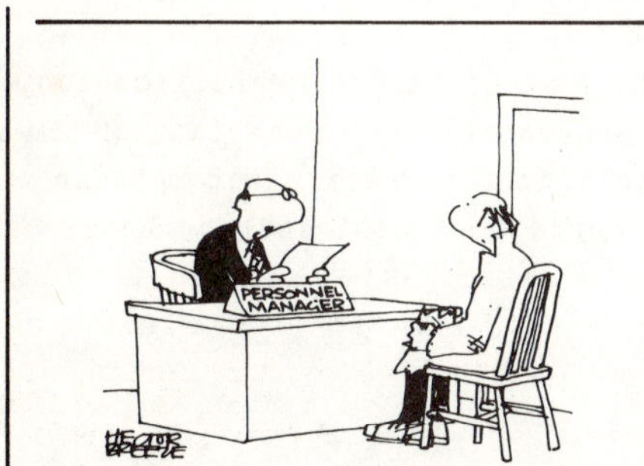

"As I understand it, your main talking point is that you're underqualified."

Breeze/Punch/London

This channelling of unprofitable labor out of the work force by means of disability pensions has created a process of "medicalization", whereby the decline in employment is treated as though it was due to individual shortcomings mainly of a medical character. Disability pensions help to aggravate inequality because they are primarily awarded to the most underprivileged--elderly single persons, the under-educated, and disabled or mentally handicapped people. Measures of labor market policy are required to avoid a further increase in disability pensions. "The principle that the labour market must be adapted to the prerequisites of people must apply all down the line. A labour market which does not presuppose that there are people with handicaps, or for instance, elderly people with impaired capacity for work, imposes obstacles."

The problem of increasing numbers of workers being eliminated from the work force is linked to the planning criteria of the enterprises in the economy. Methods of profitability and efficiency measurements in firms, public authorities and organizations make little or no allowance for external economic effects. The difference between efficiency and profitability as measured in a business enterprise and the economic consequences to the public sector and the national economy are becoming more and more obvious. For example, the greatest problems entailed by firms closing or employment cut backs occur when the firms employ a large proportion of elderly workers and local employment opportunities are limited. In these cases, the internal profit calculations preceding a closure often differ from a general economic calculation of the impact of the closure on the whole community, particularly the increase in workers moving to the disability pension rolls, and loss of tax contributions. One of the tasks of the Employment Commission is to devise means of inducing employers to take into account the implications for the national economy of their internal profitability calculations. If the disability pensions in all Sweden could be cut down to the level where it is lowest in the country,

"A conservative cost-benefit analysis of the services of U.S. vocational rehabilitation provided to Individuals Most Severely Handicapped revealed a return to society of $9.14 in 1970 and $9.13 in 1972 (in 1975 dollars) for every dollar invested in these services. This benefit-cost ratio compared to a 14.12 ratio for services provided to all groups of the disabled in 1970 and 15.94 for services provided in 1972."

Berkeley Planning Associates, Benefit-Cost Analysis of Vocational Rehabilitation Services Provided to Individuals Most Severely Handicapped, 1975.

there should be 75,000 less disability pensions. If the award of 75,000 pensions could be avoided by stepping up semi-sheltered employment and grants to employers, the public sector would save U.S. $600 million in a single year.

In many cases elimination from the labor market, particularly for people with disabilities, can best be prevented by avoiding elimination from work places. As part of this prevention focus, Sweden has introduced "adjustment groups" in the rehabilitation program. The adjustment group is a team that operates at the work place and consists of three to seven persons, representing the employer, the employee's union, and the Employment Service. The main tasks of the groups include the proposal of measures to keep elderly and handicapped persons in their jobs, measures to recruit elderly and handicapped persons, and to promote positive attitudes in working life toward elderly and handicapped persons.

The main alternative to providing a means of livelihood for occupationally handicapped persons unable to work is early retirement. Before an early retirement pension is approved, however, workers tend to sickness benefits for very long periods. During this time the individual is entitled to a sickness benefit, which as a rule amounts to 90% of the wage earned prior to the period of illness. The costs of these social insurances are financed through employers' contributions, which in turn are reflected in the final prices firms charge for their products. It is useful to examine how the costs of these measures have grown in relation to the costs of various measures to provide employment for occupationally handicapped people. (Intermingled with regular labor market opportunities for disabled persons are semi-sheltered employment (12,000 places), archive work (15,500 places) and sheltered workshops/homework (17,500 places). The development between 1970 and 1976 is illustrated on the accompanying chart. The costs for sickness benefits and retirement pensions are expressed as the employer contribution in per cent of the so-called contribution basis, i.e. largely as a percentage of the total wage sum. Each single percentage is equivalent to roughly 400 million dollars. The costs for sheltered workshops, special relief work and archive work increased fairly steeply between 1970 and 1976, whereas in contrast, the measures for rehabilitation and semi-sheltered work have shown a far more modest rise. These costs must be viewed

4.5
Growth of costs for rehabilitation, sickness benefit for more than 90 days and premature retirement pension (percent of contribution base for sickness insurance).

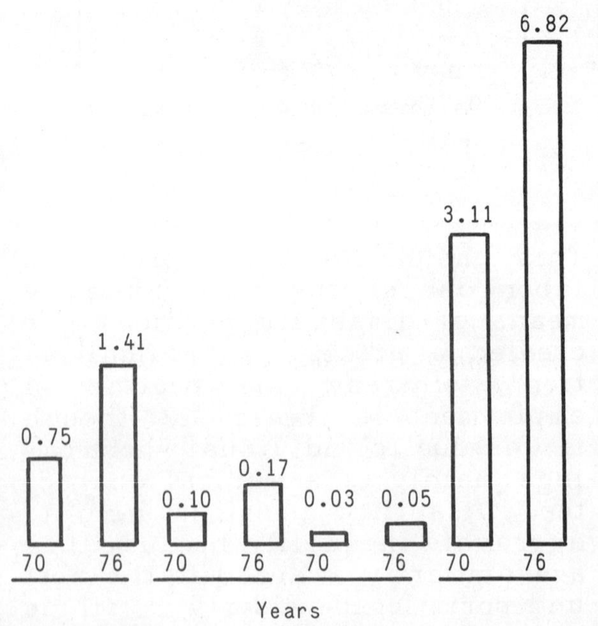

Sheltered workshop Special relief work Archive work	Rehabilitation Semi-sheltered Work	Personnel costs Labour Market Board	Sickness benefit for more than 90 days and early retirement pension

Source: Gote Bernhardsson, Employment for Handicapped Persons in Sweden, 1980.

in relation to the costs for direct inputs of personnel on the part of the Labor Market Board to work on job placement for the occupationally handicapped. The latter increase during the period was estimated at 0.015%. The increase in costs for sickness periods of more than 90 days and for early retirement pensions amounted to 3.7%. It can be seen then that insufficient resources for employment offices, rehabilitation, etc., give rise to higher costs in the social insurance sector.

The question of "benefits for whom" as a result of rehabilitation is a very relevant one. The National Labor Market Board of Sweden, recognizing the importance of early intervention and prevention of the elimination of jobs, conducted a test project in several automobile plants. The project introduced nine "technical measures" in order to try to solve the problems represented by occupationally handicapped people with physical problems. The financial evaluation of the technical measures at both the plants showed that all the experiments were financially profitable, but at different rates to different sectors of society.

The study also assessed the costs and benefits of different forms of employment provision. The average percentage of disabled workers that transferred to regular employment from semi-sheltered workplaces and archive work in Sweden was between 1% and 2%. Within this semi-sheltered rate however, those completely incorporated in the regular production process had a rate of approximately 10%, and in the separate workshop a rate of only 2%. Among those interviewed in semi-sheltered employment, two-thirds would have preferred to work in integrated production, whereas one-third preferred to work in a special workshop.

The costs of semi-sheltered and sheltered activities were as follows: In 1975 the net costs incurred by Volvo Skovde plants were estimated at approximately U.S. $2,500 per semi-sheltered workplace after state grants. This figure is comparable with the calculated costs per place for workshops for sheltered work. The average cost per filled place for 1975 in all Sweden amounted to roughly U.S.$6,500 per place excluding state grants. A comparison of the deficit at the Volvo Skovde plant for the semi- sheltered operations and the average deficit at all sheltered workshops in Sweden showed that the deficits at the sheltered workshops were nearly three times as large as at the semi-sheltered workshop at the Volvo Skovde plant.

4.6 Summary of Profitability of Implemented Technical Measures
(Recalculated to Present Value in US Dollars)

	Skovde Plants			Torslanda Plant	
	1	.2.	.3.	.4.	.1.
Financial result, community	50,700	40,900	51,800	28,900	11,600
Financial result, company	2,900	1,100	2,600	2,700	2,000
Financial result, Government	23,900	18,200	26,600	5,700	4,800

Source: Gote Bernhardsson, Employment of Handicapped Persons in Sweden, 1980.

Rate of disability pensions in the Nordic countries 1968-74. Percentage.

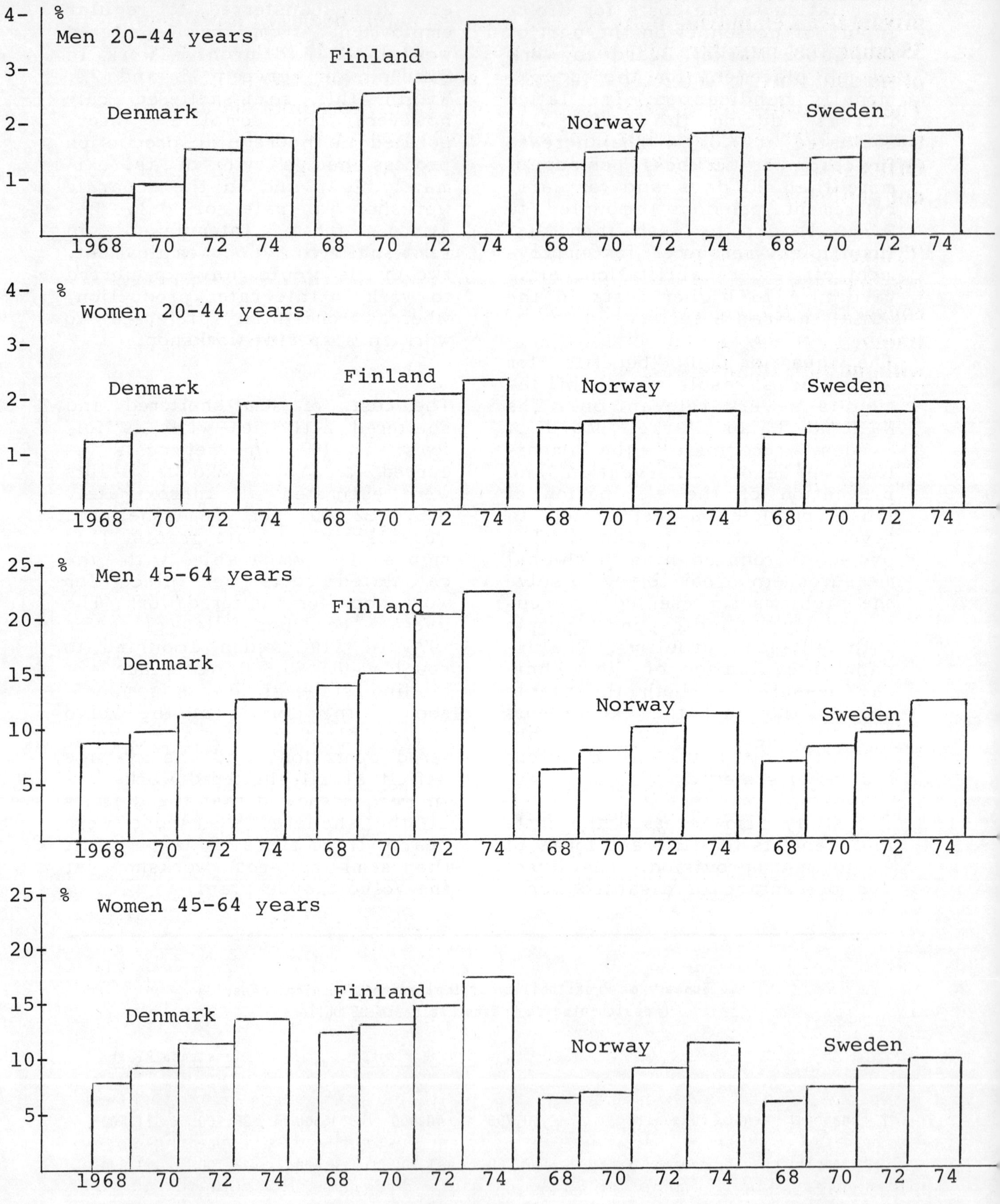

Source: Bernhardsson, Gote. Employment for Handicapped Persons in Sweden, 1980.

"In Italy, the program for the placement of disabled workers in the normal environment relied on a quota program: 15% of the total staff employed in private firms employing more than 35 workers; public bodies of more than 35 employees must hire 15% disabled workers, of which 15% must consist of manual staff, 15% in executive grades, and 40% in auxiliary positions. The law provides for sanctions in the event of failure to submit declarations (fines of 5,000-50,000 lire) or failure to submit vacancies to the Employment Office (fines of 1,000-3000 lire for each working day and each reserved job not notified.)

"These employment programs have not yielded the desired results. Not all possible jobs are filled, as some employers prefer to pay the fines rather than engage disabled applicants. Additional factors include poor vocational training, and the fact that disabled workers are often given menial jobs without hope of advancement."

Commission of European Communities, Comparative Study on the Rehabilitation of Handicapped Persons in The Countries of the Community, Volume I: Italy, 1975.

Alternatives to the employment of occupationally handicapped persons in the regular labor market, e.g. sheltered employment of various kinds and disability pensions, often entail very heavy costs. In the ultimate analysis these costs are born by production, in the form of higher prices, and coverage for them is levied in the form of payroll taxation and other contributions by employers. This means less efficiency in the overall structure of production, less coherent production, greater expense to firms, higher prices to consumers, and less satisfactory solutions from the point of view of the occupationally handicapped and their right to meaningful employment and community experience.

Among the key conclusions from the Commission's research projects are that more resources have to be allocated into efforts to employ people in the regular labor market, expand the work of adjustment teams in the work place, and reform sheltered employment by moving it closer to the regular labor market (semi-sheltered employment). The commission felt that wage subsidy is an important means of expanding regular job opportunities for the occupationally handicapped.

Levitan, Sar and Robert Taggart. Jobs for the Disabled. Policy Studies in Employment and Welfare, Number 28. Baltimore: Johns Hopkins University Press, 1977.

Though both manpower and vocational rehabilitation policymakers must decide whether to concentrate on developing human resources or on trying to change labor markets, vocational rehabilitation programs have conceptualized and measured the problems of disabled people from a medical perspective, and have paid little attention to labor markets, assuming that jobs would be available. Yet the dramatic increase in the proportion of handicapped persons unable to work regularly or at all is the result of a rapid decline in employment opportunities, and not changes in the medical or social characteristics of the severely and occupationally disabled.

The federal/state vocational rehabilitation program is the cornerstone of the vocational rehabilitation system in the U.S. The success of the vocational rehabilitation program is related to a number of factors. A key factor is the screening process, which seems to select the candidates who are potentially most successful.

The quality of services is also of great importance. What the recipient regards as helpful frequently differs from what the vocational rehabilitation system considers most important. According to one comprehensive survey, almost half the individuals who failed to be rehabilitated were dissatisfied with their rehabilitation plans; less than half remembered any counseling. A survey of a sample of disabled persons in 1972 found 71% receiving physical therapy or special devices, but only 28% received what they consider vocational services. Of this same group 67% of those with needs wanted vocational assistance, and only 20% requested physical therapy or special devices. Placement activities generally are not given a high priority.

Lower age, better education, recent work experience and male sex all are strongly related to higher rates of improvement and recovery. Yet "rates of successful rehabilitation" figures obscure the level of earnings. Studies show that many successfully rehabilitated individuals remain below minimal levels of self-support. In 1973, 15% of those successfully rehabilitated had no earnings, 10% less than $40 weekly and 28% earned between $40 and $80. Only half of those successfully rehabilitated earned the equivalent of the full-time minimum wage.

Increasing proportions of vocational rehabilitation expenditures are for administration and a declining portion for services. As the program continues to shift toward serving the most seriously handicapped, rates of successful placement will fail to provide a valid test for program effectiveness since changes in the labor market are reducing job opportunities for the severely disabled.

The most effective placement activity should focus on those members of the reserve labor supply that are least disadvantaged or disabled. The most severely disabled are likely to have transfer income which alleviates need but complicates rehabilitation efforts. Regression analysis of 1966 data suggested that (ceteris paribus--all things being equal) those with income transfers worked less. Each $100 increase in annual transfers reduced the labor force participation rate by an estimated 0.6 percent for prime age white males and by 1.1 percent for whites aged 55 to 64. Also, if the screening process favors less disabled people and gives them intensive assistance, the wage gains of this group are only marginally related to services, and the overall effectiveness of services may be overstated by success figures. A decline in the average performance of vocational rehabilitation may have adverse political repercussions.

Cost-benefit studies of the benefits of vocational rehabilitation programs have exceeded almost all the estimates for manpower programs. Yet the methodologies employed differ significantly:

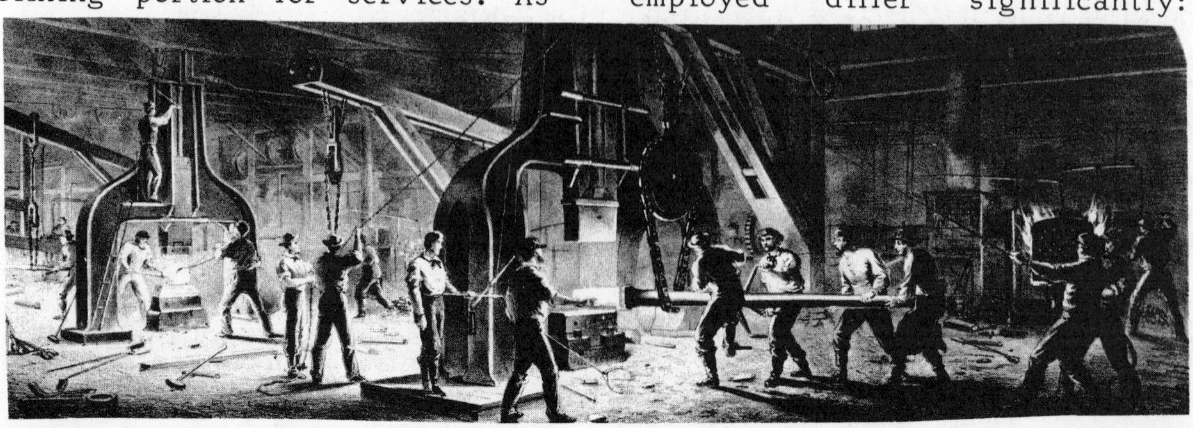

manpower studies compare employees with others with similar characteristics, while the major vocational rehabilitation studies do not include control groups. They have relied on comparisons of earnings immediately before-and-after rehabilitation, rather than comparing participants with matched samples of disabled non-participants over an extended period. Since many disabled people recover or improve their employment status without services and since those who are more likely to improve are selected for the program, before and after comparisons exaggerate the impact of rehabilitation efforts. The long run impact of services cannot be determined merely from future changes in the employment status of recipients, since there is often an initial improvement followed by a decline. Projections of the future earnings and productivity of disabled people assume that the economy does not deteriorate. For example, application of the before-and-after methodology of cost benefit studies to manpower training data resulted in a quadrupling of the cost-benefit ratio. "Lacking control groups, almost all vocational rehabilitation benefit-cost studies are seriously flawed. Studies have grown increasingly sophisticated in their efforts to get around this fundamental shortcoming, but they still overestimate the net impact of services."

Macroeconomic developments should force vocational rehabilitation policies to function more in line with general manpower policies. This would include a deemphasis of service strategies designed to increase employability, an emphasis on job creation and work experience efforts, and a higher priority on the less severely rather than the more severely disabled.

Japanese Society for Rehabilitation of the Disabled. *Rehabilitation Services for the Disabled - in Japan*. Tokyo: Japanese Society for Rehabilitation of the Disabled, 1980.

Employment of handicapped people in Japan centers on the quota system, subsidy payments to enterprises that hire physically and mentally handicapped persons, and vocational placement services. The quota system provides for a ratio of handicapped persons to the total number of employees: 1.9 percent in clerical work, 1.8 percent in non-clerical work in governmental companies and organizations, and 1.5 percent in private business. In June 1979, the employment ratio in public agencies achieved the legal employment ratio as a whole, yet the employment ratio in the private agencies did not achieve the legal employment ratio.

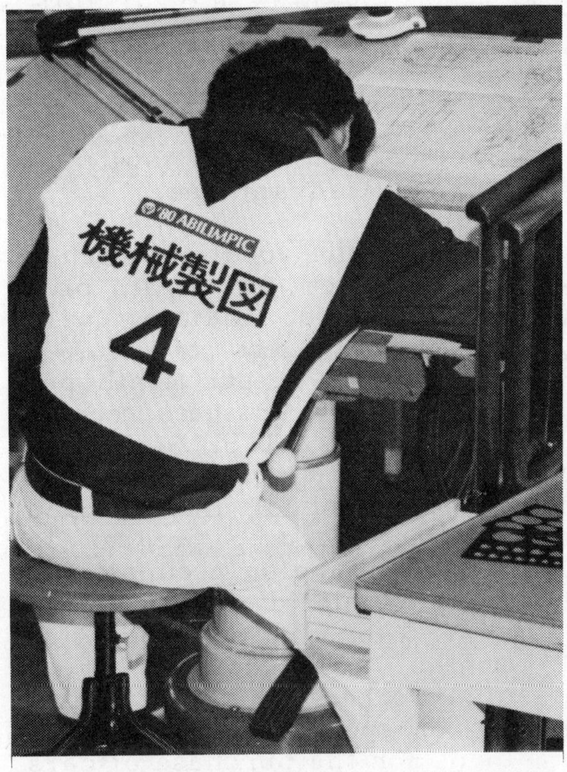

Subsidy payments are made to enterprises that hire handicapped persons and grants are made available for alterations to the workplace. In the case of employers of large numbers of disabled workers, special funds are made available for procurement of buildings and equipment, and special tax treatment is accorded. Funds are also collected "from employers who do not achieve the employment ratio, thus making available special funds to employers who are active in hiring physically handicapped persons."

Selective placement is provided by Public Employment Security Offices, which maintain a registration system of disabled individuals according to type of disability, work experience, etc. "Applicants in 1978 were 43,309 of which 24,390 were employed, that is, the handicapped employment ratio is 50.5 percent, high in spite of their many disadvantages."

In addition, the vocational rehabilitation system in Japan provides on the job training with grants to employers of Y14,000 (approx. U.S. $70) per month per trainee, and the trainees receive Y87,380 (approx. U.S. $435) per month; a bounty program to promote employment of handicapped workers is a funding program to help people changing occupations, payable in subsidies of Y15,000 (approx. U.S. $75) per month for 12 months to employers hiring disabled workers full time; and a number of special loans, including loans for the purchase of cars to provide disabled commuters with transport to work.

Organization for Economic Co-operation and Development. Centre for Educational Research and Innovation. <u>The Education of the Handicapped Adolescent: Alternatives to Work for Severely Handicapped People</u>. Paris: O.E.C.D., 1979.

Schemes to facilitate the transition of the handicapped adolescent from school to work are still inadequate in most countries both in their availability and their quality. There has been a proliferation of legislation providing for affirmative action to hire handicapped people in a number of countries. Yet while these developments will increase the <u>range</u> of work opportunities open to severely handicapped young people and adults, and help change public attitudes, there are other secular economic trends which are steadily reducing the <u>number</u> of jobs available. This decline in job opportunities is likely to bear particularly hard on people who do not fit readily into existing job categories, or are not as readily adaptable as ordinary workers.

New technology, especially micro-electronics, offers new possibilities to some handicapped people. It will be increasingly possible for people in clerical, professional, and managerial occupations to work from home. The growth of this decentralized industry will offer greater work flexibility. Yet these advantages will only benefit a small minority and even for them the gains may be partly or wholly offset by the dangers of social isolation and the ease with which "home-workers" can be and often are exploited by low pay. Chronic frictional unemployment-- short-term unemployment occurring as the unemployed search for jobs and employers search for suitable job candidates--or structural unemployment--long-term unemployment caused by a mismatch between the characteristics and skills of the unemployed and those demanded by employers, are likely to remain enduring features of most industrial countries. At the same time the improvement in welfare payments in many countries enable people to live decently, and for those handicapped people who can only obtain very low-paid jobs, the economic reward of going to work may not be great.

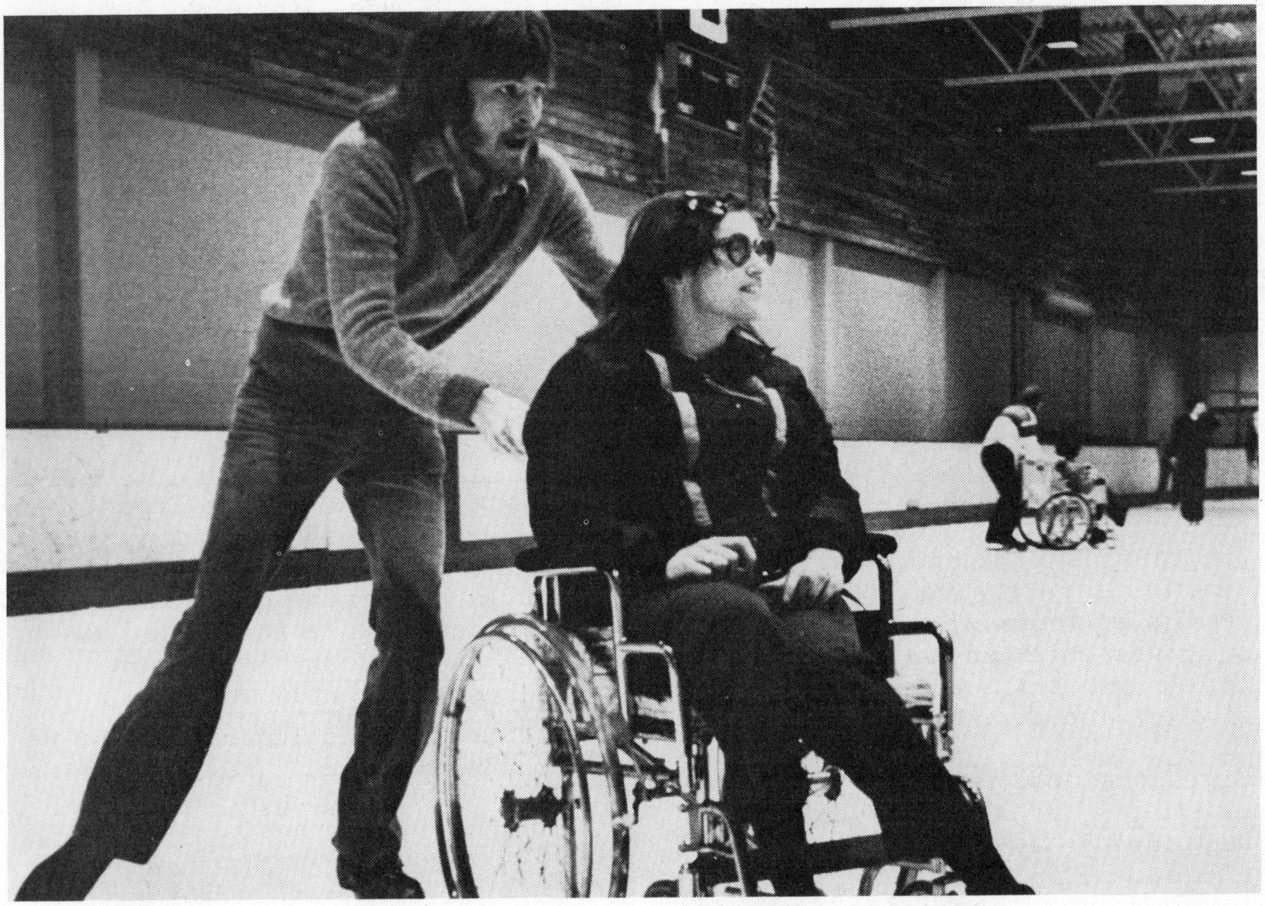

The idea of alternatives to work raises a number of profound philosophical, psychological and social issues. A central aspect is the extent to which the work ethic still predominates in industrialized western countries. The work ethic has two aspects: a moral aspect (a moral good being ascribed to work) and a financial aspect (it brings a person extrinsic rewards). However, two factors are currently weakening the work ethic. One is the structural changes in employment--reduced opportunities--and the second is the welfare programs designed to safeguard all members of society. These economic and social factors are seen to be more effective in weakening the work ethic than any philosophical arguments.

Work has a number of important psychological dimensions. A job gives a sense of personal identity, including self-esteem, responsibility, dignity, and social acceptance. Work enables an individual to feel that he or she is making an active contribution to the community, provides a structure and a regular routine for the day, and is an opportunity to widen social contacts.

Though the concept of leisure and leisure time is linked with work, the boundary between the two spheres is vague. Because the concept of leisure and its uses has been neglected, different possibilities for a life without work centered on the constructive use of leisure have rarely been seriously considered. Leisure time has too often been conceived in a negative way, as an escape from obligation. Yet chosen activities within leisure time can meet some of the psychological needs which work generally fulfills for a particular unemployed individual.

This discussion is related to the efficacy of current alternatives to work. Examination of Adult Training Centres (ATC) in the U.K.

documented a depressing catalogue of conditions. It showed mentally handicapped workers paid about L2 or L3 for a 27 or 30 hour working week. The work of snapping wheels onto toy tractors all day was described by the administrators as of "great therapeutic value," and the study pointed out that nine out of ten ATCs rely on contract work, and that contractors save on pensions, national insurance, welfare and redundancy payments, heating, etc. In such work schemes the general level of task is low, and because work is largely chosen for reasons of economy or availability it rarely reflects the interests of those who are doing it, or gives them an opportunity for developing skills such as responsibility and decision making.

Given the unsatisfactory nature of existing alternatives, ideas about meaningful life without work are needed. The potential for the involvement of handicapped people as givers rather than receivers of services has hardly begun to be explored. Schemes have been established involving moderately and severely mentally handicapped trainees in working in a local geriatric hospital with the elderly. Trainees are informed that they are completely free to participate or not in order to obviate any exploitation or forced work. Housebound adults have also been organized into telephone volunteers. Homemaking can also form a satisfying alternative to employment. These are concrete means of tapping the potential of many handicapped people.

The issue of payment for "voluntary" work is a complex one. If a trainee is capable of voluntary work, is he or she not employable and deserving of employment? Yet most volunteers, whether able bodied or disabled, provide "service" of a kind which the statutory sector provides either inadequately or not at all, usually because such services are not priorities, i.e. society cannot afford to provide them. "In helping to meet such needs, disabled people are no more being exploited than are abled bodied people who have time to give, and wish to use it in this way."

Amoako, J.B. "Socio-Economic Implications of Investments in Rehabilitation Services for the Disabled in a Developing Country," paper presented to the <u>United Nations Expert Group Meeting on Socio-Economic Implications of Investments in Rehabilitation Services for the Disabled</u>, Geneva, 1977.

Of the total population of 8.5 million in Ghana, it was estimated in 1970 that there were approximately 300,000 disabled persons in Ghana in need of rehabilitation services. A four year survey of blindness in West Africa concluded that there were at least 65,000 blind people in Ghana.

In Ghana the extended family has always been responsible for the disabled, the orphaned and the deprived. Yet social and economic changes can be seen to be breaking down traditional systems. Industrialization and urbanization are eroding the ability of the extended family to provide this support. The extended family is giving way to the conjugal family; when both parents are wage earners working away from home and non-disabled children attend school, the disabled child or adult is left to fend for himself or herself.

It has been suggested that "in the developing countries, which are less industrialized, economically disadvantaged, and have high rates of unemployment, the

"Effective rural rehabilitation need not involve paid employment."

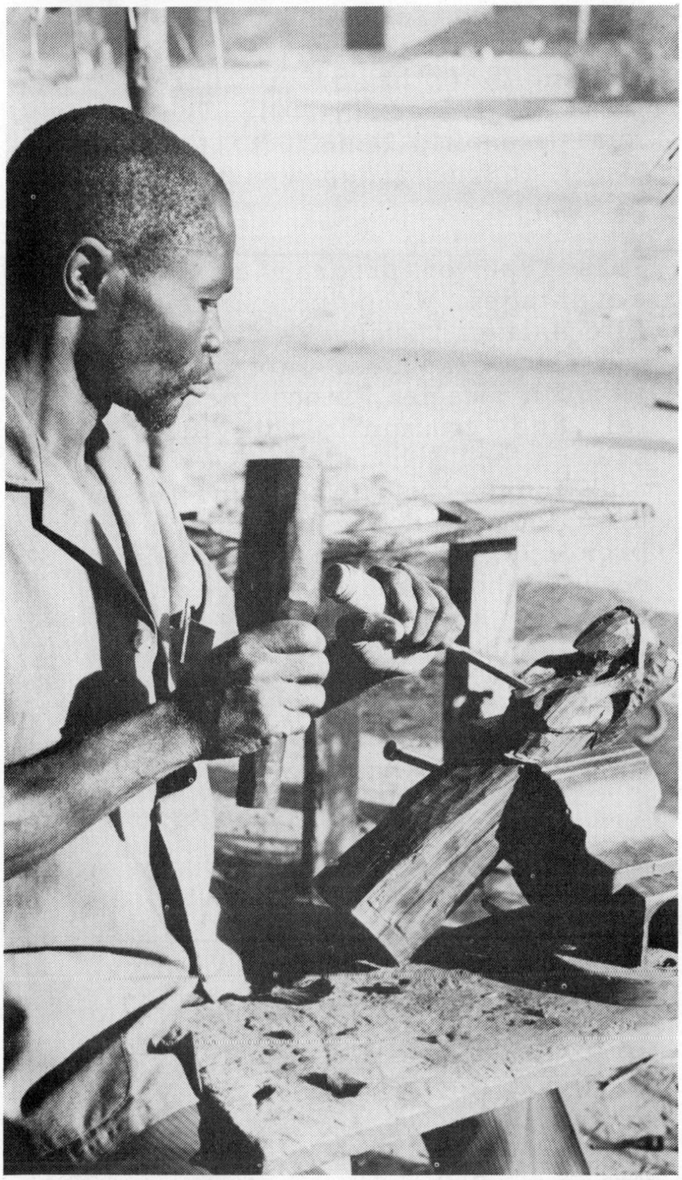

production benefits of vocational rehabilitation are low". Yet since there are fewer industries, the major aim of vocational rehabilitation is not wage earning employment. For example, in Ghana, of the total working labor force of 4,231,851 in 1970, only 693,802 were in paid employment, whereas 1,964,846 were self employed.

Therefore effective rural rehabilitation need not involve paid employment. "A disabled man in a Ghanain village will be satisfactorily rehabilitated if, instead of sitting passively at the back of his hut, he is able to take his place in the family unit as a cultivator, or as a craftsman." A disabled village woman could satisfactorily be rehabilitated if she can be trained to play her role as a competent housewife. Rehabilitation can take away the enormous burden on family members caring for the disabled, sometimes causing a reduction in their own economic performance. The value of such social gains to the individual and the family is difficult to calculate in money terms.

Symington, D.C. and M.P. Lewis. "Cost-Benefit Analysis of a Hospital and University Based Prevocational Program," Archives of Physical Medicine and Rehabilitation, Volume 54, August, 1973, pp. 341-347.

In 1968 a vocational service was established as part of the Regional Rehabilitation Centre in the Kingston (Canada) General Hospital. Approximately 40% of the patients referred were considered unable to function in an educational or work situation because of complex vocational handicaps; for them, a prevocational program was developed, utilizing the staff of the Rehabilitation Centre and the resources of the university and hospital for assessment and training purposes.

Upon entering, the patient was assigned to a counsellor who supervised his program and provided counselling as needed. When the occupational therapist and the counsellor considered that the patient had met the required standards of behavior, job performance and safety, he was promoted to a job station within the hospital. For convenience, the initial job station was usually within the hospital, taking into consideration short term goals, such as the need to build up the patients physical endurance; outside job stations came later.

One-hundred and seven patients were admitted during the first three years of operation. 52 were employed at the time of follow-up, 42 in competitive employment and 10 in sheltered work. 10 were still attending school. The vocational end result of 28 cases was in doubt, 5 lost to follow-up, and 22 classified as failures.

A cost-benefit analysis of patients discharged during the first year of the program was made since this group had reached the most stable vocational state. The total cost of the prevocational program and subsequent training from February, 1968 to June, 1971 was $29,287. Had these patients not been in the program, welfare and pension payments would have totaled $9,006 during this period, so the net cost was $20,281.

4.7 PREVOCATIONAL PROGRAM,
COST-BENEFIT ANALYSIS
1968-69

Benefit to government		
Support saved..........	$29,395	
Taxes paid............	7,108	
	$36,503	
Net cost...............	20,281	
Net savings to government.........	$16,222	$16,222
Benefit to individual		
Increased earnings......		35,826
Total benefits		$52,048

Source: David Symington, "Cost Benefit Analysis of Hospital and University Based Prevocational Program," 1973.

Two economic benefits were calculated: first, the net savings to the government, and second, the increased earnings of the group. The savings to the government in reduced welfare and pension payments was $29,395, plus the taxes payable by the group ($7,108). The government therefore recovered more than the total cost of the program through taxes and reduced financial support for the group as a whole. The annual earnings of the group increased from $15,175 to $51,001. The annual economic benefit to the patients in the group was therefore $35,826.

This type of program has many advantages when compared with alternatives such as industrial therapy workshops. Capital outlay is much smaller, since the hospital and community provide the space for job stations at no additional cost. Operating costs are low, since supervision is provided by regular supervisors on the hospital payroll, rather than by staff paid by the program. The third advantage is that the patient's performance is compared with regular employees, making for more realistic assessments of employability.

Worrall, John D. "A Benefit-Cost Analysis of the Vocational Rehabilitation Program," Journal of Human Resources, Volume 13, #2, 1978, pp. 285-298.

The many cost-benefit analyses of the U.S. Federal-State Vocational Rehabilitation Program have proven very sensitive to the assumptions employed in the methodology.

This study substitutes several of the key methodological assumptions which have tendencies to exaggerate program benefits. Wages, the usual measure of an individual's contribution to output, are generally compared at entry and closure to determine if the program has increased the client's productivity. Unlike other

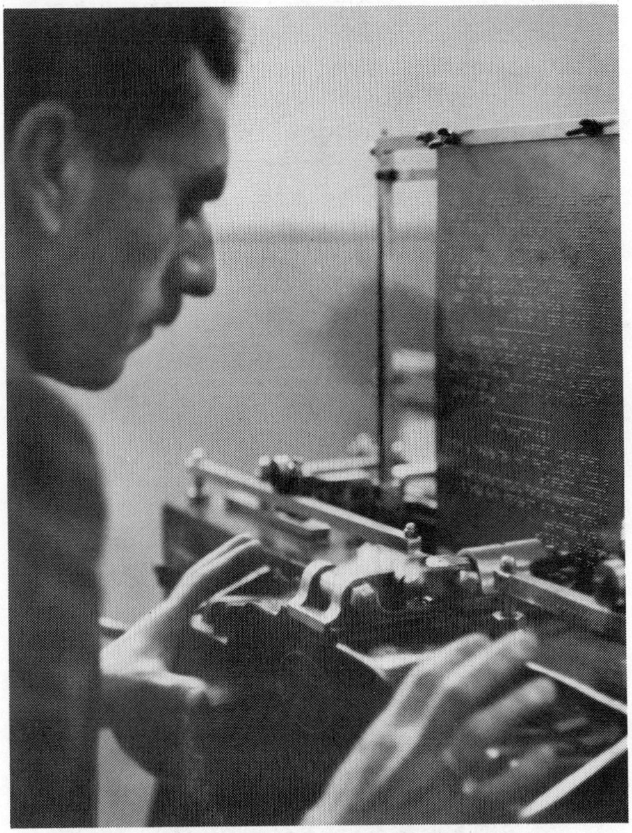

studies, wages are not reported as zero if the client was unemployed during the week prior to entering the program. Rather, clients with no earnings at opening are assigned a proxy wage based on persons in a similar cohort, adjusted for a constant 30% unemployment rate.

Wages at closure, usually based on case service records after 60 days of employment, are estimated after 30 days. Individuals rehabilitated and placed in unpaid positions are also assigned a proxy wage (cohort based), reflecting the opportunity cost of the time of unpaid workers.

The study does not assume continuous employment for successful rehabilitants, but a constant rate of unemployment of 20 percent. Wage projections are modified by an age-earnings profile technique--a cross section of wages at closure for all successful cases and stratified by race, sex, education, and disability condition.

Given these methodological changes, with a productivity factor of .025 and a social rate of discount of 10%, the vocational rehabilitation program was still found generally to be returning more in productivity gains than costs to society. Yet the study concludes that the "decision maker should not simply take empirical estimates of benefit and cost as his only criteria when making investment decisions..."

Zymelman, Manuel. The Economic Evaluation of Vocational Training Programs. World Bank Occassional Papers, #28. Baltimore: Johns Hopkins University Press, 1976.

This book presents a methodology for evaluation of various vocational programs, calculation of costs, and analyzes the economic and social factors that determine the effectiveness of each program. The study explores the factors which determine the cost effectiveness of different methods of on-the-job, off-the-job, and combined types of training--under what circumstances one type should be chosen over another. This choice will involve both economic and institutional factors. Among the key economic variables are the average cost per graduate of a training program, the scale of operation, the nature of the workshops, the nature of instruction, the cost of training and the trainee's wages, and the overall profitability to the firm. The nature of the labor market is also of great importance; high rates of unemployment among vocational school graduates may be the result of poor occupational planning rather than faulty instruction. Likewise, a high cost per graduate in formal vocational schools could result from a poor use of capacity, and should not necessarily lead to a shift to on-the-job training programs.

Among the key institutional factors that can influence the choice of vocational training programs are the rate of unemployment, level of wages, entry requirements for jobs, the quality of instruction, union policy, and the attitudes of the firms. Given these variables in program evaluation, the study found no evidence to support the superiority of one mode of training over another.

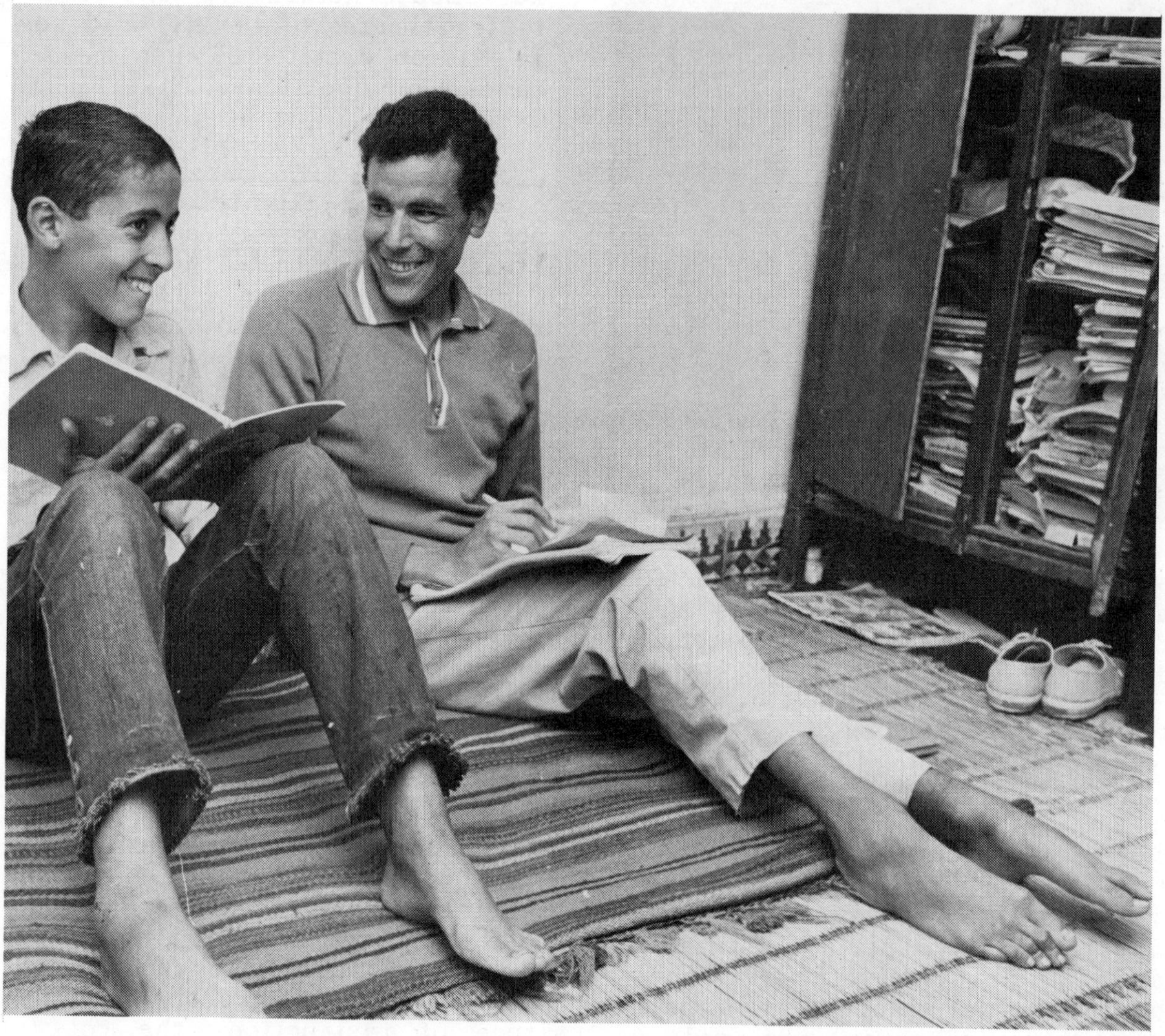

D. FACTORS ASSOCIATED WITH SUCCESSFUL REHABILITATION

Sickness Benefit Recipients in Sweden

In 1970, a study was carried out in Sweden on about 2,000 people selected by the National Health Service as being in need of rehabilitation services. 56/ The entire group was receiving sick payment benefits, and in accordance with the national insurance scheme, it is compulsory for the recipient of such benefits to undergo rehabilitation if it is prescribed, and if the recipient wishes to receive further benefits. All of the individuals in the study group were between 16 and 60 years of age, and they did not have terminal diseases. The study group included only a few individuals with severe disturbances of ability to carry out activities of daily living.

For the purposes of the study, the group was divided into matched pairs on the basis of age. Approximately 1,000 people, one person in each of the pair groups, received intensive rehabilitation services on a random basis, while the other half formed a control group which did not receive services. With the exception of the provisions of rehabilitation services, the subject and control groups were treated in like manner.

The researchers found that the control group returned to productivity at a slightly faster rate than the group receiving rehabilitation services during the first year. After the first year approximately 50 percent of the members of both groups had resumed active participation in the economically productive work force. The study concluded that, while it had been assumed that the entire study group could benefit from rehabilitation assistance, the subject group which actually received such services demonstrated no greater productivity than the control group which did not receive services. In addition, the subject group was shown to have become a greater consumer of medical care and drugs than the controls over a longer period of time.

Productivity and the Severity of Disability

As a result of findings of the type cited by the study in Sweden, rehabilitation specialists are beginning to challenge the traditional assumptions about the types of disabled people who can, through rehabilitation assistance, become most productive. It has been frequently assumed that the most effective and economical services are those that give preference to the less severely disabled rather than the most severely disabled, to the younger rather than the older worker, to males rather than females, to racially and socially dominant groups rather than minorities. Recent findings are bringing such conclusions into doubt. In the economic assessment of the United States federal vocational rehabilitation program, it was found that higher cost benefit ratios were obtained for lower rather than higher productivity groups. This resulted, in part, because the costs of service provision were lower for some of the groups. The costs of training for rehabilitants in the 45-65 year old age group were one-third of the costs for the 25-44 year olds, and one-sixth of the costs of training 18-24 year olds. It also was a result of the fact that the more disadvantaged groups demonstrated a greater increase in earnings per service dollar spent since they generally entered rehabilitation programs with significantly lower earnings. The study was led to the "unorthodox conclusion that from the standpoint of an efficient allocation of resources, it may be as desirable to assist the uneducated, the middle-aged, the unmarried, the severely disabled, and other low productivity groups as their more vocationally successful counterparts." 57/

The Rehabilitation Service of the Ministry of Social Welfare in Israel carried out a retrospective study on 1,200 disabled clients who received its services in cities and villages throughout Israel between

1966 and 1968. 58/ One of the main objectives of the study was to define the variables related to success in rehabilitation and for the purposes of the study, success was defined as termination or decrease in monthly welfare allowance, and employment for at least one full year. No decrease in welfare allowances would be made if the client was not employed for at least one year. Thus the successful rehabilitant was the person who had worked for a minimum of one year, in some cases two, when he or she was previously considered to be unemployable, and who was less dependent upon public welfare than before rehabilitation.

The study group included persons with all types of disability, with the exception of mental retardation and blindness. Recipients of services were within all of the productive age groups. Among the findings of the Israeli study were the following:

With regard to success in rehabilitation, the law of diminishing returns does not set in at any age. A person over the age of 60 has the same chance for success as a person in any other age group. In fact, the age group from 25-35 years tended to be more successful than the 36-55 year old group which is traditionally associated with the greatest productivity.

Nearly three-fourths of the successful rehabilitants had received public assistance for less than five years. The longer a client was dependent upon public support, the less his or her chance to be successfully rehabilitated.

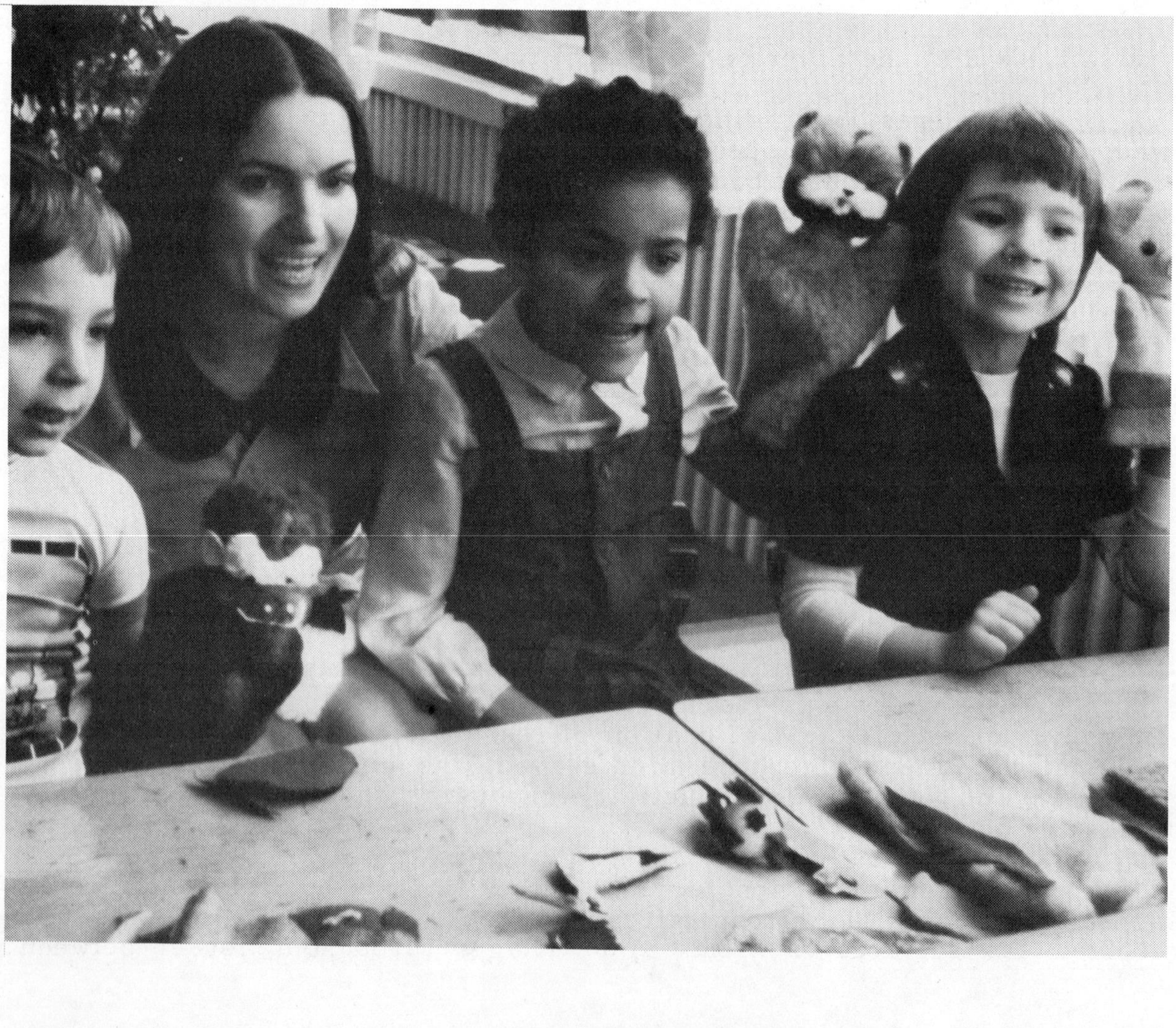

Additional References on Factors Associated with Successful Rehabilitation:

Harlem, Gudmund. "Studies on the Relation Between Impairment, Disability and Dependency," Scandinavian Journal of Rehabilitation Medicine, Supplement #4. Oslo: Kurer-Sats, 1976.

Three case studies in Norway were utilized to investigate the relationship between impairment, disability, ability to work and social adjustment. Factors analyzed that influence these relationships included type of impairment, age, sex, marital status, medical diagnosis, education, placement posibilities, psychic problems, pensions and time passed since last working. Significant findings included an inability to explain differences in successful medical rehabilitation on the basis of medical findings, severity of impairment or age. The study found no clear influence of the level of pension on long-term vocational rehabilitation results; factors observed were not highly correlated to long-term vocational results, and a large percentage of those gainfully employed were in jobs inconsistent with medical assessment. The study concluded that the distinction between objective and subjective disability is not precise.

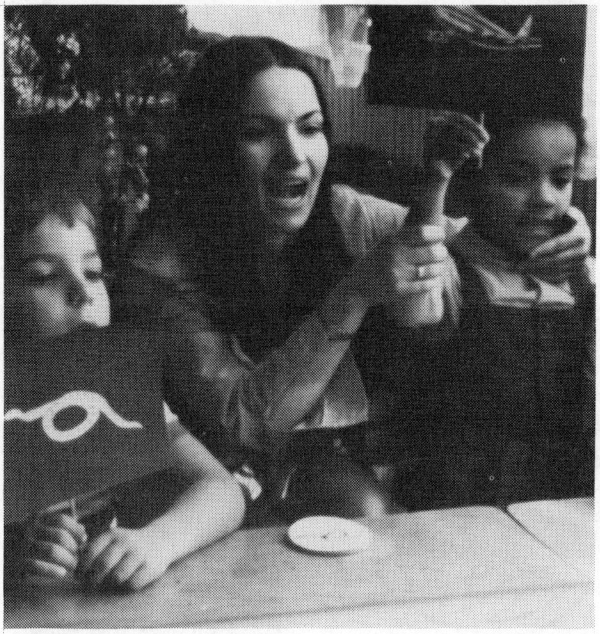

Albrecht, Gary L. and Stefan J. Harasymiw. "Evaluating Rehabilitation Outcome Cost Function Indicators," Journal of Chronic Diseases, Volume 32, #7, 1979, pp. 525-533.

The relationship between services provided and function gained by patients during hospitalization in comprehensive medical rehabilitation centers was studied in terms of cost effectiveness. A multi-dimensional outcome indicator -- a composite measure of functional gain per dollar cost of services applicable over time -- was developed. The indicator was applied to 230 patients with severe spinal cord and cerebral disabilities. The findings were: variables influencing success of rehabilitation were related to treatment and management patterns rather than demographic variables; the cost effectiveness of comprehensive medical rehabilitation centers varied significantly; and the cost effectiveness was partly dependent upon the type of disability treated.

Godstad, Anders Chr. Evaluation of Factors Determining the Results of Vocational Rehabilitation. Norway: Universitetsforlaget, 1968.

The principle aim of this study was to examine the background

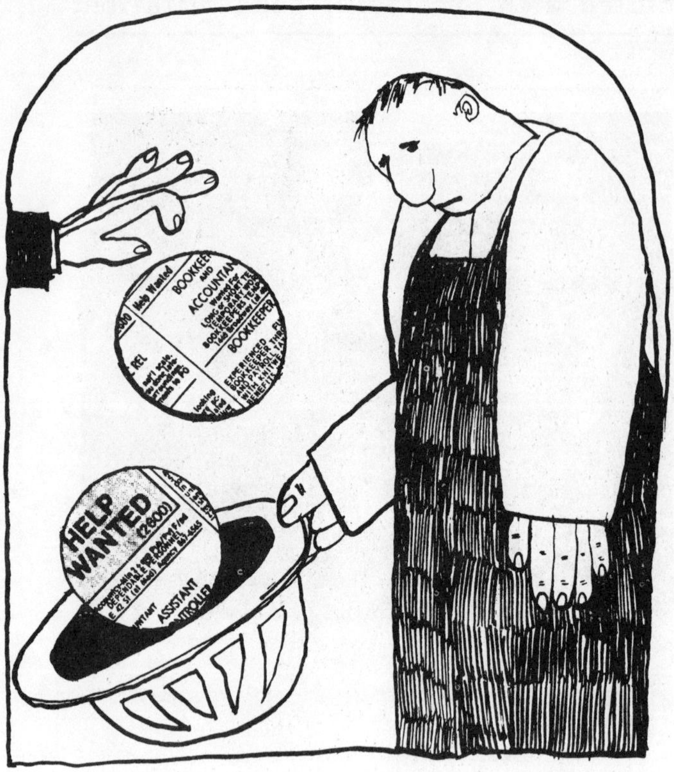

factors, apart from physical impairment, that are associated with the development of long lasting or permanent work insufficiency and social dependence in persons with enduring disabilities. The study was drawn from a regional comprehensive rehabilitation institution in western Norway. A primary concern was the degree to which multiple factors influence social and or vocational disability. The characteristics evaluated in the group that did not successfully complete rehabilitation were: old age, female sex, mental abnormalities, low intelligence, long period of unemployment, low educational status, heavy social obligations, and unfavorable employment conditions. A regression analysis demonstrated that two factors were common among unsuccessful rehabilitants: age of 45 years and older, and a registered psychiatric problem. Persons with low levels of intelligence, low levels of education, and prolonged periods of unemployment in the past were also found to have lower rates of successful social and vocational rehabilitation.

Greenblum, Joseph. "Effect of Rehabilitation on Employment and Earnings of the Disabled: Socio-demographic Factors," Social Security Bulletin, Volume 42, #8, August 1979, pp. 11-37.

An analysis of the importance of socio-demographic factors in the short-term impact of rehabilitation among disabled persons, based largely on an impact measure that compared the employment rates in 1972 of rehabilitated and non-rehabilitated clients, found virtually no difference in impact between men and women, but a greater effect among middle-aged than younger persons, regardless of sex, race, education, and type of disabling condition.

"Rehabilitation effects also varied for different minority ethnic groups. They were just as great among blacks as whites, even of the same age and sex. Among men and women of Hispanic origin, particularly those who were middle-aged and older, they were smaller. The role of education in rehabilitation impact was largely differentiated by sex. Among women, rehabilitation services resulted in a greater impact for those with more education. Among men, the impact was generally at least as great among the educationally disadvantaged. This sex-linked pattern was generally found among persons of similar age in either racial group..."

Vocational rehabilitation seemed to be a relatively successful vehicle for: middle aged men and women generally; blacks in contrast to whites, but particularly black women of all ages and teenaged black males; men and women under age 35 of Hispanic origin, compared with others of similar age; and educationally disadvantaged female black adolescents and men of both races and all ages.

V. SOCIAL SECURITY AND DISABILITY BENEFIT SYSTEMS

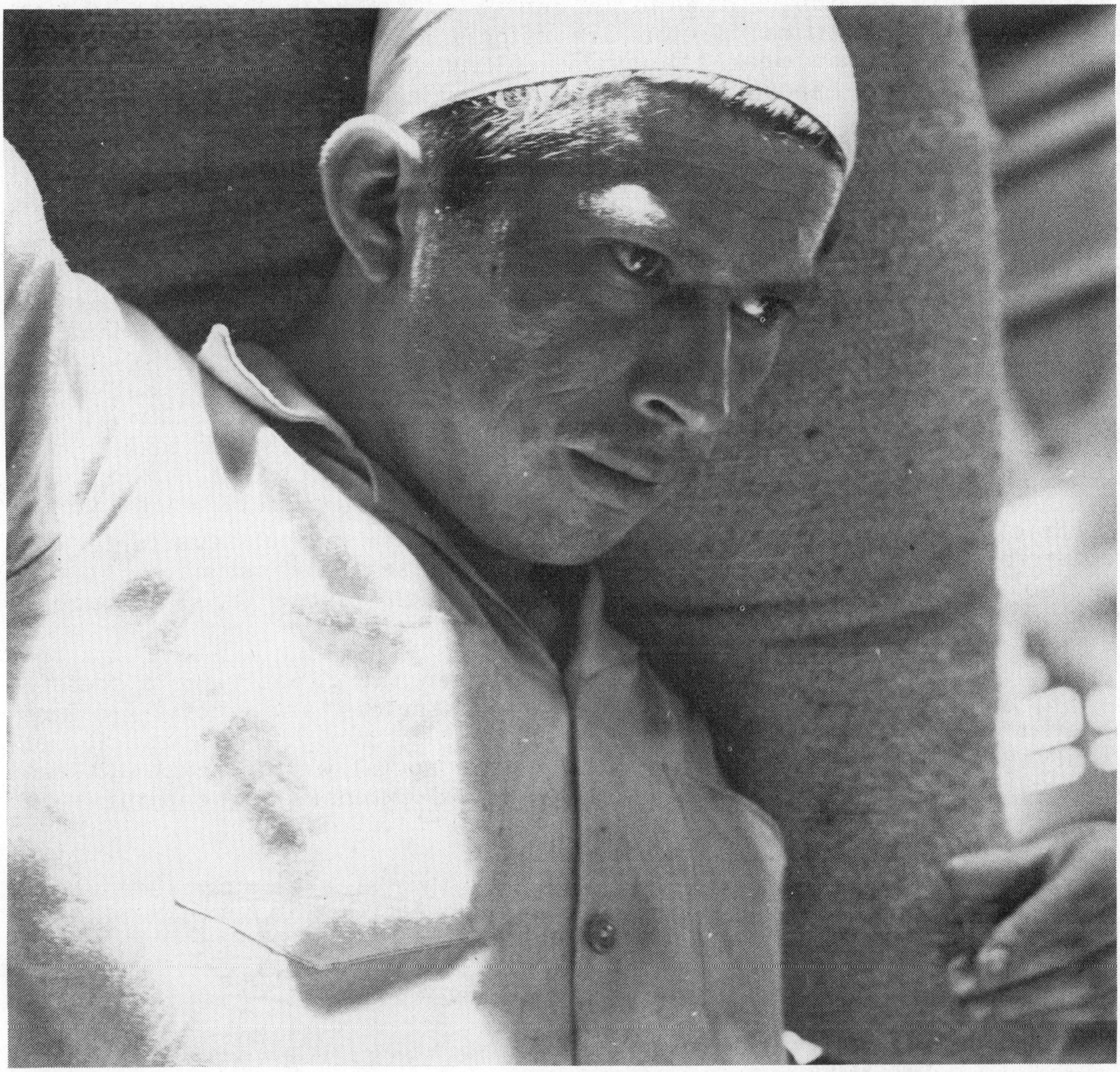

Economists and national policy planners have begun a fundamental reassessment of the traditional approach to economic development which stipulates that the growth of output is the main objective. As nations become increasingly affected by and aware of the decline in quality of life associated with increased output through its by-products, pollution, waste, noise, slums, and congestion, greater attention is being given to the environment and to man's basic relationship to nature. Increasingly, the objective is to develop technology which will not violate the harmony between man and nature and to stimulate growth and development which will improve the quality of life.

In this context, agreement is gradually being reached that the growth of output must be associated with the development of social and economic objectives. Economic growth is no longer seen as solely an objective in itself; it is a means and an instrument for achieving socio-economic goals. Governments recognize that the social objectives of economic development will not occur spontaneously, and that social objectives must be built into their basic planning models. Planners are still unable to quantify social objectives using traditional economic measures. Until now social objectives have primarily been measured by their indirect contribution to increases in productivity.

Only as public demand is generated for higher social benefits and becomes a political factor are efforts made to allocate increased resources. This has meant that the fulfilment of social objectives is assigned as much importance as other economic goals, and even in these circumstances it may be impossible to avoid conflict in choices between the claims of economic growth, and the demands of the social sector. Thus, for example, available data from centrally planned socialist countries, which advance social objectives as the primary basis for all economic efforts, do not clearly indicate how social and economic objectives are interrelated, i.e., how the degree of achievement of a particular social objective is made possible by the achievement of an economic objective, or whether there is any systematic development of such links in the central plan.

A. THE ECONOMICALLY ACTIVE WORK FORCE AND SUPPORT OF SOCIAL BENEFITS

The volume of social benefits available in any nation must ultimately depend upon the volume of national output available for redistribution. Normally economic planners base their estimates of the level of social benefits possible on factors such as the level of wages, and the numbers of economically active population.

A unique balance must exist between the capacity of a society to support a significant level of social services and social welfare benefits and the productive capacity of the citizenry. The capacity of highly productive societies to support large social welfare expenditures and still show a high benefit-cost ratio from extensive expenditures on

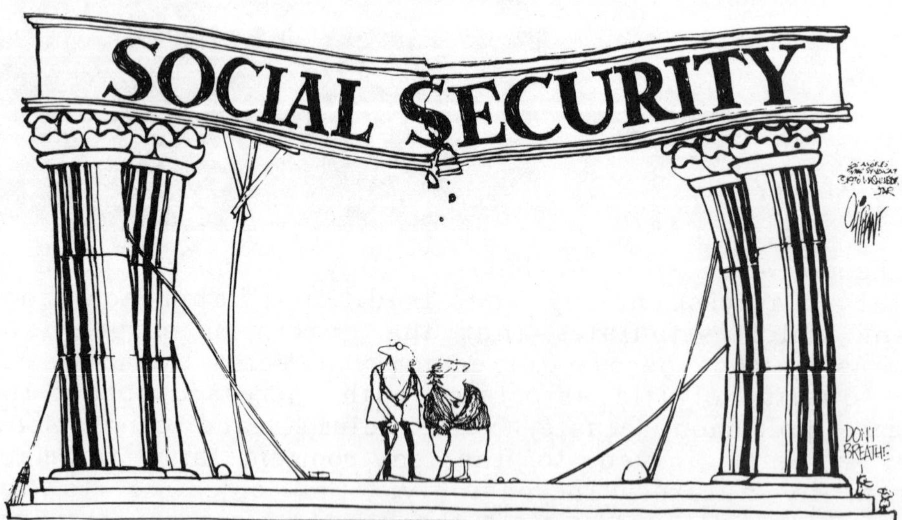

Oliphant, © 1976, *The Washington Star*/Los Angeles Times Syndicate

rehabilitation services is discussed in this chapter. There is, however, a critical and dynamic relationship between the provision of social benefits, particularly cash pensions, and the ability to add to the productivity of a nation through employment. As K.A. Jochheim, a former President of Rehabilitation International, has succinctly stated the problem:

"Regardless of the employment situation and the economic fluctuations, rehabilitation services must be available to enable all disabled persons to enjoy their rights and develop their full potentialities ... Sooner or later the development of social security will exceed the production capacity of the younger generation, which is decreasing in number, if the disabled--despite their disability and age--do not participate ... Rehabilitation is not only a humanitarian duty towards the disabled, it is at the same time the only possibility of making bearable the rapidly increasing costs for health services and social security." 59/

A rough estimation may be made of the proportions of any population which is economically active. In general, the estimate in industrialized nations without manpower shortages is:

Approximately 50 percent of the total population is made up of non-producers, such as children and adolescents receiving education and training, and the elderly beyond retirement age;

Approximately 10-20 percent of the people in productive age groups are disabled;

Approximately 20 percent of the people are providing care for dependents, or working in the educational, health and social services;

Approximately 20-25 percent sustain production. 60/

An analysis of the United States Social Security system indicated that while there were seven workers paying taxes for every person collecting social security benefits in 1955, there are less than three at present, and in 50 years there will be only two workers contributing to the scheme for each beneficiary. 61/ Similar data have emerged from the Federal Republic of Germany. In 1950 old-age social security benefits in the Federal Republic were financed by 5.2 active persons; by 1970 the figure had declined to 3.2 62/ The reduced number of active persons is attributable to longer education, lower birth rates, greater life expectancy, and the effects of an economic situation which produces a high level of unemployment. Another factor is the rising costs of social benefits, and these have been attributed to greater public awareness of available services, the rising life expectancy which has led to a growing proportion of the very old, better qualified and therefore better paid service providers, and international price inflation.

5.1 Gross national product (GNP) and social security expenditures for selected countries, 1974 [1]

[In millions of national currency units, except for percentages]

Country	GNP	Social security [2]		OASDI	
		Amount	As percent of GNP	Amount	As percent of GNP
Belgium (franc)	2,105,000	434,835	20.6	123,983	5.9
Canada (dollar)	128,050	16,940.3	13.2	4,121	3.1
France (franc)	1,324,800	287,207.4	21.7	53,858	4.1
Germany, Federal Republic (mark)	997,000	221,583	22.3	78,482	7.9
Japan (yen)	115,429,000	7,260,559	6.3	723,449	.63
Netherlands (florin)	188,130	47,439.3	25.2	11,191.6	6.3
Sweden (krona)	248,640	60,777.1	24.5	17,854.0	7.2
United Kingdom (pound)	73,620	10,426	14.2	3,320	4.5
United States (dollar)	1,381,200	164,710	11.9	54,870	4.0

[1] Data for calendar year except: Canada, Japan, and the United Kingdom data for fiscal year ending March 31, 1974; United States data for fiscal year ending June 30, 1974.

[2] Broadly defined to include expenditures under public medical care systems and cash payments under public welfare programs.

Source: GNP data from *International Financial Statistics*, International Monetary Fund, various issues; social security data derived by Social Security Administration from *The Cost of Social Security: Ninth International Inquiry*, International Labour Office, Geneva, 1978.

Additional References on The Economically Active Work Force and Support of Social Benefits:

Smirnov, S. "The Employment of Old-Age Pensioners in the U.S.S.R.," International Labor Review, Volume 116, #1, July-August, 1977, pp. 87-94.

In the Soviet Union, the number of people reaching working age is expected to decrease beginning in 1980, and according to official predictions, the number of pensioners is expected to increase from 43 million in 1975 to 80 million in the year 2000.

The case for continued employment of pensioners was based on investigations that revealed:

--"deterioration of health among working pensioners is only half as frequent as among those not employed";

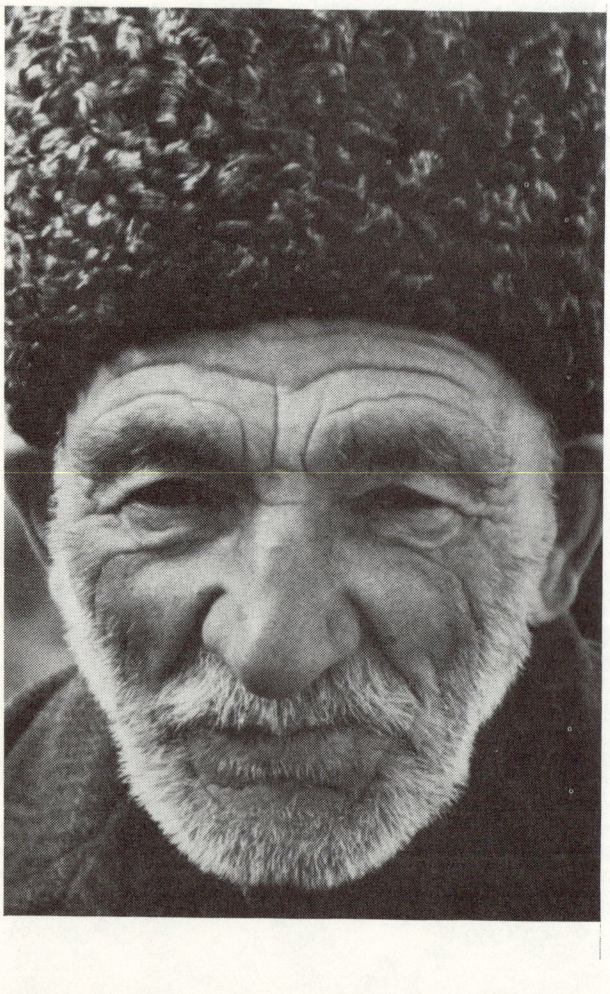

--80 percent of the old-age pensioners in the age group 60-64 have full or partial working capacity and can be considered a labor reserve;

--"sickness involving temporary loss of working capacity was significantly rarer among working pensioners than among persons of non-pensionable age";

--a survey of pensioners revealed an average productivity index of 96 percent of the overall average for the enterprise.

The potential magnitude of the U.S.S.R.'s problem led to a revision of ideas concerning the role of the people of pensionable age in the development of the country's economy. A survey of non-working pensioners disclosed that a fourth of those interviewed would have liked to continue to work part or full time. A study of what motivated pensioners to participate in the program revealed the main incentive to be economic. It was recommended that part-time workers be paid from 50% to 70% of the full amount of a pension, and that pension increments would accrue for each additional year of work.

The U.S.S.R.'s experiments with motivating pensioners to work, conducted during 1964-69, concluded: a) that it is not the size of the old age benefit but rather working conditions and wages which motivate workers to stay on the job; b) removal of the retirement test primarily motivates low-paid workers; c) non-working beneficiaries did not tend to return to work; and d) increases were registered among workers continuing on in their own specialty.

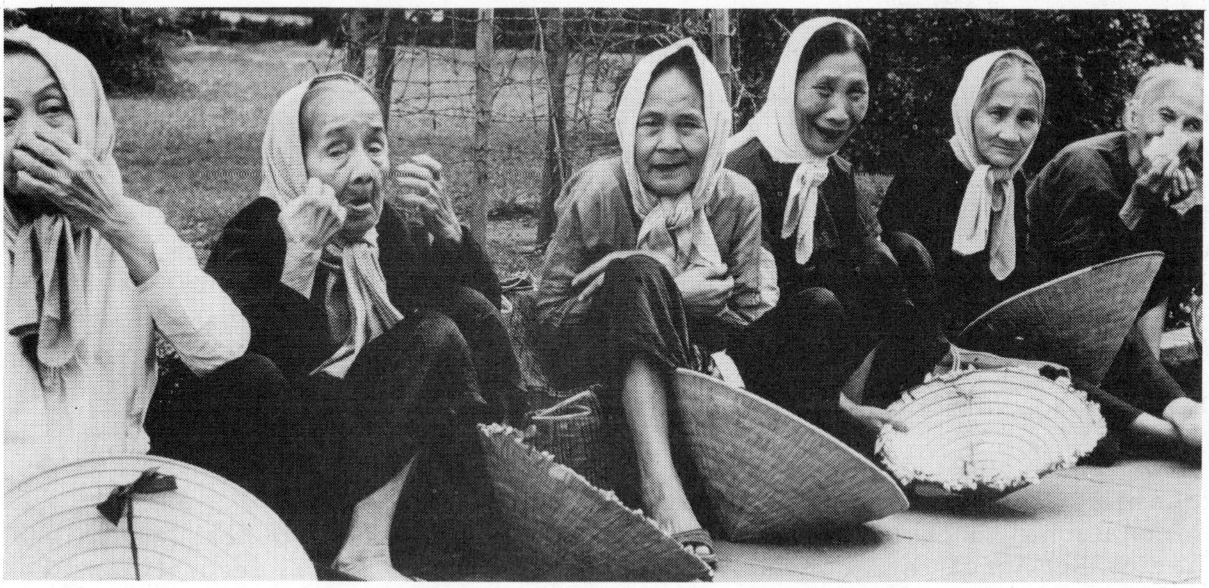

Lando, Mordechai E. et. al. "Disability Benefit Applications and the Economy," Social Security Bulletin, #10 October 1979, pp. 3-10.

This article discusses the cause of the growth in applications for disability insurance benefits in the United States, which rose from 720,000 in 1968 to a peak of 1.3 million in 1974, and declined to 1.2 million in 1979. Economic variables such as the unemployment rate and the relative value of the disability benefit were found to have a significant impact on the size of the disability program. Significant demographic variables included the size of the insured population and the proportion of the insured population aged 45 and over. It was calculated that 19% of the disability benefit applications received during the period 1970-78 were probably due to changes in the economic choices facing disabled persons.

Horlick, Max. "The Impact of an Aging Population on Social Security: The Foreign Experience," in Social Security in a Changing World. Washington, D.C.: U.S. Social Security Administration, 1979.

All of the industrial countries are experiencing a considerable increase in the proportion of older persons in the population, and a shrinking labor force contributing benefits for this population. This phenomenon is termed Rentenberg in Germany, or pension mountain.

5.2 **Number of persons in labor force under age 65 for each person aged 65 and over, selected countries, 1950–2000**

Year	Country									
	Austria	Belgium	France	(FR) Germany	Japan	Netherlands	Sweden	United Kingdom	Australia	Canada
1950	4.5	3.6	3.9	4.8	8.5	4.9	4.1	4.2	5.0	4.7
1955	4.1	3.4	3.7	4.5	8.2	4.3	3.8	4.0	4.7	4.6
1960	3.8	3.2	3.5	4.2	7.9	3.9	3.5	3.8	4.6	4.8
1965	3.3	2.9	3.3	3.7	7.6	3.8	3.4	3.8	4.7	4.7
1970	2.9	2.8	3.1	3.3	6.9	3.6	3.2	3.5	4.9	4.9
1975	2.8	2.7	3.1	3.1	6.3	3.5	2.9	3.3	4.9	4.9
1980	2.8	2.7	3.1	3.1	5.7	3.4	2.7	3.2	4.7	4.9
1985	3.3	2.9	3.6	3.6	5.4	3.5	2.7	3.3	4.6	4.6
1990	3.3	2.8	3.4	3.5	4.9	3.3	2.7	3.3	4.4	4.4
2000	3.4	2.7	3.2	3.1	3.8	3.2	3.1	3.6	4.6	4.4

Source: *Labour Force Estimates and Projections, 1950–2000*, International Labour Office, Geneva, second edition, 1977.

B. REHABILITATION IN SOCIAL WELFARE AND SOCIAL INSURANCE SYSTEMS

The extent and nature of social benefit schemes in any country, and more specifically the assistance schemes available for the disabled, are intrinsically related to the social structure of the nation, its political basis, and the beliefs and assumptions of its citizens as to the types of benefits which should be accorded to them as a right. Some discussion of the relationship of the socio-political system to the assessment of rehabilitation service costs is included in Chapter II. Differences of political philosophy and patterns of implementation have over the centuries produced distinctive differences in approach to the planning of the social welfare sector.

Organization of Social Welfare and Social Insurance Systems

An "Inventory of Measures and Services Designed to Promote Rehabilitation in Social Security Institutions" was conducted by the International Social Security Association, and analyzed for it by Dr. Charles Berlioz of the French National Federation of Social Security Bodies in 1968. The Inventory provides data on the main services, benefits and legislative bases of rehabilitation services funded through social security institutions in 35 countries. 63/

Subsequently, in 1971 the Disablement Income Group, a charitable trust in the United Kingdom, carried out a survey of financial provisions for disabled people in seven Western European countries: France, the Federal Republic of Germany, the Netherlands, Denmark, Norway, Sweden and the United Kingdom. Examining only those aspects of the general social assistance programs of these nations which were related to the needs of disabled people, the survey identified a range of variables in benefit provision which may be described as falling into the following groups:

(a) The types of coverage available -- various forms of invalidity pensions, short-term and long-term sickness benefits, special and supplemental allowances;

(b) The categories of people covered -- the war disabled, workers disabled in industrial accidents or with occupational diseases, workers' dependents, certain groups of the disabled such as the blind, all people with chronic disability regardless of the time of onset or cause;

(c) The types of benefits available -- pensions, living allowances, tax-free status, compulsory or non-contributory schemes, earnings-related or flat-rate payments, all-or-nothing and/or partial compensation, the use of means tests to determine eligibility, the duration of coverage;

(d) The measurement of disability -- the use of measures based on the kind and degree of disability, the use of measures based on the loss of functional ability, the use of measures based on the loss of employment capacity.

Patterns of financing reflected the diversity of approach to the provision of benefits. Except for the universal pension schemes in Denmark and Sweden, and the financing of social assistance programs from national and local budgets, all of the disablement schemes were founded on social insurance principles. The three main patterns for payment of contribution to the schemes which emerged were:

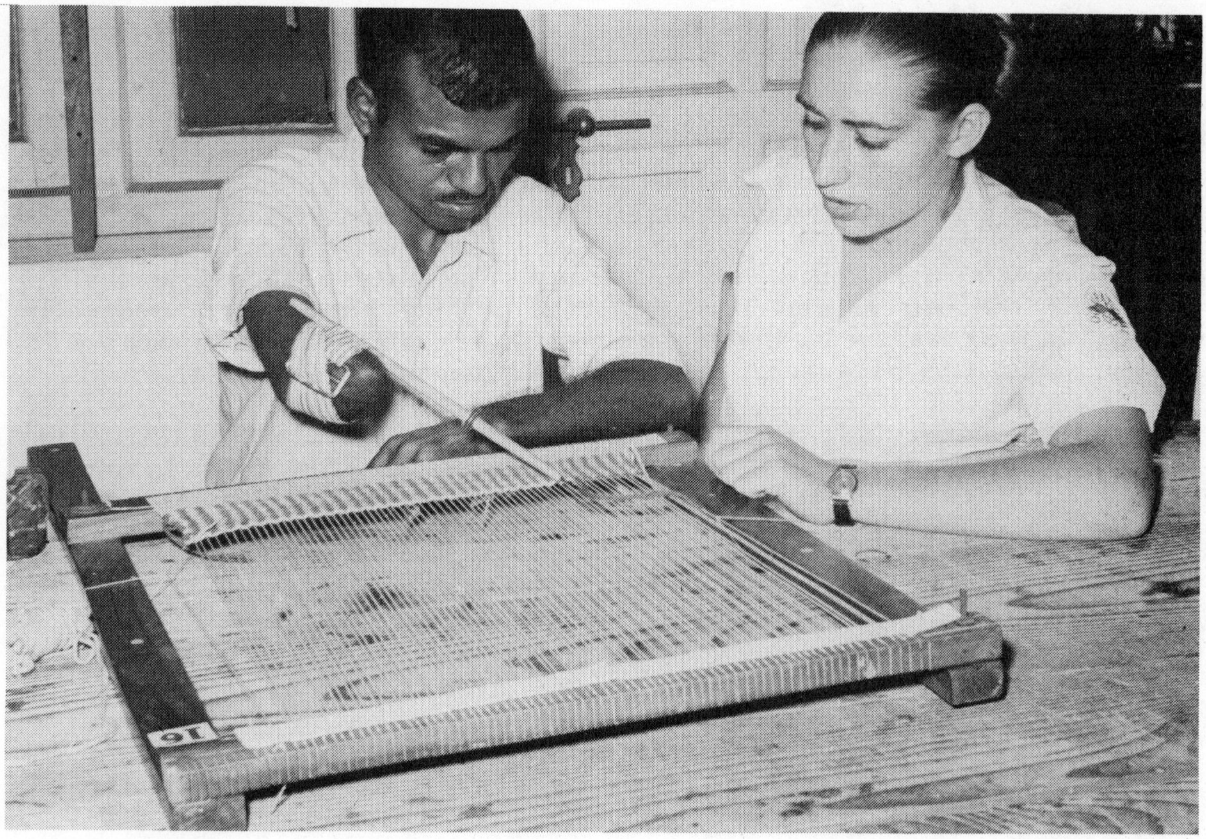

(a) Tripartite financing -- with contributions by the insured person, the employer and the Government;

(b) The joint contribution of two parties -- e.g., the insured person and the employer only, the employer and the Government only, the taxpayer and the Government only;

(c) The contribution of a single party -- the employer only. This was the case with industrial injury schemes in five of the seven countries.

It was found that all of the countries provide separate benefits for their war disabled, and all of the countries, with the exception of the Netherlands, maintain separate schemes for the award of pensions to persons disabled through industrial injury. In the Netherlands the same pension is awarded regardless of the cause of disability. In general all of the countries studied had schemes for the provision of industrial injury benefits long before disability pensions were introduced, and the disability pensions were generally an extension of old-age pension schemes which were never integrated with the industrial schemes already in existence. The only countries of those studied which guarantee pensions for all disabled persons, including those persons who have not worked and those with disabilities of a congenital nature or arising from a childhood disease, were Denmark and Sweden.

The pension schemes in Denmark and Sweden are intended to cover all members of the population whose ability to support themselves is reduced through disability. Access to allowances through general systems of social assistance for persons of insufficient means is available to provide additional allowances in those instances in which a person with reduced earning capacity may not have received a pension.

The other countries offer social assistance to disabled persons who do not fall within the pension schemes.

Comparative Status of Social Welfare and Social Insurance Schemes

The provision of social assistance creates problems of its own. In general, social assistance is regarded as "public charity for the poor" and this is especially true in countries in which the grant of assistance is discretionary and based on a means-test, often regarded as degrading by the recipients of assistance. The level of social assistance may vary with the wealth of the local community responsible for its provision. Disability pensions, on the other hand, are generally regarded as a deserved "right", and they are generally comparable in different localities because of their national regulation.

Dr. Gudmund Harlem, Director of the State Rehabilitation Institute in Oslo, Norway, has summarized the differences in historical development and approach between social service and assistance programs, and social security systems for the disabled: 64/

> "Based on existing church and voluntary efforts to aid the most needy citizens, the community develops assistance for these citizens, usually in the form of 'poor laws'. ... Assistance is given according to specific needs (food, medical expenses, shelter, clothing), in cash or in kind, and is based on decisions pertaining to the single individual, contingent upon specific conditions, and made by a committee or an administrator. The poor law system gradually becomes more flexible and comprehensive; it expands into preventing social problems ... As long as it is based upon a judgment of what ought to be given to an individual ... it is ... 'social service'.
>
> "Social security is used to mean the later development of systems covering all citizens or larger groups of citizens, giving legally defined rights (similar to rights a single individual may secure through an individual insurance, but social security may cover more than what could be covered through insurance). As long as the rules ... are clear, anyone will or may know his rights and they may be legally enforced, and in this context the concept 'social security' is used. It usually starts with workmen's compensation, next come either old age and perhaps widows' pensions or sickness (injuries) benefits, where hospital fees, other medical expenses and loss of income during illness may be covered. Social security then develops through increases in the degree to which expenses or loss of income is covered, and in the time period covered (lowering of age when old age pension starts, extension of period covered by sickness benefits until a disability pension system exists). It may include benefits in cash or in kind. The underlying value may be said to be all that citizens want to be covered automatically and definitely, if and when they are hit by difficulties they foresee they will or may meet, and this shall be a right and not something contingent upon a judgment of individual needs."

As Dr. Harlem states, social security and social assistance schemes in the different nations may eventually become responsible for the provision of funds to groups of citizens to compensate for their loss of earning capacity, to pay for their medical expenses, and to be of assistance with regard to specific needs.

Rehabilitation and Reduced Pension Payments

Given the increasing costs to society of sustaining systems of social security and social service, it is not surprising that researchers have been interested to demonstrate how rehabilitation of the disabled can not only help to reduce the number of non-productive members, but at the same time reduce the expenditures on disability pensions and public assistance.

The Commonwealth Rehabilitation Service of Australia conducted a long-term study of the post-rehabilitation history of persons provided with treatment and/or training by the Service during the years 1969-1970. 76/ The study covered all states of Australia with the exception of New South Wales, the most populous state. Data are as reported by the Research Section of the Department of Social Security, Canberra.

The Commonwealth Rehabilitation Service provides treatment and/or vocational training for persons who have a substantial handicap for employment and, except in the case of the permanently blind, have a disability wholly or partly remediable. The persons accepted must have reasonable prospects, with rehabilitation aid, of engaging in a suitable vocation within three years of beginning treatment or training.

Medical officers at each rehabilitation centre collected data relating to the personal characteristics and rehabilitation potential of all persons accepted for treatment or training during the specified period, and details of their employment, wages or other forms of income provision were kept at regular intervals following placement. Six months after placement and each 12 months thereafter, a search was made to determine if the rehabilitee had reverted to pension or benefit payments.

"Practically all of the industrialized nations... provide a constant attendance allowance or similar substitute under their old age and invalidity (disability) insurance programs. This is a cash benefit paid on behalf of permanently disabled persons who require either full or part-time care by another person at home. The benefit is normally used to hire a nurse or to reimburse family members for the costs incurred in caring for a relative. In some cases, the benefit is paid directly to the relative.... There is wide variation among countries in the qualifying conditions and benefit levels of the constant attendance allowances. Some programs require total (100%) disability; others, as in Switzerland and France, apply a means test. In France, the income of the family as well as the beneficiary is calculated in the means test.

Mary Jo Gibson, "Family Support for the Elderly In International Perspective: Policies and Programs," in Ageing International, Volume VII, #4, 1980.

A complete absence of post-placement data existed for 12 percent of the people placed in employment, 98 of 837 persons. It was assumed in the study that the characteristics of the excluded group were those of the population for whom details were available.

Almost one-half of the people placed in employment were those defined as permanently incapacitated for work, likely to remain in receipt of unemployment or sickness benefits permanently, or likely to become invalid pensioners in the absence of rehabilitative treatment or training. Return to work was estimated to have been accelerated by a period of three years or less for the balance of rehabilitees. Eighteen months following placement, the survey results indicated that 69 percent of the male rehabilitees, and 60 percent of the female rehabilitees continued to be in employment. Sixteen percent of the males and 19 percent of the females had reverted to some form of Commonwealth benefit.

The financial benefits accruing to the Commonwealth were determined to consist of two main elements: savings through non-payment of pensions and benefits, and additional personal income tax receipts. The average net annual costs of invalid pension, unemployment and sickness benefits in June 1970, plus associated fringe benefits, were calculated at A$1,050 and A$600 respectively. The amount of tax paid was based on the percentage of actual income to the rehabilitee in each case. The average weekly wage paid to adult rehabilitees at the 18-month period was A$56.10 for the males and A$43.00 for the females. The amount of pension benefit saved for persons who would not have been permanently incapacitated in the absence of rehabilitation was estimated on the basis of the amount of benefit that would have been provided during the "acceleration period," together with the tax income during that period. This type of estimation was more difficult in the case of rehabilitees judged likely to be permanently incapacitated without rehabilitation (i.e., the severely disabled). The Australian study shows that 39.1 percent of those so assessed were no longer employed within the 18 month period and 23.2 percent had reverted to pension or benefit. Further reversions were anticipated in subsequent years, the rate of which could be determined only by the continuation of the study. Thus, it was not possible for the researchers to estimate the probable length of participation of this latter group in the work force.

The researchers in this survey, therefore, estimated the total actual overall savings represented by the non-permanently incapacitated rehabilitees, and the savings represented by the "permanently incapacitated" for only the first 12 months following placement. The savings to consolidated revenue in the case of the non-permanently incapacitated placements were estimated at $250,000 in the first year after placement and $61,000 in the following year. In the case of the "permanently incapacitated" placements, the savings to the Commonwealth Government were estimated at $335,000 in the first year. It is initially assumed that a similar saving will occur for this group in subsequent years. The cost of operating the Commonwealth Rehabilitation Service for the 1969-1970 period in the five participating states was $1,633,000, excluding certain capital costs. On the basis of the above assumptions, the financial gain to the Commonwealth would result in the costs of the 1969-1970 rehabilitation program being met in four years. Subsequent to that period, the Commonwealth would earn a profit on its investment in the form of all payments of pension or benefit which would otherwise have been made to "permanently incapacitated" persons together with the receipt of income tax on their earnings.

The study cites other factors which would increase and decrease the financial gain, and, in general they were judged to offset one another. These included: employment lapses of the permanently incapacitated, a proportion of those at present on benefits who will re-enter the work force, differences in the cost of unemployment and sickness benefits and invalid pension rates, and understatement of savings calculated in terms of 1970 rates for pension and tax income since these would increase in subsequent years.

Rehabilitation and the Decline in Public Assistance

The United States of America: Data collected in the United States in connection with the analysis of pre- and post-rehabilitation service earnings of disabled clients indicated that between 1958 and 1967, the percentage of clients receiving public assistance at acceptance for service ranged from 12 to 13 percent. 77/ At closure of rehabilitation service, this was reduced on the average to between 5 and 6 percent. The estimated annual reduction in public assistance payments as a result of the federally-funded state vocational rehabilitation programs was $9.6 million in 1961, and by 1967 this figure had risen to $16.4 million. (In fiscal year 1967, more than 170,000 disabled persons were rehabilitated through the state-federal vocational rehabilitation program.) These savings were considered to be an underestimation of the total reduction in the value of the care and maintenance needed by rehabilitants.

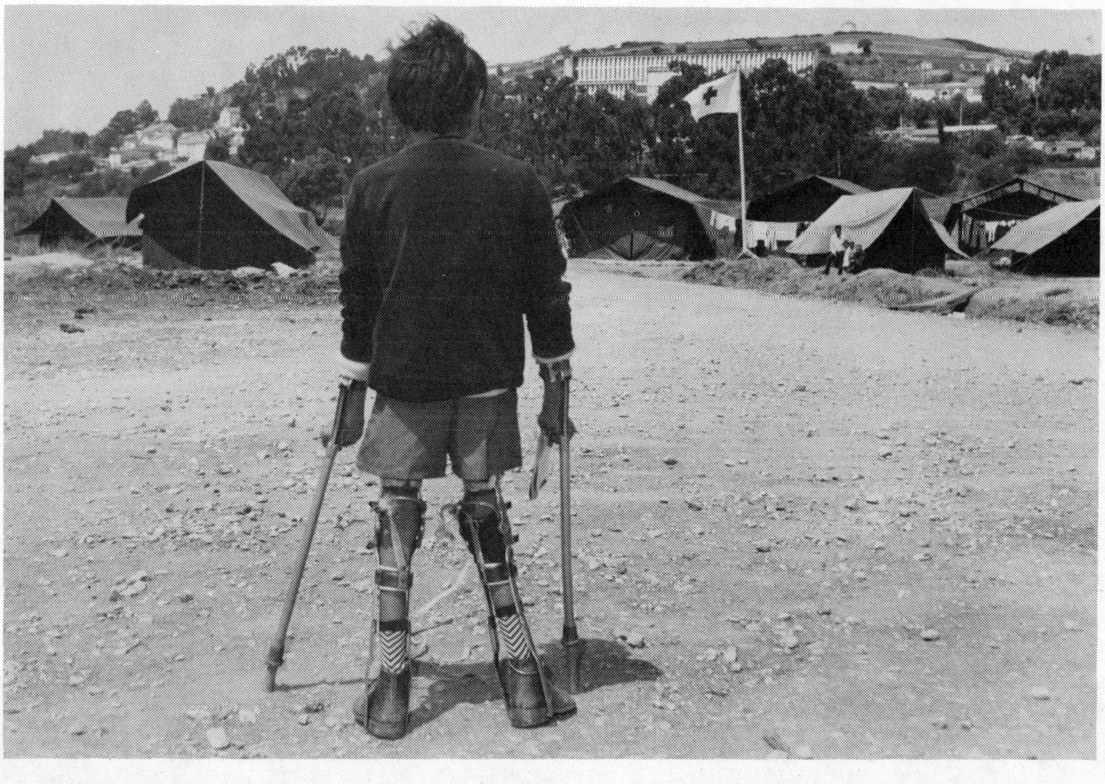

Israel: In a study by the Rehabilitation Service of the Ministry of Social Welfare in Israel, 78/ successful rehabilitation resulted in impressive savings in welfare expenditures. More than

1,300,000 Israeli pounds were being saved yearly as a result of the ministry program. These savings were computed by comparing the amount of welfare assistance received by each rehabilitant before and after rehabilitation service. In addition, the public assistance payments saved in two years covered the direct costs of service. While the rehabilitation agency's investment was a one-time expense, the saving is continuous, and may extend for generations within a family in which the dependency chain has been broken.

Over-all Economic Effect of Reduced Transfer Payments

An important limitation to this approach to demonstrating savings from rehabilitation activity is that savings in social benefits such as pension payments do not represent a saving to society as a whole, nor do they represent any increase in net income. Pensions and

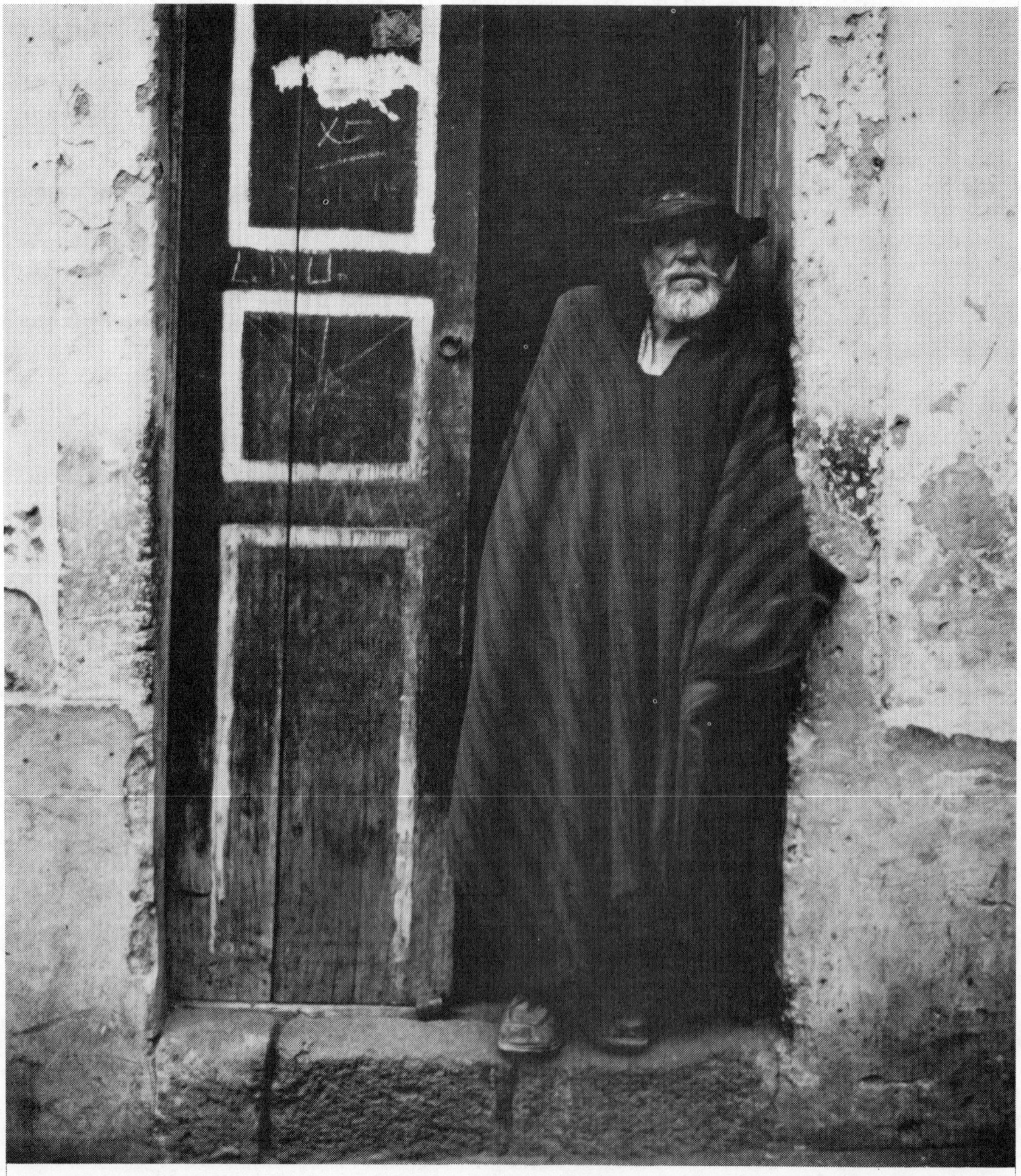

other social benefits are a type of transfer payment, a redistribution of the already existing wealth of society. The only actual saving to society as a whole inclusive of the disabled is in the cost of benefit program administration, which is generally a small percentage of the overall cost. 79/ Rather, the savings demonstrated are in relation to the agency responsible for benefit administration, and these savings must generally be demonstrated for political as compared to economic reasons.

Levels of Pensions and the Rehabilitation Process

It is widely accepted that invalidity pensions and other related benefits to assist the disabled to maintain an acceptable standard of living in their communities are an essential part of the rehabilitation process. As the participants in the European Seminar on the Contribution of Social Security and Social Services to the Rehabilitation of the Disabled (1973) observed, 65/ cash benefits in themselves serve one purpose of rehabilitation by enabling the individual to rest and recuperate when he or she should not be actively working. The meeting also urged that the patients need for longer-term assistance, in place of medical treatment and short-term benefits, be identified at the earliest possible moment.

At the same time the importance to the individual as well as to society of achieving the fullest rehabilitation was stressed. It is critical that persons who can benefit from specific rehabilitation measures be identified early. Most important:

> "The overall economic situation of the person undergoing active rehabilitation should not be worse off than it would be if he simply stayed the passive recipient of benefits: ideally it should be higher, to encourage him to choose rehabilitation." 66/

The tendency of cash benefits and other forms of social assistance to encourage an involuntary passivity and attitude of dependence is a recognized hazard. The same seminar acknowledged that there is an inevitable difference between the interests of the disabled individual as perceived by the individual, and the interests of the individual and of society as perceived by a range of administrators and practitioners. While accepting the primacy of rehabilitation, the participants emphasized the need to take account of the special needs of particular individuals and groups within a system design for the generality of people, and the fact that "compulsion is no substitute for motivation." 67/

The European seminar participants were unanimous in agreeing on the right of disabled people to cash support when unable to earn their own living. The following recommendations were made with regard to the provision of pensions to those who return to work:

"A disabled person who gives up his pension to return to work should be ensured full and prompt restoration of pension if his return to work is shortlived."

"A disabled person liable to extra expense in connection with his disablement should be assisted by services, aids, or cash benefits as appropriate, even if his pension is suspended."

"For those disabled workers whose earning capacity has been substantially and permanently reduced, consideration should be given -- according to the possibilities open to different national schemes -- to a cash benefit which would have regard to the gap between actual earnings which would have been obtained but for the disablement." 68/

Thus the meeting acknowledged the important relationship which must exist between rehabilitation and social benefits. Professionals in many countries are attempting to modify the systems which do not take adequate cognizance of the constant relationship between the two phases. They are working towards the development, instead, of graded or sliding-scale pension programs that encourage the total rehabilitation of the disabled person. It is crucial that rehabilitation not be regarded as a method whereby society can avoid an economic commitment to the disabled; experience has shown that this attitude may retard rather than foster rehabilitation.

Implications of Partial Benefits

An interesting adjunct to the experiences cited during the European seminar is provided through analysis of the results of research studies on the rehabilitation of particularly disadvantaged disabled people. One such finding was the result of a larger evaluation study of the United States Social Security Disability Insurance Program carried out by Dr. Richard Smith and Dr. Abraham Lilienfeld in 1971. 69/

At the close of 1970 approximately 2,665,000 persons were receiving monthly cash benefits through this program. The program is available to insured workers and dependents who are disabled, and who have been assessed as unable to engage in substantial gainful activity. The evaluation was based on a follow-up study of 1,564 disability applicants in one metropolitan area using personal interviews and medical examinations of persons denied and allowed benefits. The study confirmed that the system in effect for evaluation of disabled applicants did indeed differentiate the severely disabled from those less disabled in the applicant group. Its other conclusions, however, demonstrated the importance of early benefit provision cited by the European seminar. Both the applicant groups, those allowed benefits and those denied benefits, were characterized by low income and assets. Members of the denial group tended to decline after disability to a lower socio-economic level than those in the allowed group. In a reassessment of disability status, the denial group showed the greater rate of change over time; nearly one-quarter of them later became eligible for benefits. The study concluded that systematic reassessment of disability applicants is necessary to evaluate changes in their status, and more important, that identifying the disabled for benefits should not be delayed until such a critical juncture when disease and other factors have resulted in a more severe incapacity than when the applicant originally applied for assistance. By the latter point the persons' prospects for successful rehabilitation have been additionally diminished and even greater resources will be required to be of assistance.

A Special Study on the Employment of the Handicapped carried out in Finland in 1972 reached similar conclusions. 70/ This study was a follow-up survey of disabled persons placed in employment in 1970 through the counseling sections of the state labor exchanges. There were approximately 5,000 people being placed in one year. A follow-up inquiry was made two months and a further six months after job placement. The findings included that after six months, only 34 percent of the disabled were still employed. Physical illness was the obstacle for three-fourths of the unemployed group; 15 percent had problems associated with mental illness; and 10 percent had problems associated with advanced age or social maladjustment. Only 28 percent of the cases were judged to have severe disabilities, 46 percent of the cases were judged to have middle-level disability, and 24 percent slight disability. For the majority of people, earnings were insufficient to guarantee a minimum livelihood, given the low level of earned income and short duration of employment. The study concluded that it would be more economical to guarantee a minimum income for the hard-to-employ than to have repeated unsuccessful attempts at employment and self-support.

The European seminar referred to above, in affirming the need for continuing cash support in individual cases where serious residual disability remains, concluded:

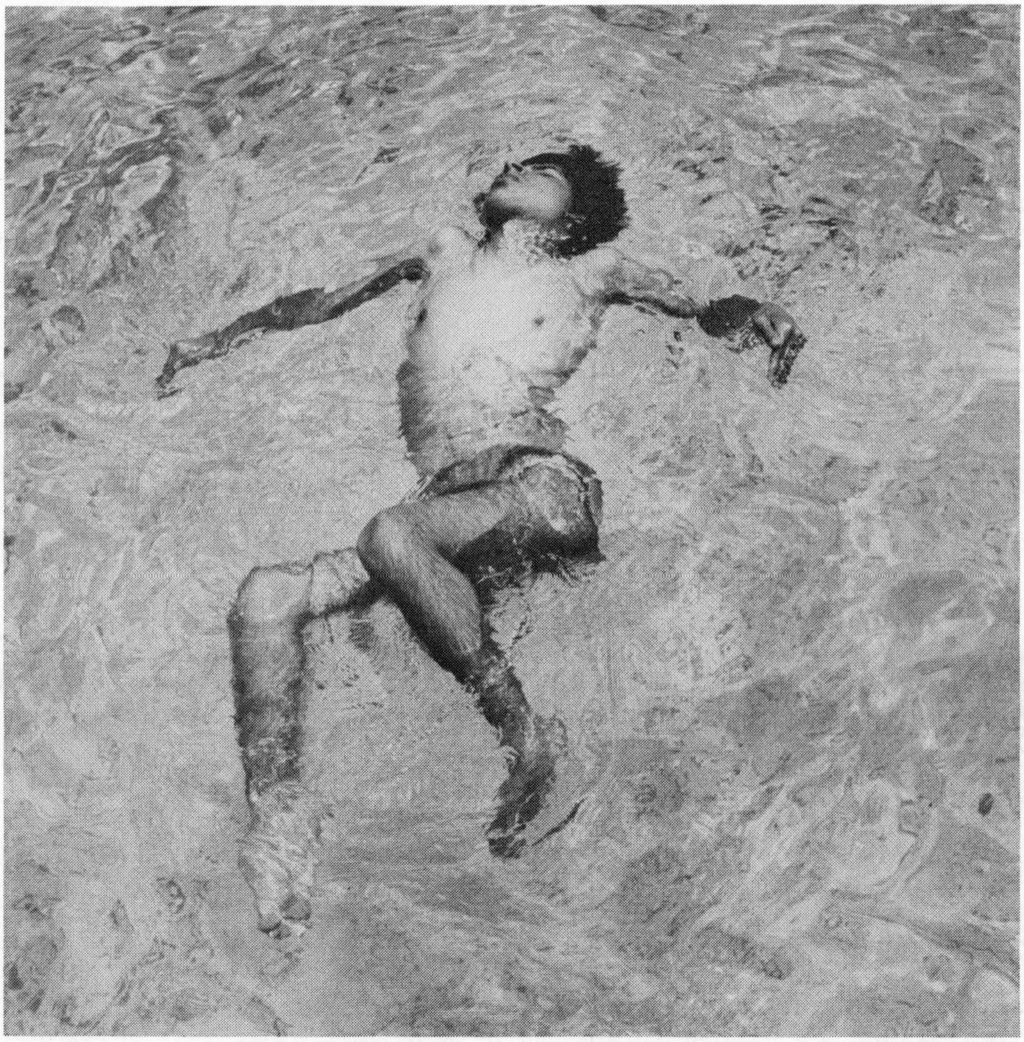

"We sometime seem better able to cope with burying the man who has drowned, or with giving swimming lessons to the man who has yet to enter the water, than with providing support and encouragement to the man who is struggling to keep afloat." 71/

Additional References on Rehabilitation in Social Welfare and Social Insurance Systems:

Haber, Lawrence D. Sickness and Injury Cash Benefits: A Proposal for Planning and Integration. Unpublished paper, 1974.

Temporary incapacity is defined in the United States as sickness, injury or incapacity which is expected to be of short duration, with the worker returning to his normal work activities with only few changes, usually within 6 months. Temporary incapacity because of sickness and injury is the most frequent cause of earning loss, yet about a third of the workers in the United States receive no wage replacement during illness and injury. Private and public programs together replace less than one-fourth of the earnings loss from temporary incapacity of wage and salary workers in private industry.

The average yearly loss per worker due to short-term sickness and injury is 7 days of work. This represents about 3% of all wages and salaries paid, or over $20 billion in 1973. 30% of the work force has a disabling illness or injury during a year. Though the period of disability is usually short (over 50% less than one week), the loss of income is accompanied by high medical care costs, and residual impairments. The burden of sickness and injury also tends to fall most heavily on those least able to afford it--low wage and unskilled workers. These factors immediately foster the development of dependency and can lead to chronic or extended disability, and application for social security disability benefits or other public assistance programs.

Another study concluded that "temporary disability is in fact the most persistent, serious and

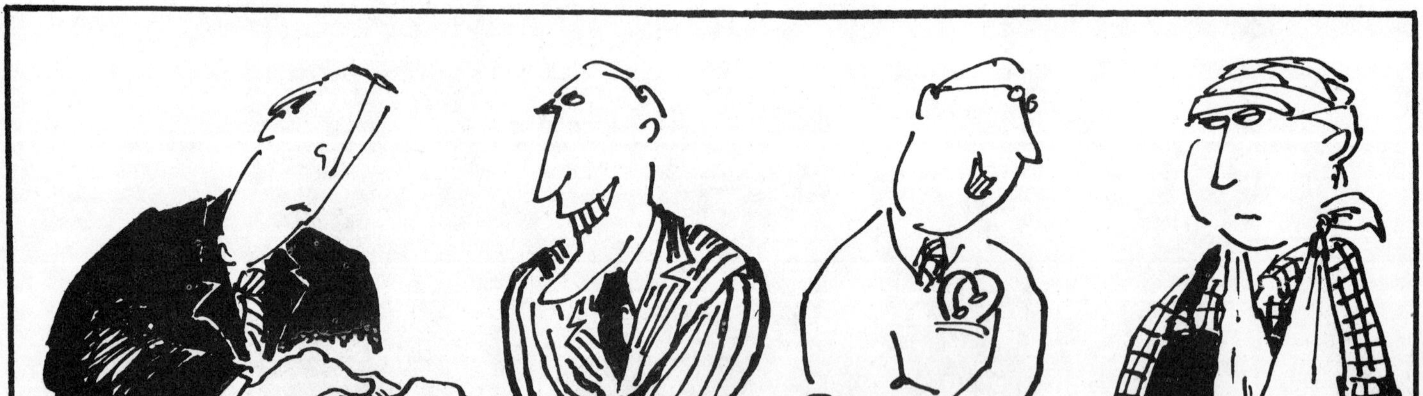

DRAWINGS BY SIGNE WILKINSON

"Some 40 to 50% of major workmens' compensation cases are contested, as opposed to only 3% of temporary disability cases. Results of this extensive litigation include high non-benefit costs of the program—only about $0.50 of every premium dollar returns to workers as benefits."

Jonathan H. Sunshine, Disability, 1979.

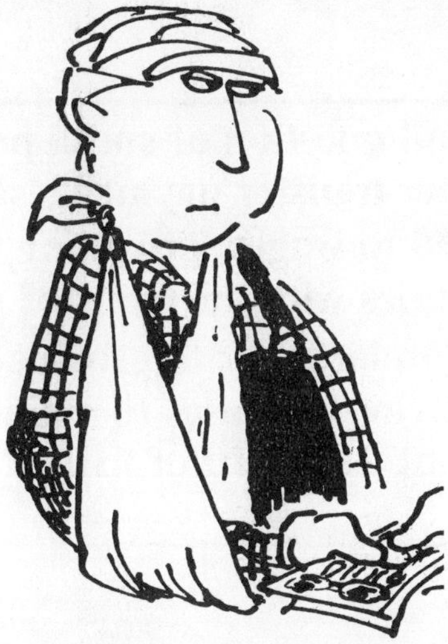

uncertain hazard confronting the mass of our working population," and pointed out that "wage loss from injury or illness of a non-occupational origin is a significant cause of the high cost of public assistance, since lack of insurance protection forces many to public relief authorities when they are disabled." Therefore the early stages of impairment or incapacity represent a crucial juncture; early referral and treatment are of the utmost importance.

The case management of services to those incapacitated must coordinate the restorative functions of guidance, rehabilitation, job adaptation, job placement, and the family maintenance functions of wage replacement and support. Weekly compensation to disabled people without this coordination is a waste of both manpower and money. (State programs have experienced administrative expenses ranging from 7-13% of total benefit costs.)

Yet the network of social insurance programs--workmen's compensation, unemployment insurance, and temporary disability benefits (in certain states) devote little attention to the prevention of disability, incentives to recovery at the onset of disability, or reemployment.

Sickness and injury cash benefits lie at the center of a coordinated approach to the problems of disability. Several studies have concluded that adequate benefits facilitate the economical utilization of human resources. To the extent that income maintenance programs fail to recognize or respond to the employability aspect of disability, they fall short of their wage replacement objectives and place a premium on incapacity.

"The provision of income maintenance for temporary incapacity and the coordination with case management service for restoration, rehabilitation and reemployment should be among the highest priorities of an adequate social policy for disability."

Palotai, K. "Problems Arising From the Low Level of Invalidity Pensions," Report X, International Social Security Association XIX General Assembly, (Madrid, 4-14 October 1977). Geneva: International Social Security Association, 1978.

"Among the benefits of social security, cash benefits in the event of incapacity to earn or incapacity to work, which make up for loss of earnings, occupy an important place... If the loss of earnings capacity continues without forseeable limit, cash sickness benefits are replaced by an invalidity pension... Under the Soviet, Polish, Romanian, Czechoslovak and Hungarian social security schemes, the accident insurance branch is integrated into the pension insurance branch, with the result that in these countries compensation for temporary or long-term incapacity to earn falls under two branches: sickness insurance and pensions insurance." In 1975, 105 countries provided compensation for both employment accidents and occupational diseases, while 22 more provided compensation only in the event of employment accidents (mostly developing countries in Africa and Asia).

A number of factors may give rise to low pensions. Low pensions may be awarded when a partial reduction in capacity for work may be offset by supplemental earnings; it may also arise when the accountable income and the period before the onset of invalidity are of low value. "In most social security systems, the minimum old age pension determines the minimum invalidity pension. This minimum normally depends on the country's economic development, and in the developing countries it is therefore extremely low. In Zaire it is 30 percent after an insurance period of fifteen years, and in the Central African Republic 50 percent of the minimum wage."

The time elapsed since the award of a pension may also reduce its value, as inflation increases the cost of living. Social security in the highly developed industrialized countries has provision for regular adjustment (indexing). Austria, France, Finland, Federal Republic of Germany, Netherlands, Norway, United Kingdom, Argentina, Bolivia, Brazil, and Uruguay adjust on the basis of changes in the wage index. These countries therefore not only maintain the real value of fixed pensions, but increase them from year to year. In the U.S.S.R., due to the stability of the consumer price index over long periods, the increases in pensions which take place from time to time mean a rise in the real value of pensions.

Another group of countries (USA, Denmark, Sweden, Luxembourg, Canada, Chile, Colombia, New Zealand, Upper Volta, Zaire) make pension adjustments on the basis of changes in the consumer price index. The original purchasing power of the pensions therefore remains unchanged. In a third group of countries (Switzerland, Portugal, Ecuador, Mexico, Poland, Czechoslovakia, Romania) adjustments to compensate for loss of purchasing power are made from time to time, but not at fixed times.

"A broad question of social policy is whether transfer payments should be linked to wages, providing beneficiaries with the fruits of rising living standards, or to provide only cost of living increases to maintain a constant standard of living."

Jonathan H. Sunshine, Disability, 1979.

Watching the Parade Go By

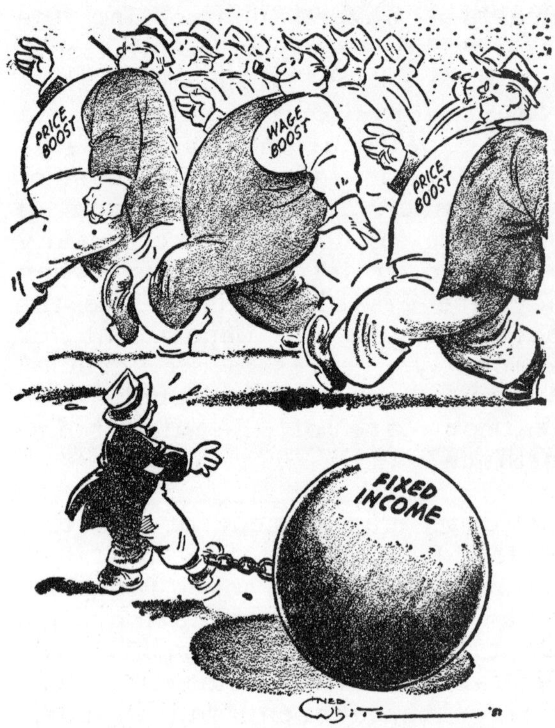

Several other problems may arise from a low level of invalidity pensions. Mere subsistence may be difficult when a person becomes disabled as a result of illness, and does not receive a pension because his period of employment is not long enough. A similar situation arises when partial pensions are not recognized in a national social security scheme, yet the individual does not qualify for a full pension. Other individuals may not be able to supplement pensions with other earnings. "In cases of pensions which do not reach the minimum subsistence level, the situation becomes worse for young people with families who become invalid." They receive a supplement for family maintenance, but it is often insufficient.

Health problems may also arise because the level is not adequate for subsistence and the pensioner's health therefore deteriorates, thereby diminishing the chances for a return to employment.

Johnson, William G. "Disability, Income Support, and Social Insurance," in Edward Berkowitz (ed.), Disability Policies and Government Programs. New York: Praeger, 1979.

Public programs for disabled people can be grouped according to three primary objectives. The first is service--programs designed to increase individual welfare. The second is income support which is designed to maintain individuals at a minimum subsistence standard of living. And third, income maintenance, which is designed to replace all or part of individual or family income lost as a result of a disabling condition.

In evaluating the administrative efficiency of a disability program, the disability benefit system as a whole must be examined. An evaluation of the adequacy of any public program must also consider the activities of all household members, not solely the disabled person.

In 1971, nearly one-half of severely disabled men and three-quarters of severely disabled women received no benefits from the U.S. disability benefits system. Most non-applicants were aware of the programs, but did not apply for benefits, presumably because of the social stigma surrounding the recipients of benefits. These non-beneficiaries often relied on the wages and transfer income of other members of the household, so that the household ended up bearing the total costs of disability.

In addition to the partial coverage of the disability benefits system, the system also supplies

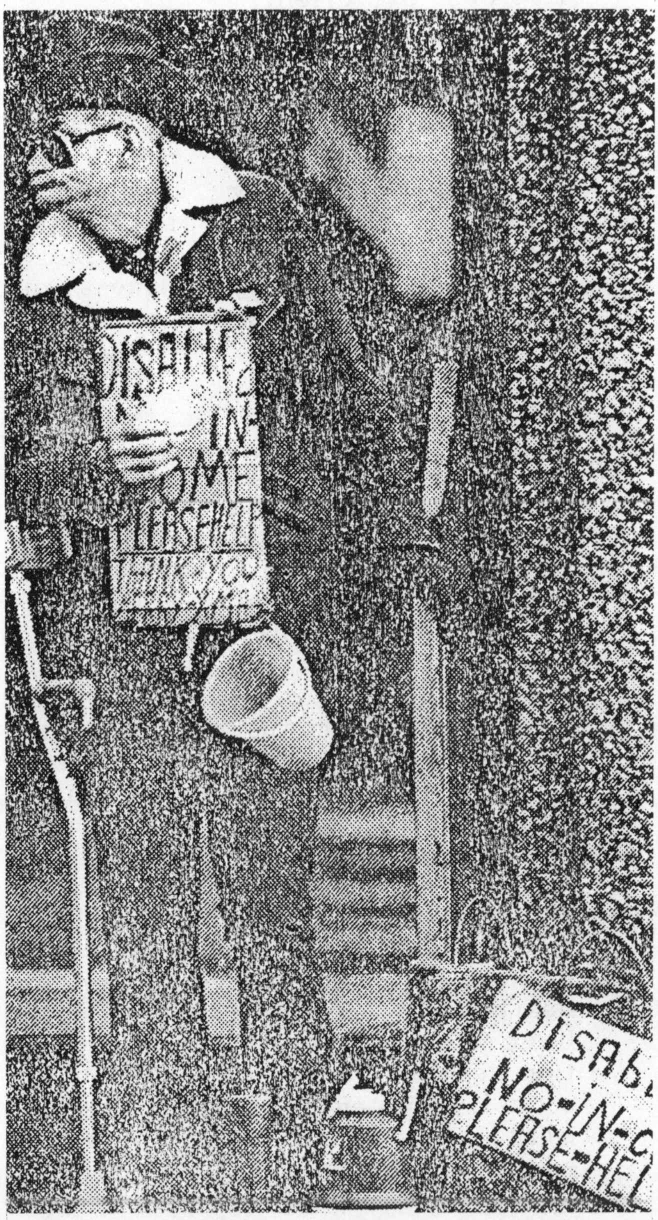

multiple benefits. "Thirty percent of severely disabled men and 18 percent of the women who received disability benefit system transfers did so from more than one program." Disparity in the treatment of women and men under the benefits systems is marked by the predominance of public assistance transfers to women.

Given the substantial degree of overlap in the provision of disability benefits to non-institutionalized disabled persons in the United States, substantial economies can be realized by program consolidation. It is possible to shift clients to the program with the minimum average administrative cost per client.

An ideal income maintenance program would feature three objectives: incentives for persons to undertake activities that are risky but socially beneficial; minimize the chance of illness, injury or disability; and minimize the costs of injury, illness or disability when they occur.

Simkins, Jean and Vincent Tickner. <u>Whose Benefit?</u> London: The Economist Intelligence Unit, 1978.

This study examines the "existing system of cash benefits and related provisions for intrinsically handicapped adults and their families in the United Kingdom." This system of benefits is a result of piecemeal legislation that has been based on a mixture of the principles of insurance, relief of destitution, and compensation. Under the insurance principle, the central feature of the social security system in the U.K., payment is made out of income while employed and benefits are paid as of right in the event of unemployment or sickness. Yet "while the insurance principle may work for a community as a whole, ability to draw benefits from the system depends on fitness for work and employment, two conditions often denied to disabled people."

The principle of the relief of destitution, consolidated under the Poor Laws in 1601, was designed to relieve poverty and

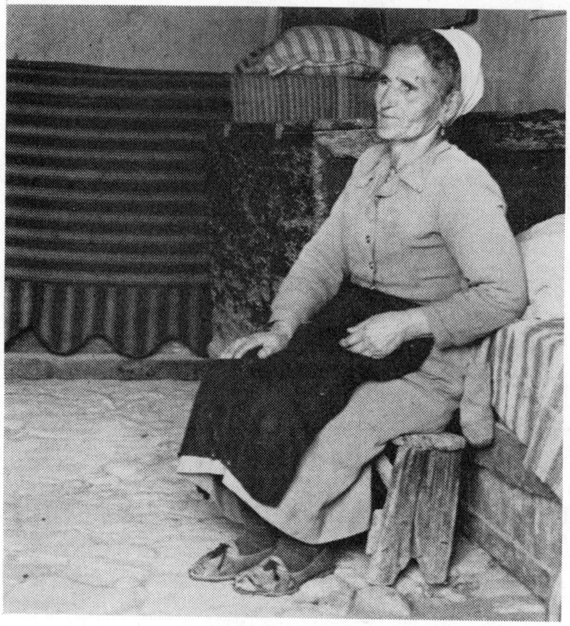

became an integral part of the Social Security system. Along with this principle was the compensatory principle - the obligation to compensate all those disabled due to defense of the country. Given these principles, there is no basis for payment <u>as of right</u> in respect of disability, unless due to war, injury at work, or prescribed industrial disease. In short, these principles do not apply to large groups of disabled people.

The many changes in provisions for disabled people have involved changes in the rates of benefit, rather than the development of a logical long-term policy. Efforts are often concentrated on controlling the rising cost of the benefit schemes, rather than the reform of the systems. Some individuals receive higher levels of benefits than others with the same disability, because of their eligibility for different systems of benefit according to where, how, and under what circumstances their disablement occurred. Even when local authorities agree on eligibility, the benefits are usually inadequate both in real terms and in money terms. The growing involvement of local authorities has resulted in a large increase of means-tested benefits (local authorities now administer over 40 different types), payment scales, and criteria for services and benefits.

As a result of the overlaps in the administration of disability payments, services, rebates, and allowances, the availability of benefits to a disabled person often depends on the "policy and pocket of the local authority." The structure of rights and benefits for disabled people has become so complex and confused that full time professionals have been created to interpret the system. "Cost and manpower usage have soared, and a new dependence on someone to guide them through the maze, rather than independence has been the result for handicapped people." The take-up of benefits and services is an important indicator of the effectiveness of a benefits system; yet because of factors such as ignorance of the existence of a benefit, severity of disability which limits mobility, and application forms oriented more to the needs of administrators than client needs, many disabled people remain impoverished. "It has on occasion seemed to be a deliberate policy to avoid efforts to achieve good take-up in order to avoid the consequent cost and associated budgetary embarrassment."

5.3 The Estimated Administration Costs of Benefits and Services For Adults With Disabilities, 1975/76

Benefit	Administration Costs as % of Total Net Expenditure on Benefits	Total Administration[1] (L million)	.Administration. Costs of Benefits Received by People with Disabilities (L million)
National Insurance Benefits	4.0	270-290	22-25
Industrial Injury Benefit Industrial Disablement Pension	10.3	22-25	22-25
War Disablement Pensions	4.2	6-7.5	6-7.5
Family Income Supplement	7.1	1	0.07
Supplementary Benefits	11.8	190	15-35 (minimum) 45-60 (probably)
Adaptations[2]	45.0	0.14-0.15	0.14-0.15
Rent Rebates[2]	6.1-6.5	7.5-8.5	n.a.
Rent Allowances[2]	11.6-16.0	2.8-3.5	n.a.
Holidays[2]	11.0	0.31-0.32	0.11-0.12
Day-care centres--Younger physically Handicapped Centres[2]	12.8	1.18-1.20	1.18-1.20
Meals-on-wheels[2]	17.5	n.a.	n.a.
Home Help Service[2]	10.5	9.85-1.00	8.88-9.50
Residential accomodation for handicapped adults[2]	13.1	1.61-1.65	1.61-1.65
Aids[2]	43.9	0.94-0.95	0.94-0.95

[1] Including overhead and central establishment charges for local authority personal social services

[2] England and Wales only

Source: EIU estimates, in Jean Simkins and Vincent Tickner, Whose Benefit?, 1978.

The costs of administration of this multiple-outlet benefits system are usually limited to personnel, salaries, and travelling time. Neglected are: the costs of administering the system for the administrators, the costs of administering the system to the potential recipients, the costs to both of duplicating assessment procedures, and the costs of providing benefits and services that are considered acceptable by the providing agency but which are unwanted by the client.

"In 1975, it was estimated that the central government expenditure on the administration of social security and miscellaneous services for the year ending 31 March 1977 would be L 424 million (at 1975 prices), compared with L 381 million for 1974/75, L 289 million for 1973/74 and L 120 million for 1966/67...In 1976/77 these administrative costs would be in the ratio of 1:22.6 with the cost of the benefits, compared with ratios of 1:17.8 in 1974/75, 1:18.8 in 1973/74, and 1:21.1 in 1966/67."

There are also costs to the client of using the system, including the time spent in finding out about benefits and services, applying, being assessed, attempting to correct errors on the part of the administration, obtaining medical evidence and collecting payments. Besides the direct costs, there are the opportunity costs associated with the time used by clients to obtain benefits and services, and the loss of income from spending this time. "The purely administrative element in the cost of dealing with an application for an aid averages L 13; the total cost of such waste due to inappropriate aids, services, and associated travel costs, could be as high as L 3.5 million (1976 prices) each year."

Mendelson, M. The Administrative Cost of Income Security Programs: Ontario and Canada. Toronto: Ontario Economic Council, 1979.

It is often thought that "a large part of the budget for income security programs is spent to pay bureaucrats rather than recipients." This paper analyzes the administrative costs of six income security programs in Canada: unemployment insurance, old age programs, and family allowances on the federal level, and provincial allowances, municipal allowances and workmen's compensation at the provincial level.

5.4
Administrative Cost as a Percentage of Total Costs (Current Dollars)

Summary of Programs

Program/Years	Mean (%)	Direction
Provincial allowances		
1960-1 - 1972-3	5.5	
1961-2 - 1966-7	6.7	None
1967-8 - 1972-3	4.2	None
Workmen's compensation (Schedules 1 & 2)		
1960 - 76	8.0	Decreasing
1960 - 65	8.9	Decreasing
1966 - 74	7.4	None
1975 and 1976	8.2	
Municipal allowances		
1964-5 - 1975-6	10.3	
1964-5 - 1971-2	8.9	None
1972-3 - 1975-6	13.2	None
Unemployment insurance		
1965-6 - 1975-6	8.9	Decreasing
1965-6 - 1971-2	10.4	Decreasing
1972-3 - 1975-6	6.3	
Old age programs		
1971-2 - 1976-7	0.43	None
Family allowance		
1971-2 - 1976-7	0.75	

Note: the mean is the average percentage of administrative costs over total costs for the period.

Adapted from M. Mendelson, The Administration Cost of Income Security Programs: Ontario and Canada, 1979.

"The distribution of supplementary benefits will always be labour-intensive so long as officials have to assess the eligibility of claimants. For every £8 paid out in benefit in 1979, it cost £1 in staff." *The Economist, September 20, 1980.*

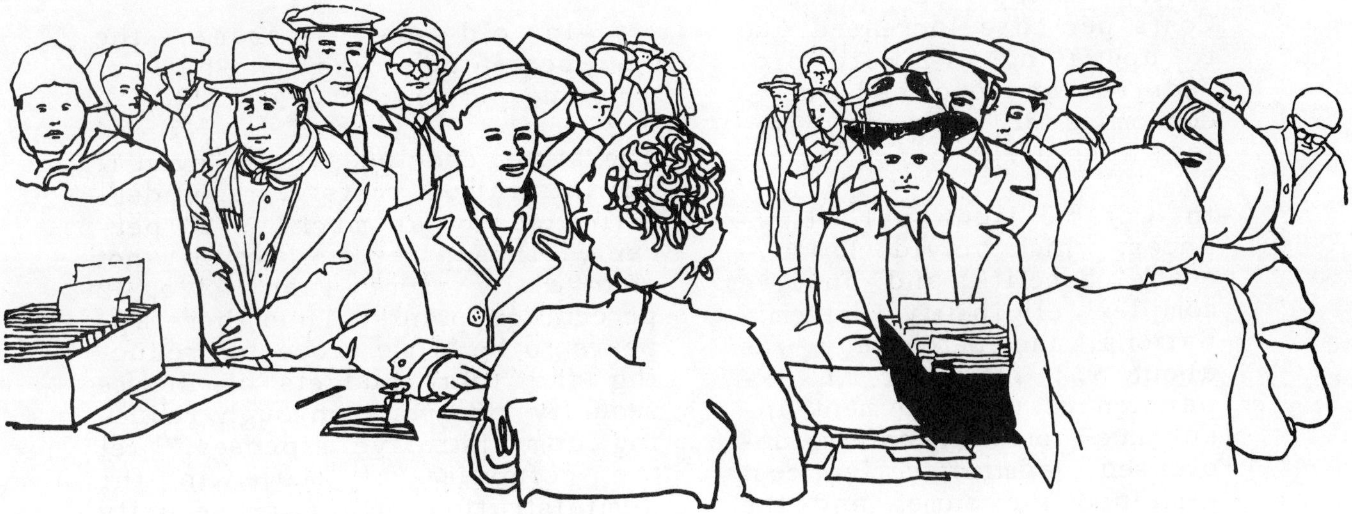

A simple measure of the cost of administration compared to the costs of the income security program is administrative costs as a percentage of total program costs (transfer payments plus administrative costs). Yet this simple measure does not assess whether the costs of administration have been increasing in relation to the size of the program. A change in percentage of administrative cost could be the result in an increase in program benefits, which automatically reduces the relative costs of administration.

An additional measure is that of administrative cost per case or caseload, measured according to stock (the average number of persons enrolled) or according to flow (the average number of persons enrolling in a given period). In addition to caseload measures, the design of the program, complexity of cases and the technical efficiency of administration also affect administrative cost.

When a program features heavy turnover of clients, flow estimates must be used; if there is little turnover, stock estimates are the best measure. In order to determine cost trends within each program, it is necessary to adjust the dollar cost for any year to constant dollars of a given year (indexing). This corrects for inflation and reflects the dollars as equivalent purchasing power. The index is derived from calculation of the increase in the labor and non-labor components of the costs of administration. Since labor accounted for 70-80 percent of these costs, the index is weighted accordingly in favor of the rate of increase in labor costs.

Using this methodology, the study found that "in general, administrative costs <u>both</u> per case and as a percentage of total costs have either remained constant or decreased in the absence of program change." The administrative costs as a percentage of total costs in each program were as follows:

- in the provincial allowance programs, which are almost entirely means-tested, the percentage remained below 5 percent in the last six years of the study, and did not exceed 7.2 percent;

-in the workmen's compensation program, with complex eligibility determinations, the percentage was consistently below 10 percent. Costs per case increased due to upgrading of award procedures, and declined due to economies of scale as caseload increased;

-in Ontario municipal allowances, which provide low average benefits and involve complex eligibility determinations, the percentage was about 9%; following an expansion of unemployment insurance total transfers decreased, administrative cost remained the same, and the ratio increased to over 13%;

-in unemployment insurance, the percentage decreased during 1965-73, largely due to increased benefits, and then remained stable at 6 percent;

-in old age programs, the percentage was one-half of one percent.

The study concludes that "even if administration costs were underestimated by as much as 20 percent, these results would not change by more than 1 or 2 percentage points. Thus there appears to be little scope for reducing the total budgets of income security programs through reducing administrative expenses." Yet the economies of scale in the administration of income security programs are seen to be significant and cost saving may be possible through centralizing decentralized programs.

D. DEPENDENCY SPENDING AND DISINCENTIVES TO REHABILITATION

As social insurance and welfare schemes have been introduced in different countries, a pattern of their increasing use has been established with time. Thus, for example, from the outset of implementation of a national disability pension system in Norway in 1962 until the end of 1971, the percentage of total population receiving disability pensions rose from 1.84 percent to 3.65 percent. Follow-up studies of 500 clients at the State Rehabilitation Institute from 1956 to 1967 indicated that the group of disabled people regularly employed remained relatively stable during that period at approximately 65 percent of the total group. There was a measurable shift in percentage between the disabled clients whose vocational adjustment was judged to be uncertain, and the group receiving disability pensions. In 1956 the two groups were approximately equal; by 1967, almost 30 percent of the Institute's clients were pension recipients and 7 percent were classified as "vocational adjustment uncertain". 72/

A similar pattern has been reported in other countries. Data from Poland show that in 1961 disability pensions made up 39.1 percent of the total number of pensions paid, and in 1965 40.3 percent of the total. This growth rate, while possibly not statistically significant, exceeded the rate of increase in the number of old-age pensions. It was estimated that the expenditure resulting from the increase in disability pensions was about 25.5 million zlotys per year. 73/

The Norwegian disabled group demonstrated in a follow-up study that the majority of those persons who had been dependent upon their families before the national disability pensions system was instituted had changed to being dependent upon pensions. In general there were three main types of dependency established: dependency upon family, dependency upon disability pensions, and dependency upon public assistance. The dependency upon public assistance tended to become a lasting pattern the longer the individual remained non-productive. The researchers did not find that persons in this dependent group could be categorized as conscious exploiters of society; they were on the contrary almost apologetic as a group for their existence. As for the other two types of dependent groups, many of the disabled living with family members did contribute to the household economy by work in the home or on the farm, and many recipients of social insurance benefits did engage in part-time or seasonal work but not in sufficient degree to lose the right to collect benefits. Thus, the study had as one of its observations that:

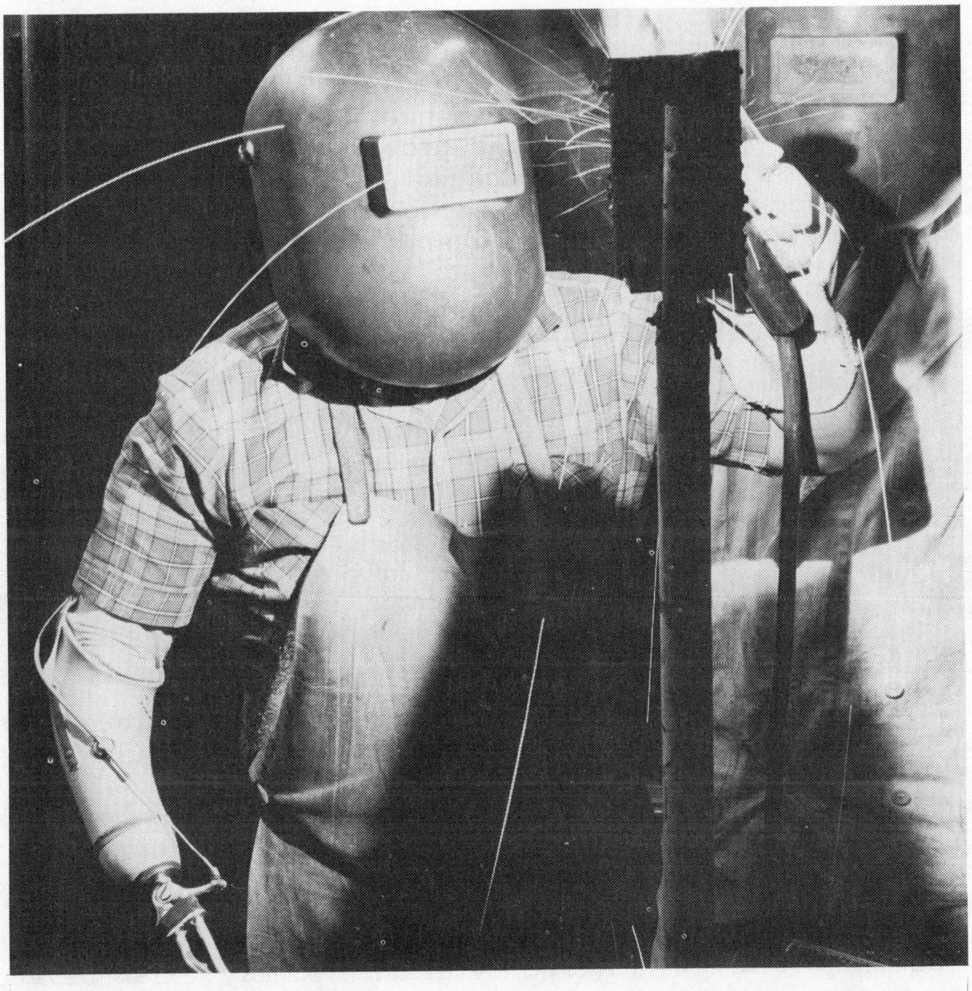

"Seven in ten of the disabled will be vocationally active. This group seems not to be influenced by a disability pension system giving fairly high coverage of ordinary income. Three in ten of the disabled do not work or seem to be poorly adjusted to work. This group is greatly influenced. Some of them obtain an economic basis they had never had (or wanted to ask for through public assistance). Some of them probably stop working. Some get their pension and go on working occasionally or working part-time, and thus get a better income." 74/

Researchers in Denmark in 1964 analyzed the various components of work activity in the normal working environment, and developed a classification scheme for the tasks involved. 75/ They then compared these tasks to the capabilities of physically handicapped people in Denmark, and concluded that the vast majority did not have impairments which significantly affect their vocational possibilities. This was found to be true with the exception of people having impairments of several physical functions, and people for whom the physical impairment was combined with psychological or social complications.

In 1965 the Danish National Institute for Social Research surveyed a representative sample of all physically handicapped people in Denmark in the 15-61 year old age groups, inclusive. Eighty percent of the 86,000 physically handicapped men were gainfully occupied and self-supporting. The majority of these people would have been entitled to disability pensions were it not for their own efforts to overcome vocational limitations. Fifteen percent of those employed had made a complete change of occupation, 14 percent worked part-time and 11 percent worked in the same occupation but had changed their working functions. Most of the handicapped were reported to have achieved the necessary adjustments themselves without substantial support from official bodies. A similar picture was provided by the women surveyed. One-third were employed, as compared to the somewhat more than one-half of all working-age women employed at that time, and most of the disabled women without paying jobs were married and fulfilling the functions of a housewife. At the time of the study the disabled in

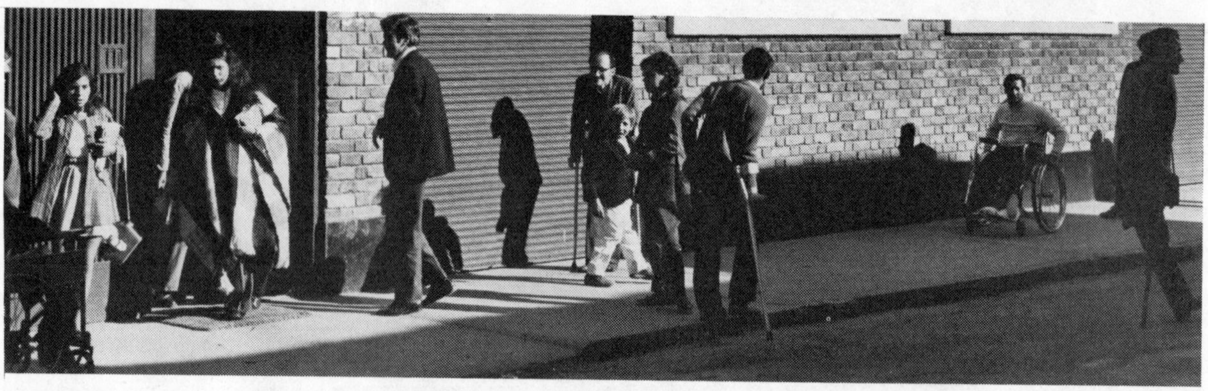

Denmark could have received almost the same amount of income through disability pensions coupled with part-time work as could be earned through full-time employment in industry. Very few people took advantage of this; the study demonstrated that the physically handicapped who could work in normal industry on equal terms with other employees preferred this course even when the economic gain was not markedly different than through receipt of a pension.

Summing up, an adverse relationship may exist between the success of rehabilitation efforts, and the provision of social benefits such as pensions, when the provision of benefits is linked to demonstration of incapacity and inability to become a productive member of society. In such circumstances, the result may be that the more successful a disabled person is within the rehabilitation process, the less likely he or she will be to receive the social benefits which permit continuation of the process, since these benefits are linked to incapacity rather than success. This, in turn, may lead to a loss in motivation to succeed in the rehabilitation process.

Additional References on Dependency Spending and Disincentives to Rehabilitation:

Better, Sybil R., et. al. "Disability Benefits as Disincentives to Rehabilitation," Milbank Memorial Fund Quarterly/Health and Society, Volume 57, #3, 1979, pp. 412-427.

"A complex relation exists among disability, disability-related benefits, and rehabilitation... In addition to income supplements, disabled individuals and/or their families in the U.S. may be eligible to receive assistance with food, health care, housing, education, employment, and training. The monetary value of such benefits may be substantial, occasionally exceeding the individuals' predisability earnings." Benefits that are tied to persisting health problems and associated unemployment may reduce the incentive to resume working.

Empirical evidence relating to the disincentive effect of disability-related benefits is unclear. Even if disability benefits were found to be consistently associated with a reduced likelihood of rehabilitation, the failure of beneficiaries to complete vocational rchabilitation may result primarily from functional limitations arising from the severity of the disability, rather than a desire to maintain disability benefits.

This study measures the disincentive effect of disability-related benefits by comparing the success rates of vocational rehabilitation clients who were receiving Social Security Insurance (SSI) and/or Social Security Disability Insurance (SSDI) benefits with clients not receiving such benefits. Two measures of rehabilitation outcome were used: the proportion of clients rehabilitated by state vocational rehabilitation agencies, and their work status at the time of closure. Rehabilitated clients were defined as those who had completed a rehabilitation program and worked successfully for a period of two months in the competitive labor market, in sheltered workshops, in self-employment, or functioned as homemakers or unpaid family workers.

Rehabilitation rates for beneficiaries and non-beneficiaries were calculated and compared. The likelihood of a successful rehabilitation was then determined for a sample of severely disabled beneficiaries and non-beneficiaries, since most SSI and SSDI benefits are eligible only to the severely disabled. Without this group or subset, the disincentive effect of disability-related benefits would be greatly overestimated.

The study found that SSI and SSDI beneficiaries were less likely to be rehabilitated than were non-beneficiaries. It revealed that severity of disability failed to account for observed differences in the corresponding rehabilitation rates.

5.5
Vocational Rehabilitation Outcome at Closure, By Beneficiary Status of Clients

Client Group	Clients Rehabilitated: Number	Percent
Beneficiaries*	7,343	55.6
Nonbeneficiaries*	54,911	71.4
Severely disabled beneficiaries**	7,106	55.7
Severely disabled nonbeneficiaries**	14,727	71.0

*A 15 percent random sample of FY 1975 vocational rehabilitation agency closures nationwide (n = 62,254).

**A subset of severely disabled clients included in the 15 percent sample (n = 21,833).

Source: Sybil R. Better, et. al. "Disability Benefits as Disincentives to Rehabilitation," 1979.

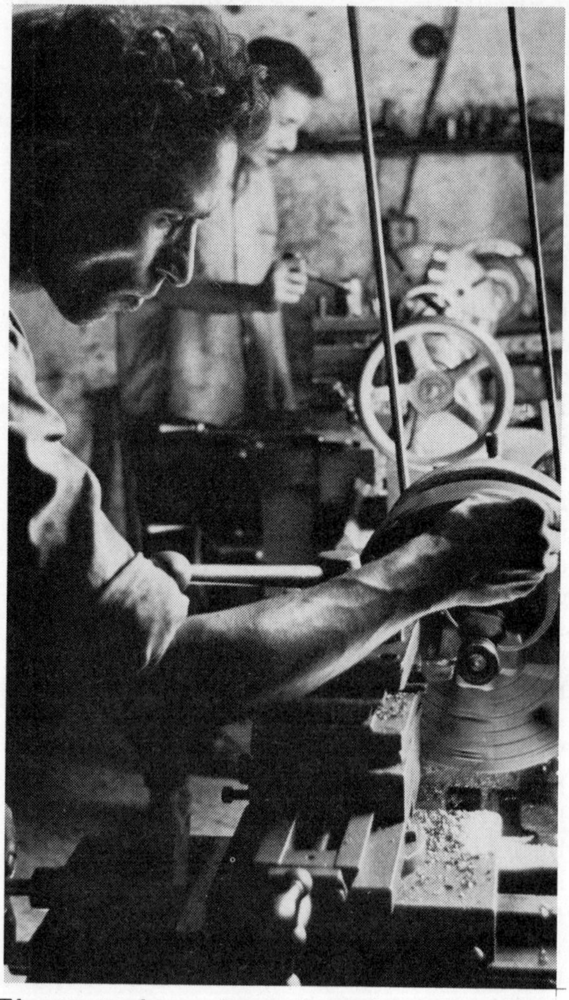

The study also found that the degree to which beneficiary status serves as a disincentive is also a function of client age and sex. Beneficiary status seemed to be more of a disincentive for men than for women, as well as for clients aged 30-45 years. Beneficiary status also affects rehabilitation outcome as measured by "work status at closure." At closure, beneficiaries were less likely to be gainfully employed. Among those in the labor force, 31% were employed in sheltered setting, and 47% in the competitive labor market. Comparable figures for non-beneficiaries and the severely disabled were 83% and 66% respectively.

Although a beneficiary who rejoins the work force may find that gross earnings substantially exceed benefits, the disparity between net earnings and benefits will be much less. Substantial work-related expenses, disqualification from Medicare (government provided medical care) and other benefits, may leave the disabled individual worse off than before employment began.

In sum, "the relation between disability benefits and rehabilitation outcome is not a simple cause and effect relation, but is influenced by a myriad of factors, including the state of the labor market and the willingness of employers to hire the disabled."

Treitel, Ralph. "Recovery of Disabled Beneficiaries: A 1975 Followup Study of 1972 Allowances," Social Security Bulletin, #4 April 1979, pp. 3-23.

This study reveals an increase in the number of persons awarded disabled workers benefits in recent years, but found no corresponding rise in the number of workers leaving the benefit rolls following rehabilitation. A comparative analysis was done of the demographic, disability, and benefit characteristics of a sample of disabled workers awarded benefits in 1972 who left the system of benefits for recovery, and the characteristics of those who remained on disability benefits. Recovery appeared unlikely for most beneficiaries, though the younger and more educated disabled workers, and those disabled by injuries, had better rates of successful rehabilitation. The level of earnings replacement--the extent to which earnings replaced benefits--appeared to have little independent effect on recovery.

Berkowitz, Monroe. Work Disincentives. Falls Church, Virginia: Institute for Information Studies, 1980.

This paper "brings together what is known about the general subject of disincentives to the rehabilitation of disabled persons and to explore the policy alternatives which may ease the disincentive problem."

Benefit programs provide income to disabled persons only if they are not employed. Benefit programs therefore may cause disabled recipients to refrain from work, making the benefit, and not the physical or mental condition alone, responsible for withdrawal from the labor market.

Functional limitations, the restrictions in activity which result from impairments, in combination with individual human resource endowment, cause withdrawal from the labor market. Education, training, on the job experience, a nd such demographic characteristics as sex and age may influence an individual's decision to enter the work force. Labor market opportunities, or lack thereof, together with the chance to receive non-employment income, may also be influential in the decision-making process.

In the United States, the principle social insurance program in the field of disability is the workplace-based DI (disability Income) program which represented a public expenditure of $11.5 billion in 1977. The principle income support program is the Supplemental Security Income (SSI) program, utilizing the same disability eligibility requirements and a needs test. Total SSI payments in 1977 were $3.4 billion.

The Disability Income and Supplemental Security Income programs both require effective withdrawal from the work force as a condition for receipt of benefits. Some minimal earnings are permitted, but receipt of income above the Substantial Gainful Activity (SGA) levels, currently set at level of $260/month, will result in the person being cut off the benefits rolls. If it is decided that he or she is able to earn or in fact does earn at a level greater than the SGA dollar limit set, eligibility for receipt of DI payments is terminated.

5.6
CALCULATION OF SSI BENEFITS AND COUNTABLE INCOME, SSI BENEFITS OF $189 a MONTH FOR A SINGLE INDIVIDUAL

Earnings	Countable Income	SSI Benefits Less Countable Income	Total Income Earnings Plus SSI Benefits
$100	$ 7.50	$181.50	$281.50
$200	$57.50	$131.50	$331.50
$259	$87.00	$102.00	$361.00
$260	--	--	$260.00

Source: Monroe Berkowitz, Work Disincentives, 1980.

A preliminary look at disincentive issues according to these rules: "Assume that an individual is entitled to the federal SSI benefit of $189 per month, has no unearned income, but earns $100 per month in the labor market. The first $85 of earned income is exempt leaving 50 percent of $15, or $7.50 as countable income. That $7.50 will be deducted from $189 in SSI benefits resulting in a monthly benefit of $181.50. That benefit combined with $100 of earned income results in total income, including SSI benefits, of $281.50. If the individual's earned income doubled to $200 per month, SSI benefit would be reduced by an additional $50 to $131.50 and total income would be $331.50. However, should earnings equal or exceed the SGA limit of $260 per month for a period which exceeds a nine month trial work period, total income would be reduced abruptly to $260 since all SSI benefits would be forfeit."

"Termination rates from the beneficiary rolls increase with increases in the wage-benefit ratio... Once the benefit ratio equals or exceeds 1, the rate of termination increases dramatically. The conclusion is that it is not enough to rehabilitate a person; she/he must also be capable of earning a wage that is greater than the Substantial Gainful Activity level but also equal to, or greater than, his/her individual monthly benefit payments. The rehabilitation counselor who fails to close out cases at wages comparable to benefit levels is fighting a losing battle if the objective is termination from beneficiary rolls."

"The obvious method for reducing work and termination disincentives is to increase the wage benefit ratio. Although that could be achieved by lowering benefits, the opposition would be great on equity grounds. Improving the wages can be achieved by liberalizing the provision of the trial work period, by improving the performance of rehabilitation counselors, and by a long term strategy of making the labor market more receptive to the rehabilitated population."

5.7 **Wage/Benefit Ratio and the Rate of Termination**

Wage/ Benefit Ratio	Category Total[1]	Nonterminations	Terminations	Rate of Terminations
0.00-0.25	2,342 (27.9)	2,239	103	4.4
0.25-0.50	525 (6.3)	452	73	13.9
0.51-0.75	463 (5.5)	360	103	22.2
0.76-1.00	513 (6.1)	305	208	40.5
1.01-1.25	511 (6.1)	252	259	50.7
1.26-1.50	506 (6.0)	235	271	53.6
1.51-1.75	468 (5.6)	179	289	61.8
1.76-2.00	365 (4.4)	129	236	64.7
Greater than 2.00	1,653 (19.7)	503	1,150	69.6
Insufficient data	1,040 (12.4)	794	246	23.7
	8,386 (100.0)	5,448 (65.0)	2,938 (35.0)	

[1]Percentage figures are in parenthesis

Monroe Berkowitz, 1980.

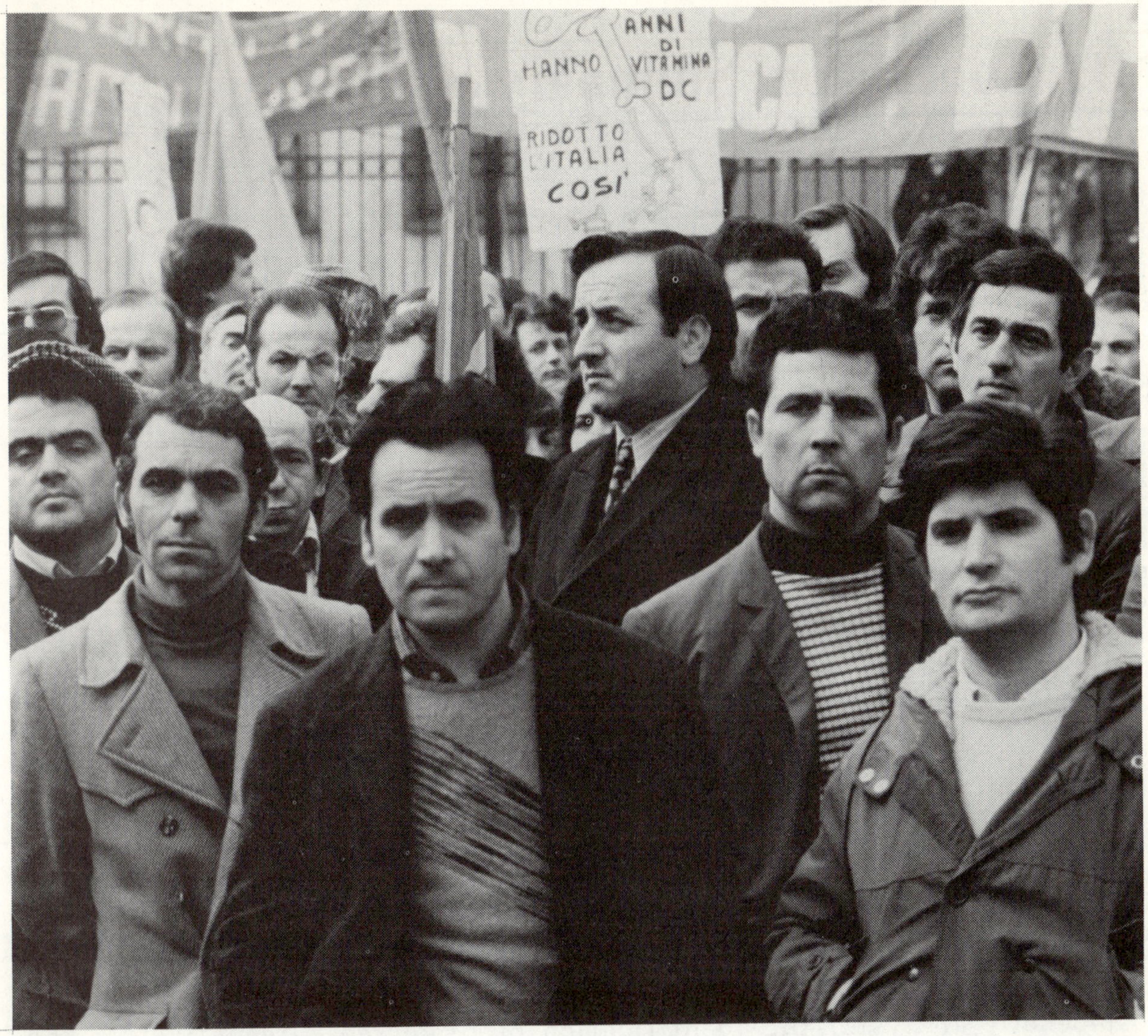

Franklin, P.A. and J.C. Hennessey. "Effect of Substantial Gainful Activity Level on Disabled Beneficiary Work Patterns", Social Security Bulletin, #3 March 1979, pp. 3-17

An examination of disabled beneficiaries earnings records over a 15-year period indicated that increases in the substantial gainful activity (SGA) level in 1966, 1968, and 1974 were not followed by incremental increases in beneficiary earnings. The recovery rate of disabled worker beneficiaries dropped steadily during the late 1960's and early 1970's. The earnings pattern indicates that about 10 percent of the beneficiaries were employed, and about 3 percent had earnings above the SGA level. Median annual earnings remained well below $1,000, whatever the SGA level. Findings of the study suggest that policy considerations on changing the SGA level should not center on the implications for marginal part-time employment. Most of the evidence from beneficiary work and earnings patterns indicates that the SGA level has not operated as an effective work incentive. The study findings suggest that a gradual earnings allowance process rather than termination of benefits for recovery after sustained work is the key to controlling program growth.

VI. Conclusion: Summary of Findings

A. SUMMARY OF FINDINGS

The Need For "Socio-Economic" Development

Governments are becoming increasingly aware that economic development based upon the growth of output alone can be detrimental. The by-products of accelerated growth - pollution, waste, noise, slums and congestion - are evidence of the growing challenge to man's ability to coexist harmoniously with nature. National planners are beginning to recognize the interdependence of social and economic objectives and the fact that their linkage provides the only hope of preserving and improving the quality of life. They also recognize that inclusion of social objectives within economic development plans will not occur spontaneously and requires governmental leadership. Strategies for unified socio-economic development inclusive of social benefit schemes are increasingly being incorporated within national development plans.

Economists and social planners are collaborating in this development of integrated models for socio-economic development. As yet, effective methods do not exist for measuring the achievement of social goals. Traditionally the methods of assessment have been linked to the direct or indirect demonstration of productivity, and they have been ineffective in assessing values and gains that cannot be quantified monetarily. None-the-less, some powerful economic assessment tools do exist which have potential application to social phenomena, once their methodological and conceptual limitations are taken into account. Cost-benefit analysis, the identification of preferred alternatives on the basis of the costs and benefits possible from each alternative action, is one such tool. Each cost-benefit analysis may be undertaken from many different points of view, such as that of the individual, the social institution and society as a whole. The choice of perspective will alter the preferability of the alternatives. Economists and social scientists agree that cost-benefit analysis may be of great use but that, in the determination of policies based on alternative actions of incommensurate value, it can be only one element in the total pattern of decision making.

Social Benefit Systems and Productive Capability

Social benefit systems may be divided into two main categories: social insurance schemes, including social security systems, which are based on the contributions of one or more parties and which are available to all participating citizens on a legally defined basis, and social welfare schemes which are administered on a discretionary basis depending upon the individual's demonstration of insufficient means. The types of benefits available, the patterns of financing and the eligibility requirements of the schemes will vary from country to country depending upon the overall socio-economic conditions and the political philosophy. Social benefits are a form of transfer payment, a redistribution of the wealth of a nation. Savings in transfer payments do not represent an increase in net national income although such savings may have

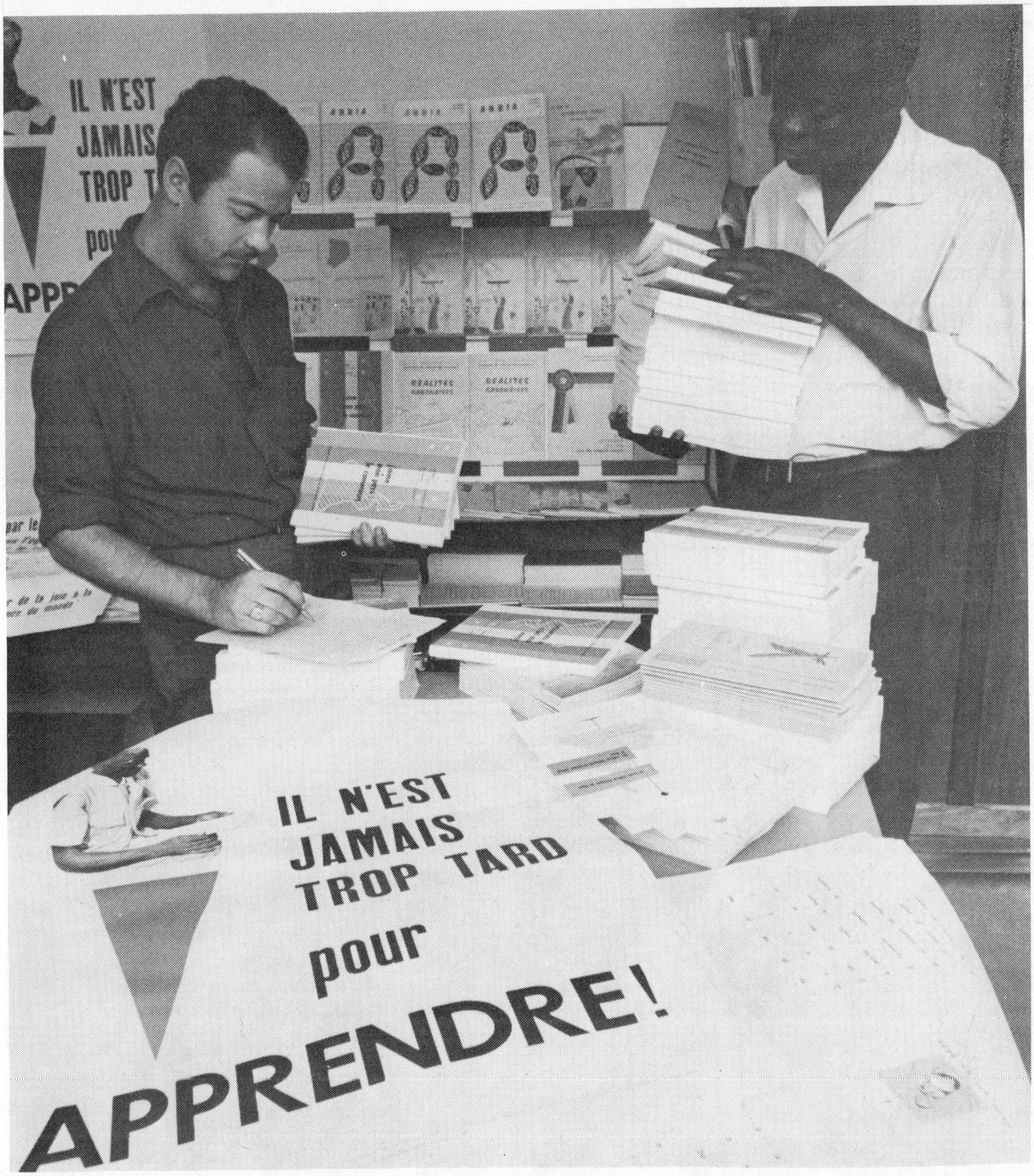

important social and political implications. It is important to recognize that savings in social benefit payments do not represent a savings to society as a whole. The only real savings to society are in the cost of benefit programs administration and these costs may be shown to be a minimal proportion of the overall cost of providing transfer payments.

Nations which have instituted comprehensive systems of social benefits and have had a sufficiently long-term experience with them to begin to assess trends in their use, have found that the utilization of available benefits by the public increases with time and that the costs of maintaining the benefit system increase exponentially. This has been attributed to such factors as growing public awareness of available benefits, increased longevity, better trained service providers and, consequently, higher service costs.

The economic process may be considered as a constant interaction of three main phases: the generation of the national product which produces income; the distribution of income to various groups--the active work force, the recipients of transfer income -- to needs designated by the Government, and the consumption of income for goods and services, and for savings and investments. Ultimately, the volume of social benefits any nation may extend to its citizens will depend upon the productive output and the character of the economically active work force.

In nations without manpower shortages, the active work force responsible for sustaining production may be only 20 to 25 per cent of the total population. As a result of technological developments and changing population characteristics, particularly the increasing number of older retired citizens in industrialized countries, nations with long-established systems of social benefits have found that there are increasingly fewer active workers to support the benefits for each recipient. Thus, for example, whereas in 1950, old-age social security benefits were financed by 5.2 active persons per benefit recipient in the Federal Republic of Germany, by 1970 the figure had declined to 3.2. In the United States, less than three workers support benefits for each recipient at present; within 50 years there will be only two contributors for each beneficiary.

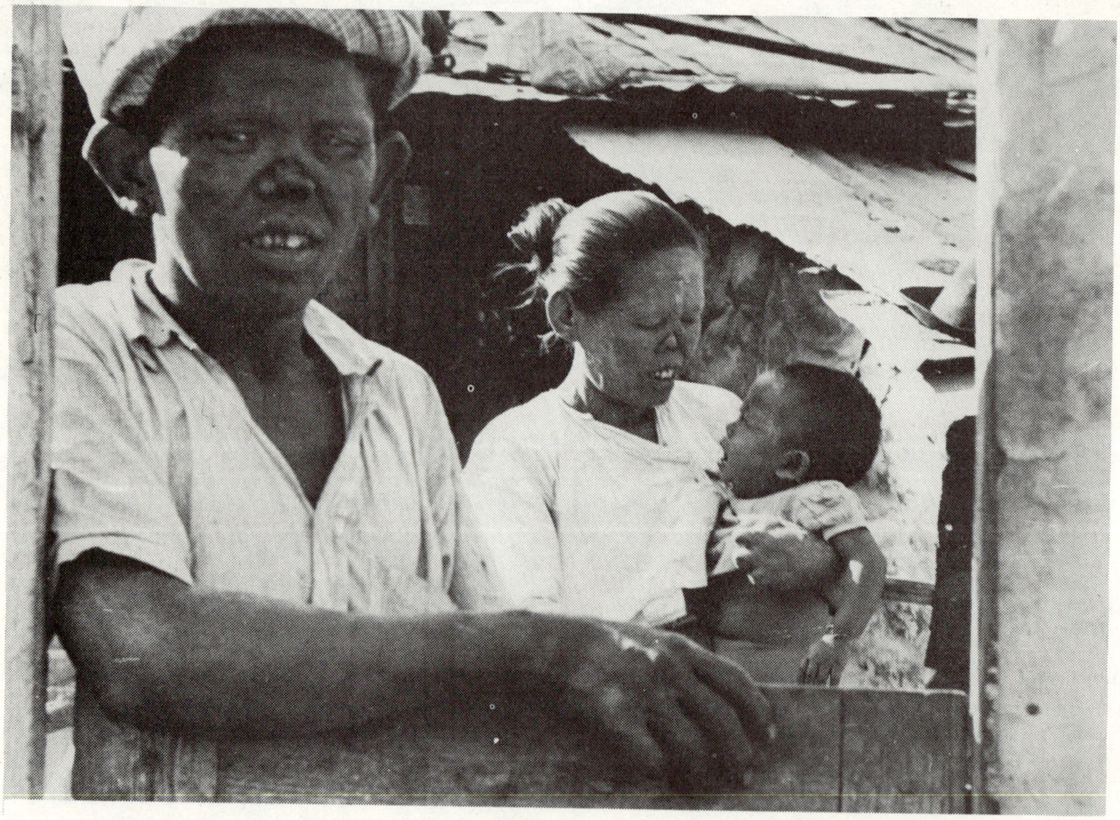

Disability can result in serious reductions in the active work force. Research has shown that disability may exist in close relationship with such significant problems as unemployment and underemployment, early retirement, non-participation in the labor force, and poverty. In addition, disabled people are at much greater risk of losing their residual working capacity because of their disability. They are less adaptable than the non-disabled and their recovery from a loss in productivity will extend over a much longer period of time. People may be considered to be "operational capital", the element in the production triad of land, labour and capital, without which production may not take place. The greater the investment in machines that are dependent upon people, and in the technical training of people, the greater is the loss associated with any reduction in the capacity of people to apply their skills and knowledge. It becomes increasingly important to preserve, maintain and generate the work capacity of all available manpower. Whereas disability can severely reduce the working capacity of a nation, rehabilitation of the disabled can provide one of the most important sources of reserve worker strength within an economy. The importance of such strength may often only become apparent as a nation moves from an economy based on a surplus of manpower to one of a shortage of manpower, or as technological changes occur.

Nations which do not as yet maintain extensive systems of social benefits but plan to establish such systems in the future must take into account the long-range relationship of disability to the base of social system support.

The Costs of Disability and the Provision of Rehabilitation Service

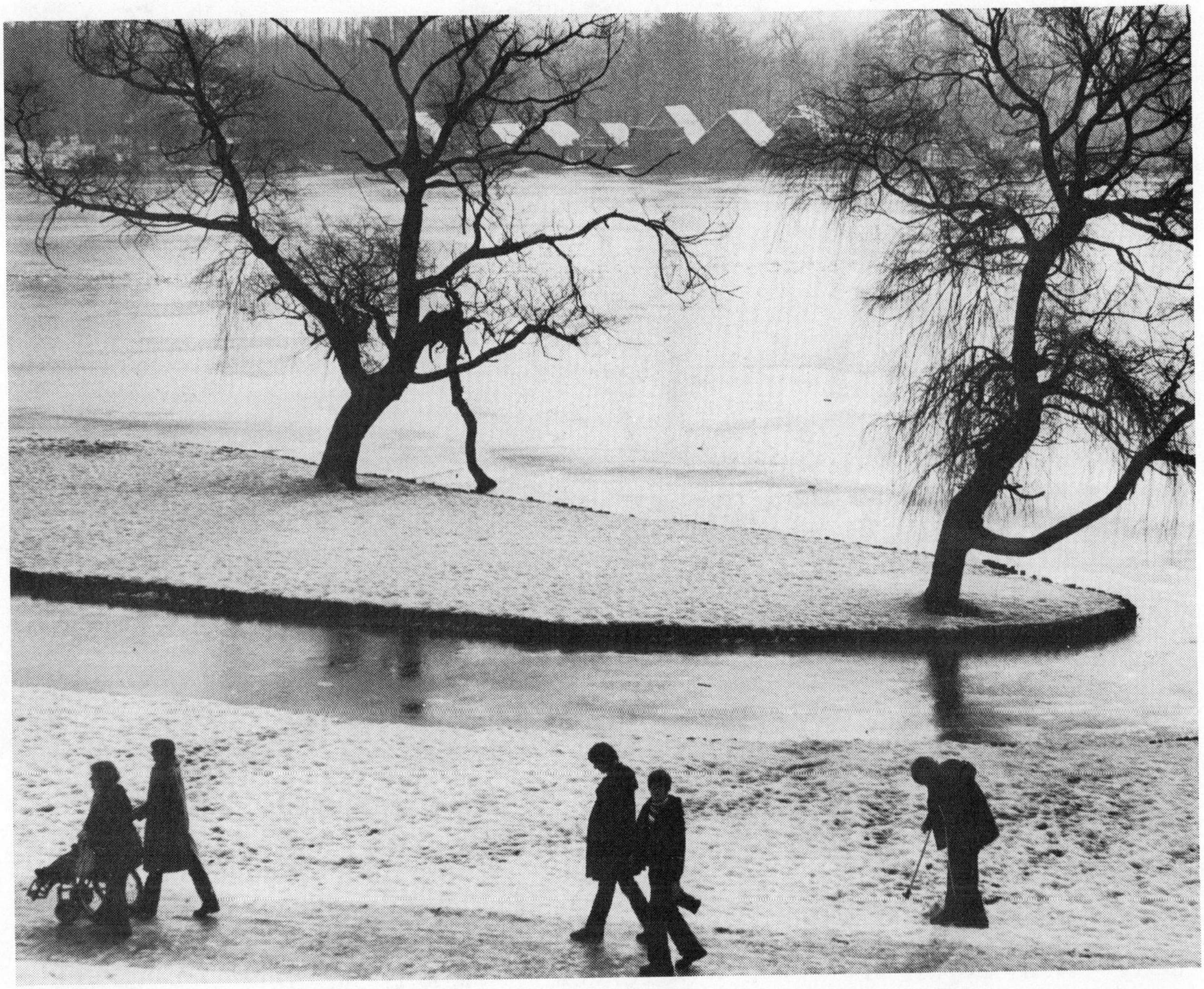

Disability may have lifelong implications for the disabled person and his or her family members and friends. Disability can reduce the capacity of the individual to function independently, to absorb education and to be productive in work. Those who must care for the disabled, particularly in the absence of comprehensive rehabilitation and care services, may experience a significant reduction in their own productive capacity. Disability may result in marital instability, family dislocation and property losses. Its effects may reach into the future to reduce the health, well-being and productive capability of children whose parents, siblings or close relatives were disabled. In general, the costs of these effects of disability are either unknown or not measurable using present techniques.

The direct costs of providing rehabilitation service are generally considered to include the expense of personnel to provide the necessary services, the capital costs of buildings, equipment and facilities, and the cost of their depreciation in value with time, and the operating expenses and overhead maintenance costs for all facilities and services. Transfer payments in the form of disability pensions, social assistance allotments, and sickness benefits are not a net cost to society since the costs to the community are offset by the gains to the disabled. They represent a redistribution of the overall wealth and as such have social and political, as opposed to economic, costs.

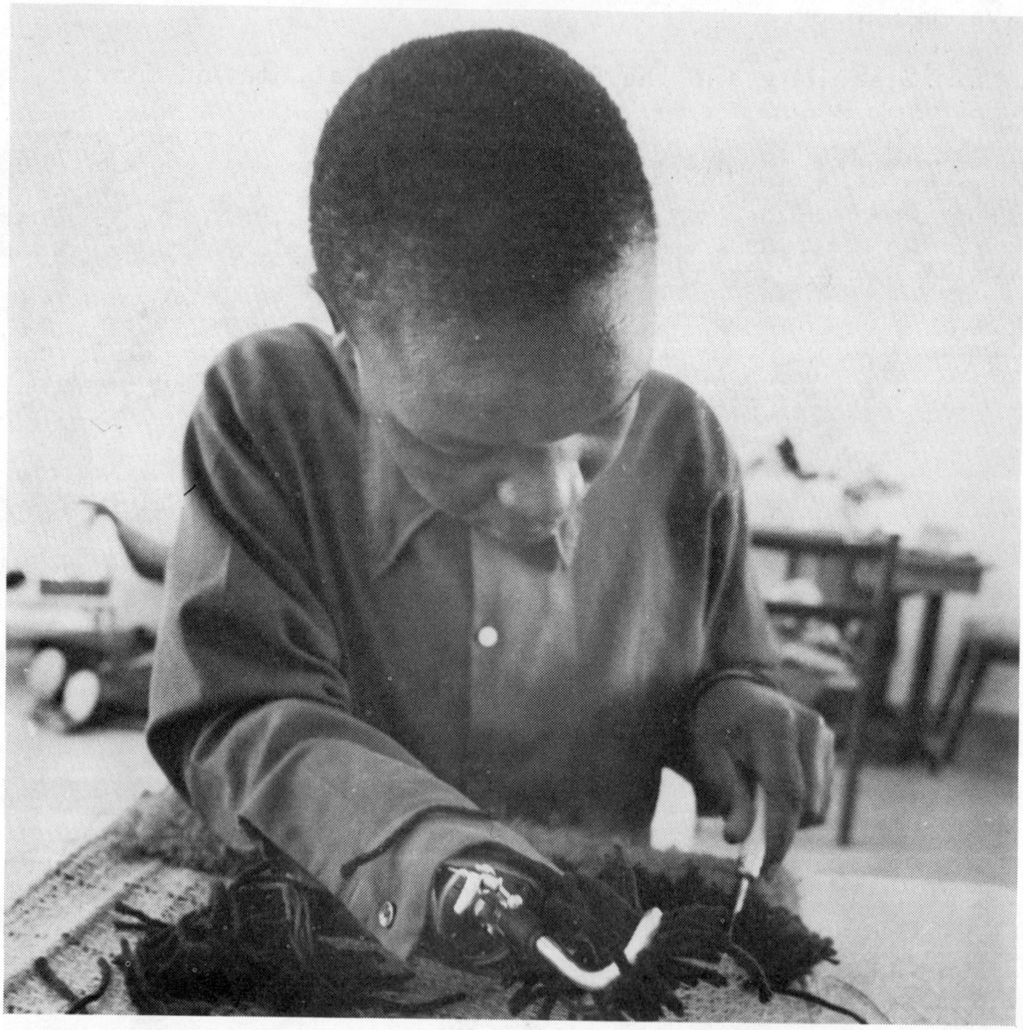

It is extremely difficult to measure the exact costs of providing rehabilitation service, just as it is most difficult to measure many other types of social service costs. This is in part due to the special nature of the rehabilitation process. Rehabilitation requires the complex interaction of disabled people, their family members and friends, with specialists from the medical, social, educational and vocational fields. All elements of the rehabilitation process are interdependent and all are utlimately linked to the removal of physical and social barriers in the community. It is extremely difficult to isolate the costs of any one element in the rehabilitation process; the costs and success of each element are dependent upon all the others.

The difficulty in measurement is also related to the prevailing system of social benefits in each nation. Disabled people, like all other people, will incur expenditures for food, clothing, shelter, education,

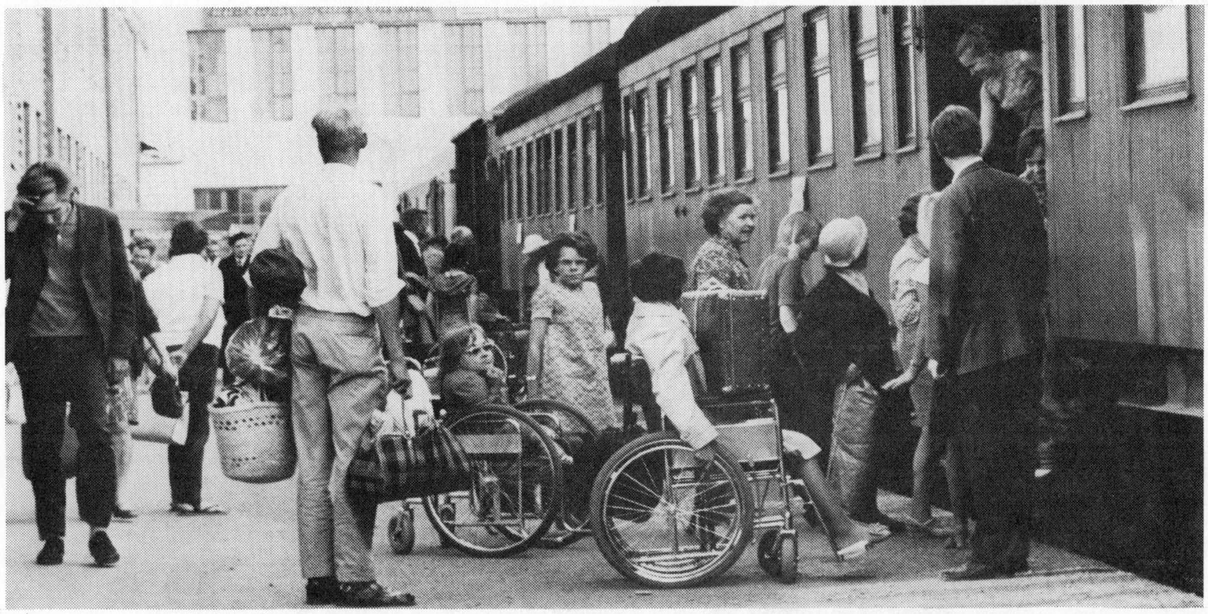

medical care, transportation, work and recreation. These expenses will exist whether or not rehabilitation services are present. The level of service costs utilized by disabled people in excess of normal consumption levels is very difficult to define. This is especially true in nations in which the State assumes responsiblity for the provision of services to meet the basic needs of all citizens, including health care, education and employment. In such circumstances, the level of generally available services will be expected to reduce the need for specialized services, and the actual costs of services to the disabled will be obscured by the general public's use of many of the same facilites. Societies which offer a range of highly specialized services for the disabled and make these available according to principles of individual choice and self-help, through a broad framework of social institutions, may demonstrate a higher overall level of cost per disabled person since the service utilization has a much narrower basis.

Neglect of the disabled also exacts an economic cost. In general, if society does not provide rehabilitation services and a sufficient system of social benefits to encompass the needs of the disabled, a transfer of initiative will occur from public authorities to private resources, such as the family or private voluntary organizations. Private initiatives may, or may not, be adequate to deal with the total disability problem. The experience in most countries, and the consequent evolution in service structure which has occurred throughout the world, indicates that major societal measures are necessary. Data do not exist on the costs to society of the transfer for the care of the disabled to private individuals and institutions which may take place when rehabilitation services in a nation are grossly inadequate.

It is possible to provide rehabilitation services at a variety of levels according to the technical and manpower resources available within each nation and region. There has not been sufficient study of the possible types of phased approaches towards the provision of rehabilitation services nor of the potential of integrated community level services to reduce service delivery costs. It is most important that the levels of expenditure based upon the experience of the past in industrialized nations not be utilized as the sole basis for prediction of the needs of the future.

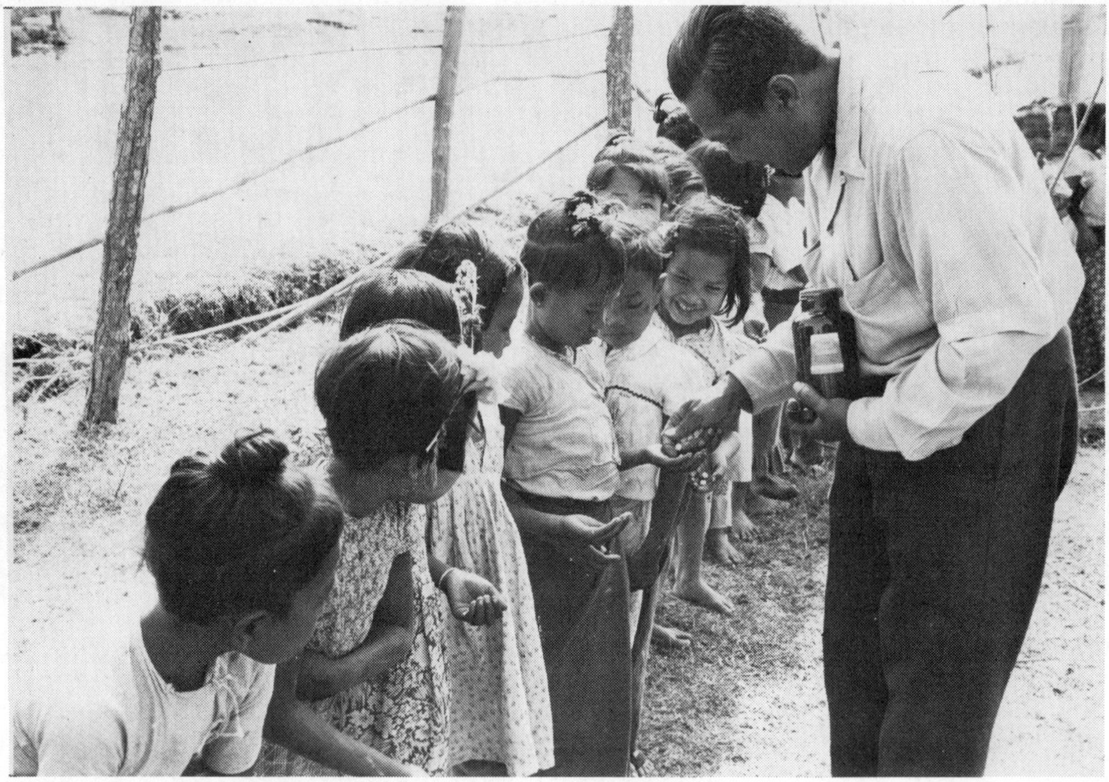

Rehabilitation and Savings in Health Care Costs

Research studies have indicated that effective implementation of rehabilitation services, through patterns of comprehensive service delivery, and early intervention and assistance, can reduce overall expenditures for health care delivery. These savings can be of significant magnitude, and may continue on a long-term basis. For example, it has been estimated that a reduction in the mean length of stay of patients in a Dublin hospital by only one day each, through the provision of rehabilitation services, could result in an annual savings of L1 million. In addition, effective rehabilitation may reduce the need for expensive services which might have been forgone. Especially dramatic savings may be demonstrated in reduced costs for institutionalization.

Production Benefits of Rehabilitation

Production benefits of rehabilitation, those benefits which add to the national output, have been demonstrated in countries representing the three main economic structures in the world: developed market economies, centrally planned economies, and developing country economies. They have been demonstrated in conditions of full employment, underemployment and unemployment, and they have been seen to be of particular importance in countries shifting from one type of manpower base to another. Countries which have recently shifted from economies based on manpower surpluses to labor scarcity or from primarily agricultural to industrially based economies fall in the latter category.

Available research studies demonstrate that it is possible to have a range of approaches towards the identification of the production benefits of rehabilitation. The approach taken and the benefits demonstrated will depend upon the structure of rehabilitation activity in each country, as well as on the entire pattern of social services and economic development. The methods, definitions and assumptions of each study become additional variables which alter the outcome.

In general, rehabilitation of the disabled can add to the national product through:

The individual disabled person, who demonstrates an increase in lifetime earnings and a decline in post-disability income loss. This effect is extended to the family of the disabled;

The rehabilitation institution, social security or social welfare agency -- which may demonstrate a reduction in transfer payments and a return of tax income to governmental bodies;

Society as a whole -- which acquires increased goods and services as a result of the productivity of disabled workers.

Additional benefits of rehabilitation may be realized through the potential reduction of national expenditures for foreign currency when locally consumed goods are produced locally. Small-scale business enterprises for disabled people in developing countries have been most useful in this regard.

Cost-Benefit Ratio

When the sum of all of the categories of production benefit is compared to the total costs of rehabilitation service provision, it is possible to demonstrate a very positive benefit to cost ratio for services for the disabled. In general the repayment to society of the costs of rehabilitation occurs over a much shorter period than the productive period of the disabled worker. A nation may thus regain the costs of its rehabilitation services through benefits such as returned tax income, reduced transfer payments and added production output, in a period of three to five years whereas the disabled worker may be productive for an average of 12 to 16 years after rehabilitation. In order to demonstrate benefits of this type, it must be assumed that society does

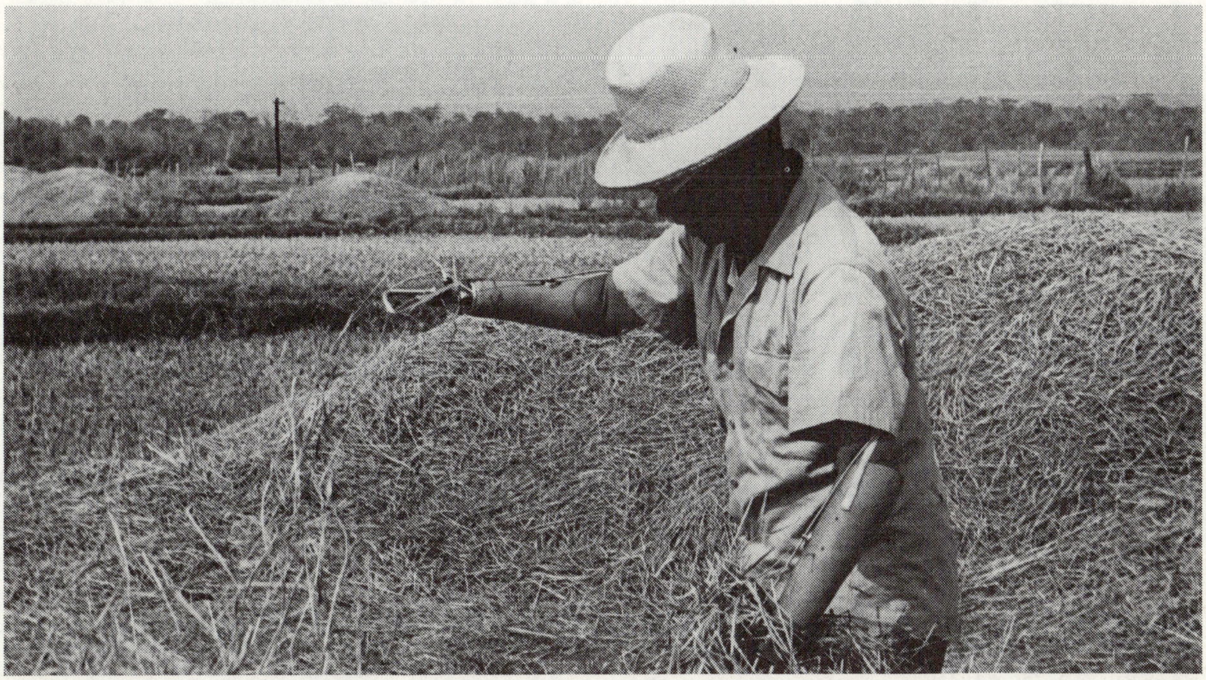

not neglect the disabled and that it is taking some actions to provide disabled people with a socially acceptable level of living. The social subsidy may take many forms, ranging from the provision of an extensive scheme for transfer payments to the availability of special privileges, incentives or monopolies, and the cost-benefit analysis must be undertaken from the perspective of everyone in society other than that of the disabled and their families.

Rehabilitation and the Social Benefits System

It is possible to demonstrate significant reductions in disability pension and public assistance payments to disabled people who, as a result of the provision of rehabilitation services, re-enter the labor force and are no longer dependent upon public funds for their livelihood. As in the case of production benefits, it is possible to demonstrate that these savings in social benefit expenditures can repay the costs of rehabilitation service in a relatively short period of time compared to the overall period of anticipated productivity for each rehabilitant.

The large majority of disabled people are economically active, and prefer to function independently without recourse to social benefit schemes. Studies of disabled people have shown that the proportion economically active tends to remain stable regardless of the existence of schemes offering a high coverage of ordinary income. The economically active disabled have accounted for between 60 per cent and 80 per cent of the total surveyed in different countries, and research has confirmed that those disabled people who can work in ordinary work settings prefer to do so even when the economic gain may not be markedly greater than through receipt of a pension. Major patterns of dependency change have been demonstrated within the remaining groups of disabled. These less economically active disabled people generally demonstrated an uncertain vocational adjustment and often had been dependent upon family members for support prior to the inception of social benefit schemes. They tended to become more dependent upon benefit schemes once such benefits were available.

The availability of social benefits may serve as an important stimulus to the success of rehabilitation. Through early intervention, it is frequently possible to break a pattern of dependency which may have existed for generations within a family, and, at the same time, it is possible to prevent deterioration in the physical and psychological status of the disabled individual. Rehabilitation specialists are increasingly urging the development of graded social benefit systems which encourage the disabled person to participate in rehabilitation programs and return to an active producer status rather than remain as a passive receiver of benefits.

Human and Social Gains of Rehabilitation

Human and social gains add another dimension to the impact of rehabilitation on the social and economic development of a nation which must be considered by national planners. They remain, for the most part, unmeasured and excluded from socio-economic assessment. Human gains may include the feelings of well-being and satisfaction, the improved ability for independent self-care and the capacity for more harmonious relationships with other people that accrue to the disabled and their family members as a result of the provision of rehabilitation service. The cumulative effects of human gains become social gains for society as a whole.

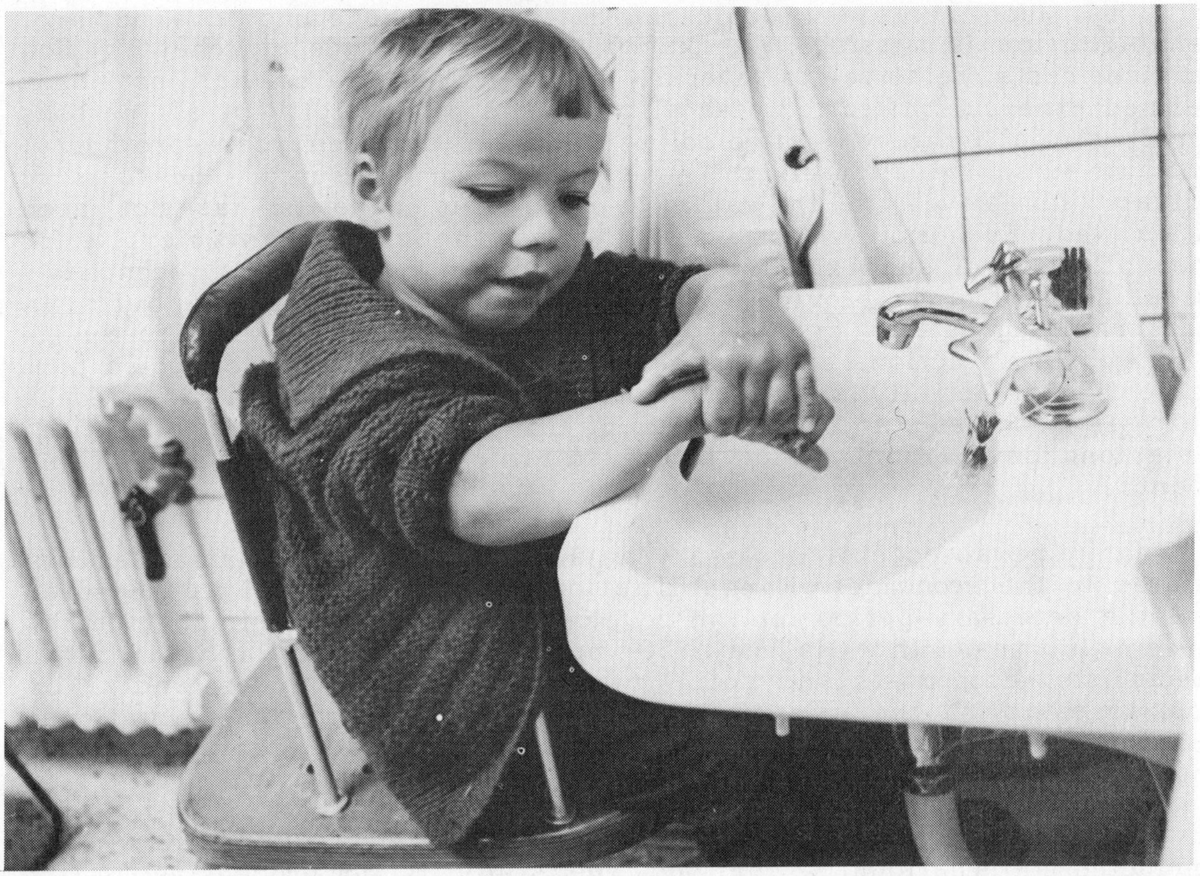

The presence of rehabilitation services may also provide social gains which are present without regard to the disabled. Their availability may assure all members of society of the possibility of re-entering active life should disability occur. In this sense, rehabilitation can "not only remove the pains of the sick but also the fears of the healthy".

Limitations of Data at Present Available

Serious limitations exist in currently available data on the socio-economic implications of investments in rehabilitation, particularly on an international basis. Cross-national comparisons on this subject are inhibited by all of the usual complications: the differences in population sampled, the definition of disability, the time period of the study, the data collection techniques and additional factors directly related to the nature of the area of study.

As previously noted, methods for the economic assessment of social phenomena are not well-developed, and in fact are in a state of evolution. Aside from the many methodological differences, and differences of professional opinion with regard to the interpretation of data, there is a basic inability to quantify costs and benefits which cannot be assigned monetary values. In general, these factors have been excluded from present studies. The fact of their exclusion should not lead to any presumption of a limitation on their relative magnitude of worth, yet there is some truth in the adage "Out of sight; out of mind". Since the so-called "non-economic" factors of rehabilitation are rarely taken into account, they are somehow thought of as being of lesser overall value. Without complete data, it is obviously impossible to come to a conclusion of that kind.

Much necessary basic information on the economic aspects of rehabilitation is missing. As examples, the magnitude of rehabilitation service costs relative to overall social expenditures has not been defined; the full effect of disability on the productivity of all persons directly and indirectly affected -- spouses, children, care-providers, and the disabled themselves -- has not been measured; the costs of private initiatives in the absence of public benefits has not been calculated. Even more important is the fact that no mechanism exists for the collection of such kinds of information. In recent years, economists have been urging providers of rehabilitation services to build in measurable objectives and valid measurement techniques when formulating programme actions so that the necessary data can be collected from the outset of activity and for as long a follow-up period as is needed. There is much resistance to concepts of this kind. As a result, there will be a long development period before suitable data are available in any country.

The absence of necessary data, the exclusion of major elements related to the economics of rehabilitation which are difficult to measure, and the necessary period for the development of such data in the future: these all mean that it may be many years before rehabilitation specialists, economists and social planners will fully understand or be able to establish the role of disability and rehabilitation in national economic planning unless a concerned effort is made to identify and obtain the needed categories of data.

It can also be seen from the research which has been conducted internationally that no one study is comprehensive in its outlook, and most can be subject to serious methodological criticism. Each study is an examination of only one or some few aspects of rehabilitation activity from some limited point of view: that of society, of a particular social institution or more rarely, of the disabled person and his or her family circle. National planners require data on all possible implications of their actions relative to the disabled. As yet, in the area of economic concern, rehabilitation specialists have been either unable or uninterested in creating such a composite picture.

Predicating the Future On The Past

Reference has been made throughout the study to factors which may alter our ability to collect data on the economic and social impact of disability and rehabilitation, and which may alter the significance of these data for overall socio-economic planning. These factors may be considered in three broad groupings:

Developments in socio-economic assessment methodology

The conceptualization of techniques that will give appropriate value to production, human and social gains that are not measurable in monetary terms, and the increase in understanding of the effect of such gains on total socio-economic development.

Changing patterns of productivity and consumption

Certain trends are already evident: the increasing consumption of social services, the decreasing work-force base for support of such services, the changing population structure in the world's different regions, the diminution of the world's available natural resource supplies which foretells radical alterations in consumption and development patterns, particularly in those countries most heavily dependent

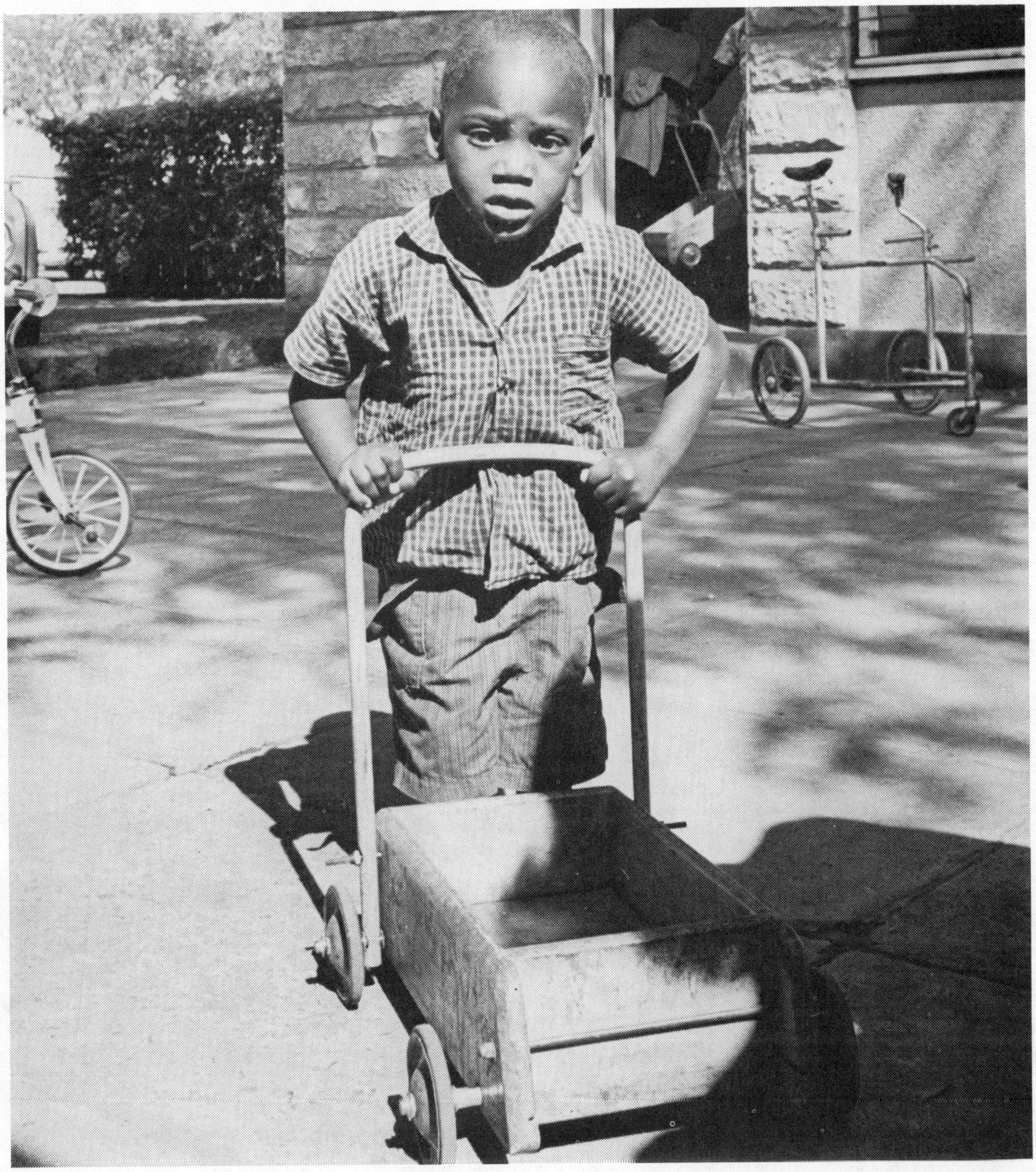

upon natural fuels and resources. The potential of "intermediate technology", based upon lessened natural resource consumption and increased use of people-power, is being studied in many fields ranging from agriculture to health care delivery, and it is quite likely that significant implications will be gleaned for the provision of rehabilitation services as well.

Changing patterns of assessment of disability and delivery of rehabilitation services

It is known that current patterns of assisting the disabled will never be adequate to deal with the present dimensions of the world-wide problem, nor do they offer adequate solutions for the growing numbers of unserved disabled. Promising possibilities to alter the situation have been demonstrated by programs which make use of services integrated within already existing community-level programs, and which are based upon the skills of community, auxiliary and professional workers. The prevention of disability, at the primary level through elimination of the controllable causes, and at the secondary level through early intervention and remediation, is being better understood and given greater priority. Factors associated with success in rehabilitation are subject to continuing analysis, and increasingly rehabilitation specialists are able to identify those groups of people for whom the rehabilitation process is least effective. This in turn will lead to an improved capability to assist the individuals who are now continual "repeaters" of service programs. There is also a growing recognition that not all disabled people will be productive in traditional work-oriented terms. The important benefits of useful recreation and leisure are beginning to be understood, especially in their relationship to the development of a capability for independent self-care.

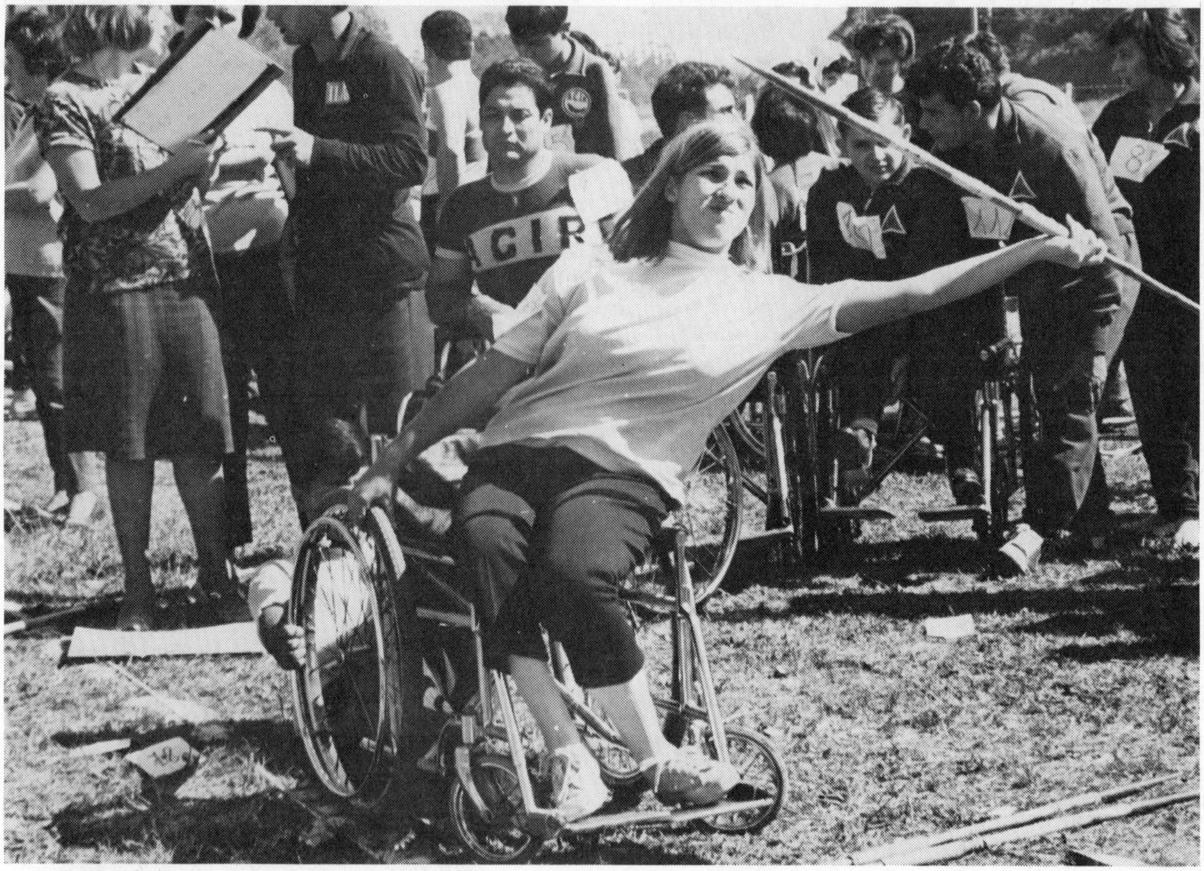

RESEARCH NEEDS AND AREAS FOR FURTHER ACTION

Expanded research is greatly needed on the socio-economic significance of disability to permit a basic understanding of its total effects. Some areas of special importance are:

The effects of disability on the economically active work force, and the effect of rehabilitation services on the preservation of reserve working capacity; a forecast of the applicability of preserved working capacity on the normal labor market as a result of technological, population and economic changes;

The effects of disability and rehabilitation services on the economic and emotional conditions in the families of the disabled, particularly with regard to the productivity of the non-disabled family members;

The effect of rehabilitation services on the children and dependents of disabled people, with regard to their health and educational development, and their potential productivity;

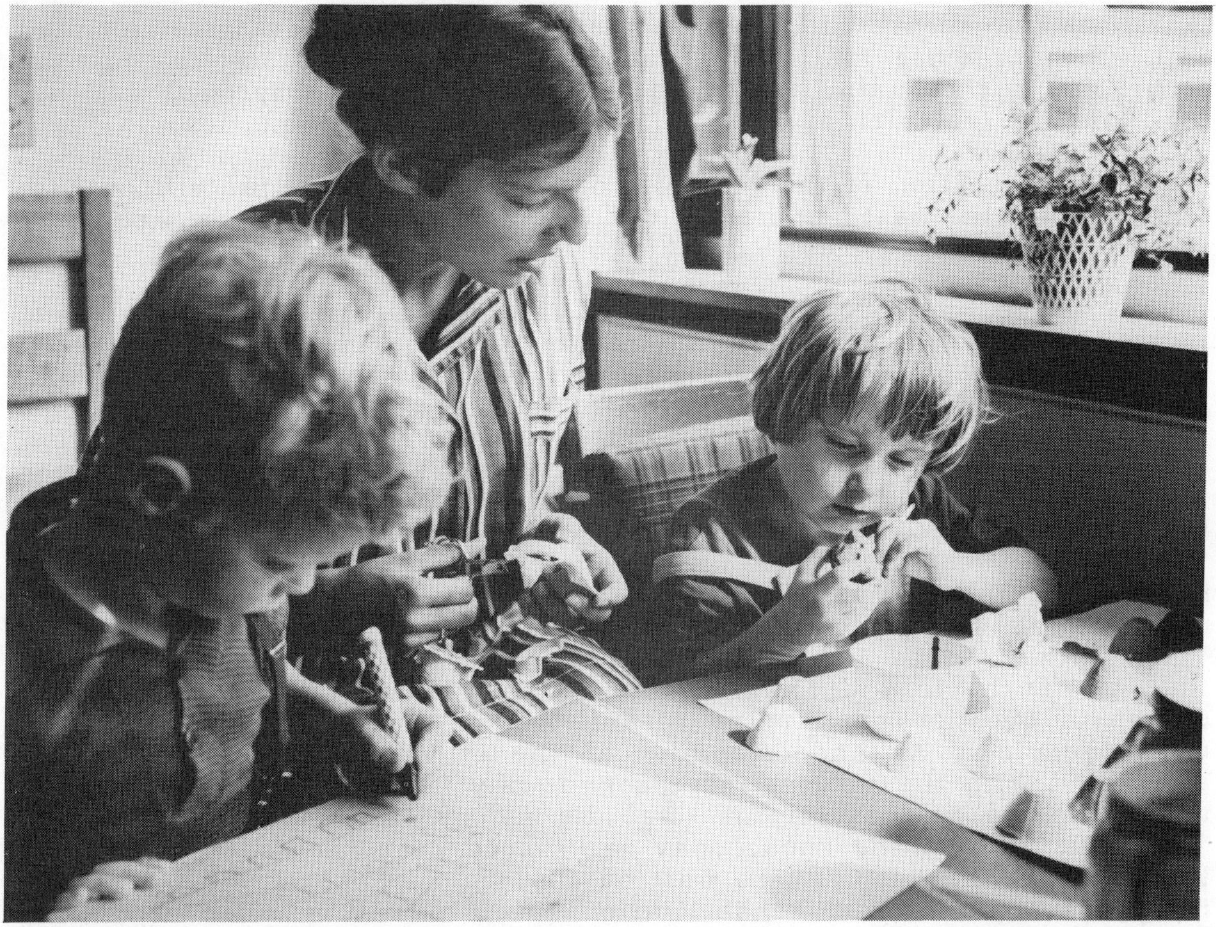

Identification of the basic costs of providing rehabilitation services within differing socio-economic structures, and particularly in situations which utilize simpler levels of service provision;

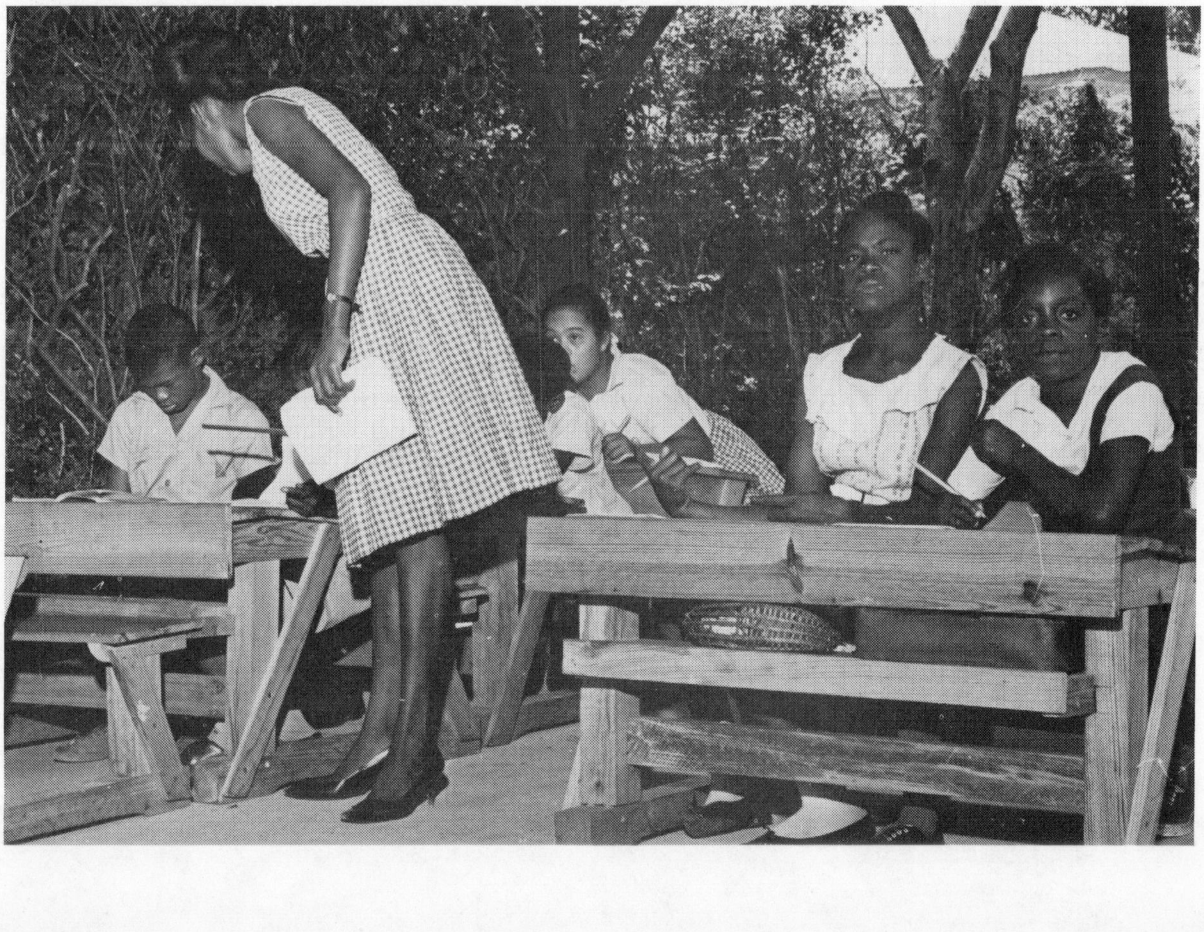

The identification of methods to quantify factors associated with the presence of rehabilitation services, such as feelings of security, psychic gain, increased independence, and improved well-being, and the inclusion of such factors in the economic equation.

Estimation of the relative costs to society of reliance upon care for the disabled based primarily upon private initiatives as compared to public-supported services;

The limits of rehabilitation in economic terms; i.e., the point, if any, at which expenditures on rehabilitation service provision begin to demonstrate a negative benefit/cost ratio for society as a whole, particularly within different systems of socio-economic organization;

Implications of disability and rehabilitation service provision in developing economies, taking into account the utilization of appropriate service delivery patterns including simpler methods, the use of auxiliary workers, mobile units and other innovative approaches, and recognizing the differing levels of social benefit system coverage which may exist as well as the differences in manpower levels and capacity.

Economic and social planners need to be involved to a greater degree in questions concerning disability and the provision of rehabilitation services. As understanding of the effect of all of the factors associated with the process increases, it may become apparent that until now only a small part of the total dimensions of the problem has been measured. In fact the impact may far exceed even current expectations. Economic and social planners must be encouraged to take this possibility into consideration, and rehabilitation specialists very much need their help in determining the best ways to collect the needed data. Governments must be encouraged, particularly in the developing countries, to include from the outset measures for the assessment of economic factors in their disability prevention and rehabilitation programs.

The United Nations Universal Declaration of Human Rights asserts that: "All human beings are born free and equal in dignity and rights", and the United Nations Declaration on Social Progress and Development declares that "Social progress and development shall be founded on respect for the dignity and value of the human person."

These essential humanitarian principles must be the basis for all social planning and development. They establish the equality of rights among all people as a universal ideal, and in so doing, provide each person with the hope of social justice. Disabled people have an equal right to all of the benefits of society. The fear has often been expressed that emphasis upon the economic implications of assistance for the disabled could result in an abrogation of these basic rights. It is feared that cost/benefit analysis, and other forms of economic assessment can persuade that no care for the disabled is preferable to any care.

"The goal of economic development is to improve the well-being of people. Health for all is not just a by-product of development. It is a primary lever for initiating the development process itself."

Halfdan Mahler, "People," Scientific American, September 1980.

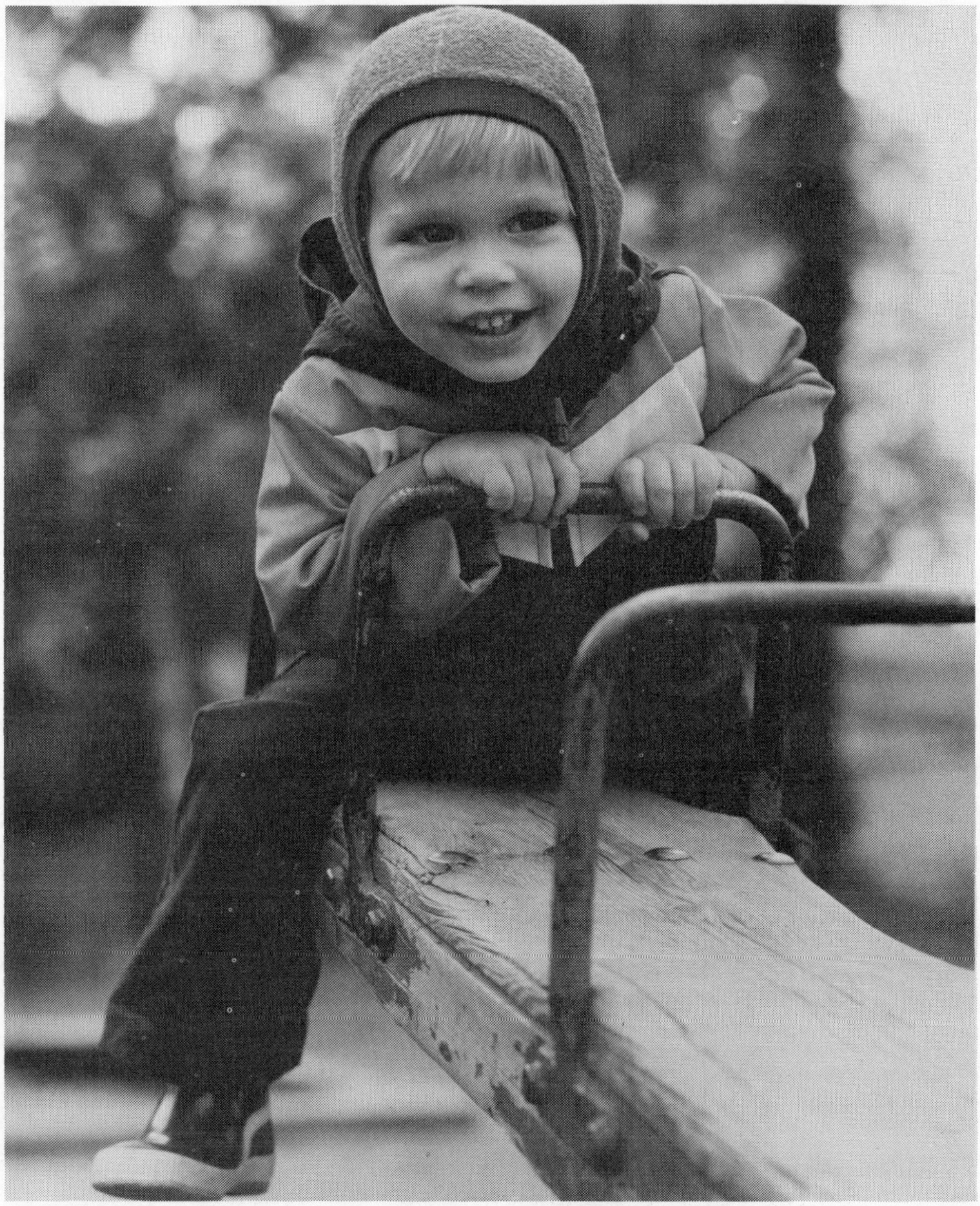

The results of available research studies do not appear to demonstrate any conflict between the humanitarian basis for rehabilitation service provision, and the basic principles of socio-economic planning. Disability will create a cost to society regardless of whether or not rehabilitation services exist. In fact, it appears that the more a society recognizes these costs, and the more it attempts to ameliorate them through the provision of adequate disability prevention and rehabilitation services, the greater is the overall economic return that may be expected. It is thus apparent that we have been too cautious in evaluating the full impact of disability and rehabilitation service provision in economic terms, and that a greater understanding of these forces will serve to strengthen governmental motivation to implement the most essential humanitarian principles.

Footnotes

Rehabilitation for the Disabled

1 World Health Organization, "Reports on Specific Technical Matters: Disability Prevention and Rehabilitation." A29/INF. DOC/1. (Geneva, 1976), p. 18.

2 "Rehabilitation of Disabled Persons; Report of the Secretary-General," E/CH.5/500.

3 "Report of the Secretary-General on an International Programme for the Rehabilitation of the Physically Handicapped." E/CN.5/259.

4 Rehabilitation International, Rehabilitation Guidelines for the Future in the Medical, Vocational, Educational, and Social Fields (New York, 1972), pp. 35-36.

5 Wilf Race, "Social Action," in Proceedings Preview of the Twelfth World Congress, Sydney, Australia, 27 August - 1 September 1972 (Sydney, 1972), p. 222.

6 World Health Organization, "Disability Prevention and Rehabilitation," p. 24.

7 Rehabilitation International, The Development of Rehabilitation Services in Relation to Available Resources, Report of a Meeting of Experts (New York, 1969).

8 Monroe Berkowitz et. al., "Cost-Benefit Analysis in Rehabilitation and Rehabilitation Research," in An Evaluation of Policy-Related Rehabilitation Research (New York, 1975).

9 Charles Berlioz, Inventory of Measures and Services Designed to Promote Rehabilitation in Social Security Institutions (Geneva, 1968), p. 9.

10 Thomas Teas, "Organization and Administration of Services to Meet Patient Needs," in Proceedings Preview of the Twelfth World Congress, Sydney, Australia, 27 August - 1 September 1972 (Sydney, 1972), p. 409.

11 Ronald W. Conley, The Economics of Vocational Rehabilitation (Baltimore, 1965), p. 99.

12 Thomas Teas, op. cit., p. 409.

13 Louis Nau and Jerry Turem, "The Comprehensive Needs Study" in American Rehabilitation (November - December 1975), p. 12.

14 Finnish Committee of Rehabilitation International, "Data On Government Assistance to the Maintenance of Rehabilitation Services, on the Quantitative Needs of Rehabilitation, and on the Costs of Individual Rehabilitation Benefits," Unpublished Documents compiled by Aulikki Kananoja, Helsinki, 1975.

15 Alexander Hulek, Legislative Aspects of Rehabilitation Services for the Disabled in Poland (Warsaw, 1972), p. 37.

16 J. Fourastie, "Quelques Considerations Economiques," Strategie Institutionnelle, Seconde Seance, 4 December 1971, Les Cahiers de l'Institut de la Vie, 1972-1973, (19:287-298).

17 Lawrence Haber, "Defining the Scope of the Problem: Social Planning for the Disabled" in Issues in Social Planning for the Physically and Mentally Disabled, Rehabilitation International Seminar on Social Planning for the Disabled, Brisbane, Australia, 20-24 August 1972; (unpublished seminar papers).

18 Ibid., p. 28.

19 U.P. Katzenstein, "The Rehabilitation of Severely Disabled Young People as a Humanitarian, Medical, Social and Economical Concern," Doctoral Dissertation. (Berlin, Humboldt University, 1970).

20 J. Silberstein, "The Costs of Non-Rehabilitation of Patients Hospitalized because of Cerebro-Vascular-Accident or Heart Disease," in Rehabilitation Research in Israel (Tel Aviv, 1972), pp. 115-118.

21 Permanent Inter-American Committee on Social Security, Mesa Redonda OIT-CISS: Seguridad Social y Recursos Humanos, 24-29 Noviembre 1969 (Mexico City, 1970), pp. 186-193.

22 B.T. Legge, "The Effects and Economics of Vocational Rehabilitation," in Report of the Seminar on the Economics of Vocational Rehabilitation, Galway, Ireland, 5 September 1969 (Dublin, 1969), pp. 48-55.

23 B. O'Donnel, "The Economics of Rehabilitation as seen by Doctors Responsible for the Administration of Medical Services," in Proceedings Preview of the Twelfth World Congress, op. cit., p. 28.

24 J. Paul Thomas, "Treating Spinal Cord Injuries" in Social and Rehabilitation Record (1972, 1:4), pp. 16-20.

25 Study conducted by Wolfgang Presber, Director of the Rehabilitation Hospital of Berlin, and reported in an interview for the study.

26 Alexander Hulek, op. cit., p. 37.

27 Finnish Committee of Rehabilitation International, "A Summary of the Findings of the Study on Brain-Injured Patients' Rehabilitation," (Doctoral Dissertation by Mikael Relander, Helsinki, 1969).

28 National Fund for Research into Crippling Diseases, Care with Dignity: An Analysis of Costs of Care for the Disabled (Sussex, 1973).

29 Sven-Olof Brattgard, "Social-Psychological Aspects of the Situation of the Disabled," in Proceedings Preview of the Twelfth World Congress, op. cit., p. 118.

30 Research Utilization Branch, United States Social and Rehabilitation Service. "From Institutional to Community Living," Research Brief, 1972, V:3, in Summary of "A Transitional Program for Institutionalized Adult Retarded" (Elwyn Institute, Pennsylvania).

31 John Kenneth Galbraith, Economics and the Public Purpose (Boston, 1973), p. 4.

32 Catherine Girardeau, "Towards a System of Social Statistics," Social Science Information (XI:3/4:189-202).

33 Ibid.

34 Bent Anderson, Work or Support: An Economic and Social Analysis of Substitute Permanent Employment (Paris, 1966), p. 31.

35 Ibid., p. 34.

36 Ida C. Merriam, "The Objectives of Social Security Research and Evaluation," International Social Security Association Research Conference (Vienna, 10-13 September 1975, Background Paper) ISSA/RDS/Conf/3.

37 Ronald W. Conley, "Issues in Benefit-Cost Analysis of the Vocational Rehabilitation Program" in American Rehabilitation (November - December 1975), pp. 19-23.

38 G.G. Somers and W.D. Wood, eds, Cost-Benefit Analysis of Manpower Policies, Proceedings of a North American Conference (Madison, 1970).

39 Ibid.

40 Anton Heering, "Legislation for Compulsory Employment of the Handicapped and its Economic Effects," in Report of the Seminar on theEconomics of Vocational Rehabilitation, Galway, Ireland, 5-12 September 1969 (Dublin, 1969), pp. 61-63.

41 Ronald W. Conley, "Issues in Benefit-Cost Analysis of the Vocational Rehabilitation Program" in American Rehabilitation (November - December 1975), pp. 19-23.

42 Richard Sterner, Social and Economic Conditions of the Mentally Retarded in Selected Countries, published for the United Nations by the International League of Societies for the Mentally Handicapped (Brussels, 1976), p. 9.

43 Ronald W. Conley, "Issues in Benefit-Cost Analysis of the Vocational Rehabilitation Program," in American Rehabilitation (November - December 1975), pp. 19-23.

44 Bent Anderson, op. cit., p. 100.

45 Anton Heering, The Social Policy of Industrial Companies in Respect of Handicapped Workers (The Hague, 1975).

46 A. Radner, "Sozialokonomische Aspekte der Rehabilitation" in *Rehabilitation* (1975, 14:42-50).

47 Bent Anderson, *op. cit.*

48 *Ibid.*

49 International Labor Office, *ILO/UNDP Regional Seminar on the Organization and Development of Disabled Persons' Cooperatives.* Warsaw, 16 September - 5 October 1974 (Geneva, 1974).

50 Invalids' Cooperatives Union, *The Cooperative Movement of the Disabled in People's Poland* (Warsaw, 1972), p. 13.

51 International Labor Office, *Report to the Government of Ethiopia on the Vocational Rehabilitation of the Disabled* (Geneva, 1967).

52 Ronald W. Conley, "A Benefit-Cost Analysis of the Vocational Rehabilitation Program," *Journal of Human Resources* 1969, Volume 4, #2, 226-252.

53 *Ibid.*, p. 243.

54 *Ibid.*, p. 248.

55 B.T. Legge, *op. cit.*

56 Einar Helander, *Rehabilitering av Lagvarigt Sjukskrivna*, Report to the Swedish Medical Research Board, Stockholm, 1975 (as orally reported to Susan Hammerman, Assistant Secretary General of Rehabilitation International).

57 Ronald W. Conley, "A Benefit-Cost Analysis of the Vocational Rehabilitation Program," p. 249.

58 Yehuda Schiff, "Social and Vocational Rehabilitation of the Chronically Unemployed Public Assistance Recipient," in *Issues in Social Planning for the Physically and Mentally Disabled*, *Rehabilitation International Seminar on Social Planning for the Disabled*, Brisbane, Australia, 20-24 August 1972 (unpublished seminar papers).

59 Kurt-Alphons Jochheim, "Rehabilitation in the Framework of Modern Social Policy" in *Rehabilitation after Central Nervous System Trauma* (Stockholm, 1974), pp. 15-23.

60 *Seminar on the Contribution of Social Security and Social Service to the Rehabilitation of the Disabled, within the Framework of Comprehensive Social Policies*, Warsaw, Poland, 16-26 September 1973 (United Nations Publication, SOA/ESDP/1973/74), p.51.

61 Warren Shore, *Social Security: The Fraud in Your Future* (New York, 1975).

62 Council of Europe. *Welfare Expenditure - Who Is To Pay?*, A Colloquy, Berlin, 11-13 November 1975 (unpublished working papers).

63 Charles Berlioz, op. cit.

64 Seminar on the Contribution of Social Security and Social Service to the Rehabilitation of the Disabled, pp. 48-49.

65 Australia Department of Social Security, "Survey of Persons Placed in Employment During 1969-1970 Following Rehabilitation: An Interim Report" Canberra.

66 Ronald W. Conley, "A Benefit-Cost Analysis of the Vocational Rehabilitation Program," p. 244.

67 Yehuda Schiff, op. cit.

68 Wilbur Cohen, "Social Security Reaches Age 40," New York Times (18 August 1975), p. 25.

69 Seminar on the Contribution of Social Security and Social Services to the Rehabilitation of the Disabled, p. 62.

70 Ibid., p. 64.

71 Ibid., p. 65.

72 Ibid., p. 67.

73 Richard T. Smith and Abraham Lilienfeld, The Social Security Disability Program: An Evaluation Study (Washington, D.C., 1971).

74 Markku Lehto and Ruuska Tauno, "Employment of the Handicapped," Official Statistics of Finland, Special Social Studies (Volume 32, Helsinki, 1972).

75 Seminar on the Contribution of Social Security and Social Services to the Rehabilitation of the Disabled, p. 66.

76 Seminar on the Contribution of Social Security and Social Services to the Rehabilitation of the Disabled, pp. 52-55.

77 Alexander Hulek, op. cit., p. 40.

78 Gudmund Harlem, Studies on the Relation Between Impairment, Disability and Dependency (Oslo, 1976).

79 Bent Anderson, op. cit., pp. 23-26.

Bibliography

Akehurst, R.L. and Sally Holtermann. "Application of Cost-Benefit Analysis to Programmes for the Prevention of Mental Handicap," in Major Mental Handicap: Methods and Costs of Prevention, Ciba Foundation Symposium 59. Amsterdam: Exerpta Medica, 1978. 226 pp.

Albrecht, Gary L. and Stefan J. Harasymiw. "Evaluating Rehabilitation Outcome Cost Function Indicators," Journal of Chronic Diseases, Volume 32, #7, 1979, pp. 525-533.

Amoako, J.B. "Socio-Economic Implications of Investments in Rehabilitation Services for the Disabled in a Developing Country," paper presented to the United Nations Expert Group Meeting on Socio-Economic Implications of Investments in Rehabilitation Services for the Disabled, Geneva, 1977. Mimeo.

Alberta Committee of Action Groups for the Disabled. Recommendations Relating to the Government of Alberta's Transportation Policy. Edmonton: A.C.A.G.D., 1974.

American Society of Landscape Architects Foundation. Barrier-Free Site Design. Washington, D.C.: United States Department of Housing and Urban Development, 1977. 82 pp.

Anderson, Bent. Work or Support: An Economic and Social Analysis of Substitute Permanent Employment. Paris: Organization for Economic Cooperation and Development, 1966. 122 pp.

Australia Department of Social Security. "Survey of Persons Placed in Employment During 1969-1970 Following Rehabilitation: An Interim Report." Canberra.

Australian Council for Rehabilitation of Disabled. Proceedings Preview of the Twelfth World Congress of Rehabilitation International. Sydney, Australia: Australian Council for Rehabilitation of Disabled, 1972. 852 pp.

Australian Council for Rehabilitation of Disabled. Issues in Social Planning for the Physically and Mentally Disabled. Rehabilitation International Seminar on Social Planning for the Disabled. Brisbane, Australia: Australian Council for Rehabilitation of Disabled, 1972. Unpublished papers.

Australian Government Commission of Inquiry into Poverty. The Relationship Between Poverty and Disability in Australia. Canberra: Australian Government Publishing Service, 1977. 72 pp.

Barnum, H.N. et. al. "Cost-Effectiveness of An Immunization Programme in Indonesia," in Bulletin of the World Health Organization, Volume 58, #3, 1980, pp. 499-503.

Beckerman, Wilfred. Poverty and the Impact of Income Maintenance Programmes. Geneva: International Labor Organization, 1979. 90 pp.

Berkeley Planning Associates. Benefit-Cost Analysis of Vocational Rehabilitation Services Provided to Individuals Most Severely Handicapped. (IMSH). Berkeley: Berkeley Planning Associates, 1975. 83 pp.

Berkowitz, Edward ed. Disability Policies and Government Programs. New York: Praeger, 1979. 185 pp.

Berkowitz, Monroe, W.G. Johnson and Edward H. Murphy. Public Policy Toward Disability. New York: Praeger, 1976. 150 pp.

Berkowitz, Monroe and W.G. Johnson. "Towards an Economics of Disability: The Magnitude and Structure of Transfer and Medical Costs," Journal of Human Resources, Volume 5, #3, 1970, pp. 271-297.

Berkowitz, Monroe and Jeffrey Rubin. The Costs of Disability: Estimates of Program Expenditures for Disability, 1967-75. New Brunswick, New Jersey: Bureau of Economic Research, 1977. Mimeo. 26 pp.

Berkowitz, Monroe. Work Disincentives. Falls Church, Virginia: Institute for Information Studies, 1980. 78 pp.

Berkowitz, Monroe et. al. An Evaluation of Policy-Related Rehabilitation Research. New York: Praeger, 1975. 229 pp.

Berlioz, Charles. Inventory of Measures and Services Designed to Promote Rehabilitation in Social Security Institutions. Geneva: International Social Security Association, 1968.

Bernhardsson, Gote and Anne-Marie Qvarfort. Employment for Handicapped Persons. A Report to the O.E.C.D. on the Work of the Swedish Government Commission on Long-Term Employment. Paris: Organization for Economic Cooperation and Development, 1980. 66 pp.

Better, Sybil R., et. al. "Disability Benefits as Disincentives to Rehabilitataion," Milbank Memorial Fund Quarterly/Health and Society, Volume 57, #3, 1979, pp. 412-427.

Blaxter, Mildred. The Meaning of Disability. London: Heinemann Educational Books, 1975. 258 pp.

Bowe, Frank. Rehabilitating America: Toward Independence for Disabled and Elderly People. New York: Harper and Row, 1980. 203 pp.

Brown, Joan C. A Hit and Miss Affair: Policies for Disabled People in Canada. Ottawa: Canadian Council on Social Development, 1977. 508 pp.

Casarin, Arlindo. Avaliacao de Beneficio e de Custo na Reabilitacao Profissional Do INPS. (Evaluation of Benefits and Costs of Professional Rehabilitation of the National Institute for Social Welfare). Rio de Janeiro: INPS, 1979. 90 pp.

Chaplain, Marie Therese. "Perinatality: French Cost-Benefit Studies and Decisions on Handicap and Prevention," in Major Mental Handicap: Methods and Costs of Prevention, Ciba Foundation Symposium 59. Amsterdam: Excerpta Medica, 1978. 226 pp.

Chigier, E. ed. Rehabilitation Research in Israel. Tel Aviv: Gomeh Scientific Publications, 1972. 208 pp.

Cohen, Wilbur. "Social Security Reaches Age 40," New York Times, 18 August 1975, p. 25.

Commission of the European Communities. Directorate-General for Social Affairs. Comparative Study of the Rehabilitation of Handicapped Persons in the Countries of the Community. Volume I: Belgium, France, Italy, Luxembourg (207 pp.); Volume II: Federal Republic of Germany, Netherlands (96 pp.); Volume III: Denmark, Republic of Ireland, United Kingdom (104 pp.). Luxembourg: C.E.C., 1975.

Conley, Ronald W. "A Benefit-Cost Analysis of the Vocational Rehabilitation Program," Journal of Human Resources, Volume 4, #2, 1969, pp. 226-252.

Conley, Ronald W. "Issues in Benefit-Cost Analysis of the Vocational Rehabilitation Program," in American Rehabilitation, November-December 1975, pp. 19-23.

Conley, Ronald W. The Economics of Mental Retardation. Baltimore: Johns Hopkins University Press, 1973. 377 pp.

Conley, Ronald W. The Economics of Vocational Rehabilitation. Baltimore: Johns Hopkins University Press, 1965. 177 pp.

Copeland, Lois S. Defining Disability: A Cross-Country Study. Washington, D.C.: U.S. Social Security Administration, 1977. 46 pp.

Council of Europe. Welfare Expenditure - Who Is To Pay?, A Colloquy, Berlin, 11-13 November 1975 (unpublished working papers).

Coventry Home Help Project. Costs and Benefits: One Day Workshop. Report of Proceedings. Coventry, United Kingdom: Coventry Social Services Department, 1978. 52 pp.

Creese, A.L. and R. Fielden. "Hospital or Home Care for the Severely Disabled: A Cost Comparison," British Journal of Preventive and Social Medicine, Volume 31, 1977, pp. 116-121.

Creese, A.L. and R.H. Henderson. "Cost-Benefit Analysis and Immunization Programmes in Developing Countries," Bulletin of the World Health Organization, Volume 58, #3, 1980, pp. 491-497.

DeJong, Gerben. The Movement for Independent Living: Origins, Ideology, and Implications for Disability Research. East Lansing: University Centers for International Rehabilitation, 1979. 85 pp.

Disability Alliance. Poverty and Disability. London: The Disability Alliance, 1975. 20 pp.

Disablement Income Group. Social Security and Disability -- A Study of the Financial Provisions for Disabled People in Seven West European Countries. Surrey: DIG Charitable Trust, 1971. 61 pp.

Djukanovic, V. and E.P. Mach, eds. Alternative Approaches to Meeting Basic Health Needs in Developing Countries. Geneva: World Health Organization, 1975. 116 pp.

Economics Division, South Australia Department of Economic Development. "Community Care and Institutional Care: A Discussion," in National Rehabilitation Digest, Volume 3, # 3/4, 1979, pp. 30-36.

Enthoven, Alain C. "The Behavior of Health Care Agents: Provider Behavior," paper delivered at the World Congress on Health Economics, September 9-11, 1980, Leyden University, The Netherlands.

Finnish Committee of Rehabilitation International. "Data on Government Assistance to the Maintenance of Rehabilitation Services, on the Quantitative Needs for Rehabilitation, and on the Costs of Individual Rehabilitation Benefits," Unpublished documents compiled by Aulikki Kananoja, Helsinki, 1975.

Finnish Committee of Rehabilitation International. "A Summary of the Findings of the Study on Brain-Injured Patients' Rehabilitation," Doctoral Dissertation by Mikael Relander, Helsinki, 1969.

Fourastie, J. "Quelques Considerations Economiques," Strategie Institutionnelle, Seconde Seance, 4 December 1971, Les Cahiers de l'Institut de la Vie, 1971-1973, Volume 19, pp. 287-298.

Franklin, P.A. "Impact of Disability on the Family Structure," Social Security Bulletin, #5 May 1977, pp. 3-18.

Franklin, P.A. and J.C. Hennessey. "Effect of Substantial Gainful Activity Level on Disabled Beneficiary Work Patterns," Social Security Bulletin, #3 March 1979, pp. 3-17.

Frohlich, Philip. "Income of the Newly Disabled: Survey of Recently Disabled Adults," Social Security Bulletin, #9 September 1975, pp. 3-18.

Galbraith, John Kenneth. Economics and the Public Purpose. Boston: Houghton Mifflin Co., 1973. 334 pp.

Gennard, John and M. Wright. "A Sheltered Workshop," United Kingdom Department of Employment Gazette, September 1978, pp. 1028-31.

Gibson, Mary Jo. "Family Support for the Elderly in International Perspective: Policies and Programs," in Ageing International, Volume 7, #4, 1980, pp. 13-19.

Girardeau, Catherine. "Towards a System of Social Statistics," Social Science Information, Volume 11, #3/4, pp. 189-202.

Godstad, Anders Chr. Evaluation of Factors Determining the Results of Vocational Rehabilitation. Norway: Universitetsforlaget, 1968. 154 pp.

Greenblum, Joseph. "Effect of Rehabilitation on Employment and Earnings of the Disabled: Socio-demographic Factors," Social Security Bulletin, #8 August 1979, pp. 11-37.

Greenleigh Associates Inc. The Role of Sheltered Workshops in the Rehabilitation of the Severely Handicapped. New York: Greenleigh Associates Inc., 1975. 365 pp.

Haber, Lawrence D. "Some Parameters for Social Policy in Disability: A Cross National Comparison," Health and Society, Summer 1973, pp. 319-340.

Haber, Lawrence D. Sickness and Injury Cash Benefits: A Proposal for Planning and Integration. Unpublished paper, 1974.

Harlem, Gudmund. "Studies on the Relation Between Impairment, Disability and Dependency," Scandinavian Journal of Rehabilitation Medicine, Supplement #4. Oslo: Kurer-Sats, 1976. 119 pp.

Haveman, Robert H. A Benefit-Cost And Policy Analysis of the Netherlands' Social Employment Program. A Report Submitted to the Ministry of Social Affairs of the Netherlands. Madison, Wisconsin: Institute for Research on Poverty, 1977. 197 pp.

Heering, Anton. The Social Policy of Industrial Companies in Respect of Handicapped Workers. The Hague: Ministry of Social Affairs, 1975. 22 pp.

Helander, Einer. Rehabilitering av Lagvarigt Sjukskrivna, Report to the Swedish Medical Research Board, Stockholm, 1975 (as orally reported to Susan Hammerman, Assistant Secretary General of Rehabilitation International).

Horlick, Max. "The Impact of an Aging Population on Social Security: The Foreign Experience," in Social Security in a Changing World. Washington, D.C.: U.S. Social Security Administration, 1979. 136 pp.

Hulek, Alexander. Legislative Aspects of Rehabilitation Services for the Disabled in Poland. Warsaw: Ministry of Health and Social Welfare, Department of Rehabilitation, 1972. 117 pp.

Hyman, Mavis. The Extra Costs of Disabled Living. London: National Fund for Research into Crippling Diseases, 1977. 196 pp.

Intagliata, James C., et. al. "Cost Comparison of Institutional and Community-Based Alternatives for Mentally Retarded Persons," Mental Retardation, June 1979, pp. 154-156.

International Labor Office. ILO/UNDP Regional Seminar on the Organization and Development of Disabled Persons' Cooperatives. Warsaw, 16 September - 5 October 1974. Geneva: ILO/UNDP, 1974. 186 pp.

International Labor Office. Report to the Government of Ethiopia on the Vocational Rehabilitation of the Disabled. Geneva: International Labor Organization, 1967.

International Labor Organization/Swedish International Development Agency. ILO/SIDA African Regional Seminar on the Organization of Cooperatives for Handicapped Persons. Geneva: International Labor Organization, 1978. 119 pp.

International Labor Organization. The Cost of Social Security: 9th International Inquiry, 1972-74. Geneva: International Labor Organization, 1979. 111 pp.

Ison, Terence G. Human Disability and Personal Income. Kingston: Industrial Relations Centre, 1978. 33 pp.

Invalids' Cooperatives Union. The Cooperative Movement of the Disabled in People's Poland. Warsaw: Publishing House of the Central Agricultural Union, 1972. 48 pp.

Jain, Harish C. Disadvantaged Groups on the Labour Market and Measures to Assist Them. Paris: Organization for Economic Cooperation and Development, 1979. 68 pp.

Japanese Society for Rehabilitation of the Disabled. Rehabilitation Services for the Disabled in Japan. Tokyo: Japanese Society for Rehabilitation of the Disabled, 1980. 150 pp.

Jarvikoski, Aila and Eero Lahelma. Early Rehabilitation at the Work Place. New York: World Rehabilitation Fund, 1980. 79 pp.

Jochheim, Kurt-Alphons. "Rehabilitation in the Framework of Modern Social Policy," in Rehabilitation after Central Nervous System Trauma. Stockholm: Nordisk Bokhandelns Forlag, 1974, pp. 15-23.

Kaim-Caudle, P.R. Comparative Social Policy and Social Security: A Ten Country Study. London: Martin Robertson and Company, 1973. 357 pp.

Katzenstein, U.P. "The Rehabilitation of Severely Disabled Young People as a Humanitarian, Medical, Social and Economical Concern," Doctoral Dissertation. Berlin, Humboldt University, 1970.

Krute, Aaron and Mary Ellen Burdette. Chronic Disease, Injury and Work Disability: 1972 Survey of Disabled and Non-Disabled Adults. Report #10. Washington D.C.: U.S. Social Security Administration, 1978. 18 pp.

Lando, Mordechai E. et. al. "Disability Benefit Applications and the Economy," Social Security Bulletin, #10 October 1979, pp. 3-10.

Lehto, Markku and Ruuska Tauno. "Employment of the Handicapped," Official Statistics of Finland, Special Social Studies, #32 Helsinki, 1972. 147 pp.

Levitan, Sar and Robert Taggart. Jobs for the Disabled. Policy Studies in Employment and Welfare, Number 28. Baltimore: Johns Hopkins University Press, 1977. 129 pp.

Mayor's Task Force. Report on the Disabled and Elderly. Toronto, 1973.

McManus, Leo A. The Effects of Disability on Lifetime Earnings. Paper No. 30. Washington, D.C.: U.S. Social Security Administration, 1978. 30 pp.

Mendelson, M. The Administrative Cost of Income Security Programs: Ontario and Canada. Toronto: Ontario Economic Council, 1979. 118 pp.

Merriam, Ida C. "The Objectives of Social Security Research and Evaluation," International Social Security Association Research Conference, Vienna, 10-13 September 1975, background paper ISSA/RDS/Conf/3. 18 pp.

Mezerville, Gaston de. Disability and Rehabilitation in Rural Costa Rica. East Lansing, Michigan: University Centers for International Rehabilitation, 1979. 46 pp.

Mikkelsen, Margareta and Gert Nielson. Cost-Benefit Analyses in Prenatal Diagnosis. Glostrup, Denmark: Danish National Board for Social Welfare, 1974. 20 pp.

Morgan, P.L. and Peter Makeham. Economic and Financial Analysis of Sheltered Employment. Research Paper #5. London: United Kingdom Department of Employment, 1978. 29 pp.

Nagi, Saad Z. Disability and Rehabilitation: Legal, Clinical, and Self-Concepts and Measurement. Columbus: Ohio State University Press, 1969. 329 pp.

National Fund for Research into Crippling Diseases. Care with Dignity: An Analysis of Costs of Care for the Disabled. Sussex: National Fund, 1973. 180 pp.

National Labour Market Board. Labour Market Policy 1975/76. Stockholm, Sweden: National Labour Market Board, 1976.

Netherlands Central Bureau of Statistics. The Physically Handicapped in the Netherlands 1971/1972. The Hague: Staatsuitgeverij, 1976. 73 pp.

Nau, Louis and Jerry Turem. "The Comprehensive Needs Study," in American Rehabilitation, November-December 1975, pp. 10-14.

Noble, John H. Jr. "Rehabilitating the Severely Disabled: The Foreign Experience," Journal of Health Politics, Policy and Law, #4 (Summer, 1979), pp. 221-249.

Noble, John H. Jr. "The Limits of Cost-Benefit Analysis as a Guide to Priority Setting in Rehabilitation," Evaluation Quarterly, Volume 1, #3 August 1977, pp. 347-380.

Noble, John H. Jr. and Ronald W. Conley. "The Search for Fact Amidst Conjecture in the Policy of Deinstitutionalization," Health Policy Quarterly, 1981. In press.

Office of Health Economics. Physical Impairment: Social Handicap. London: Office of Health Economics, 1977. 32 pp.

Organization for Economic Cooperation and Development. Centre for Educational Research and Innovation. The Education of the Handicapped Adolescent: Alternatives to Work for Severely Handicapped People. Paris: Organization for Economic Cooperation and Development, 1979. 50 pp.

Palotai, K. "Problems Arising From the Low Level of Invalidity Pensions," Report X, International Social Security Association XIX General Assembly, (Madrid, 4-14 October 1977). Geneva: International Social Security Association, 1978. 9 pp.

Pan-American Health Organization. Medical Auxiliaries: Proceedings of a Symposium Held during the Twelfth Meeting of the PAHO Advisory Committee on Medical Research. Washington, D.C.: PAHO/WHO, 1973. 62 pp.

Permanent Inter-American Committee on Social Security. Mesa Redonda OIT--CISS: Seguridad Social y Recursos Humanos, 24-29 Noviembre 1969, Mexico City, 1970. 267 pp.

Pollitt, Ernesto. Early Childhood Intervention Programs. New York: The Ford Foundation, 1979. 302 pp.

Radner, A. "Sozialokonomische Aspekte der Rehabilitation," in Rehabilitation, Volume 14, 1975, pp. 42-50.

Region II Rehabilitation Research Institute. Rehabilitation, Sheltered Workshops, and the Disadvantaged: An Exploration in Manpower Policy. Ithaca, New York: Cornell University Press, 1970. 251 pp.

Rehabilitation International. Barrier Free Design. New York: Rehabilitation International, 1975. 36 pp.

Rehabilitation International. Rehabilitation Guidelines for the Future in the Medical, Vocational, Educational, and Social Fields. New York: Rehabilitation International, 1972.

Rehabilitation International. The Development of Rehabilitation Services in Relation to Available Resources. Report of a Meeting of Experts. New York: Rehabilitation International, 1969. 26 pp.

"Rehabilitation of the Physically Handicapped," in International Social Service Review, March 1957, p. 10.

Report of the Independent Commission of International Development Issues (Brandt Commission). North-South: A Program for Survival. Cambridge, Massachusetts: MIT Press, 1980. 304 pp.

Report of the Snowdon Working Party. Integrating the Disabled. Surrey, United Kingdom: National Fund for Research into Crippling Diseases, 1976. 71 pp.

Research Utilization Branch, United States Social and Rehabilitation Service. "From Institutional to Community Living," Research Brief, 1972, V:3, in Summary of "A Transitional Program for Institutionalized Adult Retarded," Elwyn Institute, Pennsylvania.

Rideau, Y. "Enquete Economique A Propos de la Readaptation," In Readaptation (Paris), #264, November 1979, pp. 3-6.

Roth, William. The Uncounted Poor: An Excursion to an Institution. Madison, Wisconsin: Institute for Research on Poverty, 1977. 29 pp.

Sainsbury, Sally. Measuring Disability. London: Social Administration Research Trust, 1973. 125 pp.

Shore, Warren. Social Security: The Fraud in Your Future. New York: Macmillan, 1975. 238 pp.

Simkins, Jean and Vincent Tickner. Whose Benefit? London: The Economist Intelligence Unit, 1978. 245 pp.

Simkins, Jean. The Value of Independent Living: Looking at Cost-Effectiveness in the U.K. New York: World Rehabilitation Fund, 1979. 86 pp.

Smirnov, S. "The Employment of Old-Age Pensioners in the U.S.S.R.," International Labor Review, Volume 116, #1, July-August 1977, pp. 87-94.

Smith, Richard T. and Abraham Lilienfeld. The Social Security Disability Program: An Evaluation Study. Washington, D.C.: United States Department of Health, Education and Welfare, 1971. 295 pp.

Somers, G.G. and W.D. Wood, eds. Cost-Benefit Analysis of Manpower Policies. Proceedings of a North American Conference. Kingston: Industrial Relations Centre, Queens University, 1970. 272 pp.

Sterner, Richard. Social and Economic Conditions of the Mentally Retarded in Selected Countries, published for the United Nations by the International League of Societies for the Mentally Handicapped. Brussels: International League, 1976. 58 pp.

Study conducted by Wolfgang Presber, Director of the Rehabilitation Hospital of Berlin, and reported in an interview for the study.

Sunshine, Jonathan H. Disability. Washington, D.C.: United States Office of Management and Budget, 1979. 128 pp.

Symington, D.C. and M.P. Lewis. "Cost-Benefit Analysis of a Hospital and University-Based Prevocational Program," Archives of Physical Medicine and Rehabilitation, Volume 54, August, 1973, pp. 341-347.

Thomas, J. Paul. "Treating Spinal Cord Injuries," in Social and Rehabilitation Record, Volume 1, #4, 1972, pp. 16-20.

Treital, Ralph. Benefits and Costs of Cost-Benefit Analysis of Vocational Rehabilitation Programs. Paper presented at the International Sociological Association Conference, Upsala, Sweden, August 1978.

Treital, Ralph. "Recovery of Disabled Beneficiaries: A 1975 Followup Study of 1972 Allowances," Social Security Bulletin, #4 April 1979, pp. 3-23.

United Nations. Economic and Social Council. Childhood Disability: Its Prevention and Rehabilitation. Report of Rehabilitation International to the Executive Board of UNICEF. New York: UNICEF, 1980. 31 pp. (E/ICEF/L.1410)

United Nations. European Social Development Program. Seminar on the Contribution of Social Security and Social Services to the Rehabilitation of the Disabled, within the Framework of Comprehensive Social Policies. (Warsaw, Poland 16-26 September, 1973). New York: United Nations, 1973. SOA/ESDP/1973/74. 88 pp.

United Nations Educational, Scientific and Cultural Organization. Economic Aspects of Special Education: Czechoslovakia, New Zealand, United States of America. Paris: UNESCO, 1978. 152 pp.

Walsh, Julia A. and Kenneth S. Warren. "Selective Primary Health Care: An Interim Strategy for Disease Control in Developing Countries," New England Journal of Medicine, Volume 301, #18, November 1979, pp. 967-974.

Ward, Nicholas. "Malawi: EEC/NGO Anti-Polio Campaign," Courier, #65, January-February 1981, pp. 30-32.

Werner, David. "Health Care and Human Dignity--A Subjective Look at Community-Based Rural Health Programmes in Latin America," in Contact, #57, August 1980, pp. 1-17.

Wood, Mary M. et. al. "The Economics of Special Education in a Developing Country," in International Perspectives on Future Special Education. Reston, Virginia: The Council for Exceptional Children, 1978. 318 pp.

World Bank. Health. Sector Policy Paper. Washington, D.C.: The World Bank, 1980. 85 pp.

World Bank. World Development Report 1980. New York: Oxford University Press, 1980. 166 pp.

World Commission on Vocational Rehabilitation. Report of the Seminar on the Economics of Vocational Rehabilitation. Galway, Ireland, 5-12 September 1969. Dublin: National Rehabilitation Board, 1969. 84 pp.

World Health Organization. "Reports on Specific Technical Matters: Disability Prevention and Rehabilitation." A29/INF. DOC/1. Geneva, 1976. 53 pp.

World Health Organization. International Classification of Impairments, Disabilities, and Handicaps. Geneva: World Health Organization, 1980. 205 pp.

World Health Organization. Cost/Benefit Analysis in Mental Health Services. Report on a Working Group. The Hague, 21-25 June 1976. Copenhagen: World Health Organization, 1976. 76 pp.

Worrall, John D. "A Benefit-Cost Analysis of the Vocational Rehabilitation Program," Journal of Human Resources, Volume 13, #2, 1978, pp. 285-298.

Zymelman, Manuel. The Economic Evaluation of Vocational Training Programs. World Bank Occasional Papers, #28. Baltimore: Johns Hopkins University Press, 1976. 122 pp.

Index, by Country

Publication Resources

INTERNATIONAL ORGANIZATIONS

Commission of European Communities
Luxembourg, Luxembourg

Vocational Rehabilitation Section
International Labor Office
CH 1211 Geneva 22
Switzerland

International Social Security Association
Case Postale 1
CH 1211 Geneva 22
Switzerland

International League of Societies
for the Mentally Handicapped
12 Rue Forestiere
1050 Brussels
Belgium

Organization for Economic Cooperation
and Development
2 Rue Andre Pascal
75775 Paris, France
or
1750 Pennsylvania Avenue N.W.
Washington, D.C. 20006 U.S.A.

Rehabilitation International
432 Park Avenue South
New York, New York 10016 U.S.A.

United Nations Educational, Scientific,
and Cultural Organization
Place de Fontenoy
75700 Paris, France

United Nations International
Children's Fund
866 United Nations Plaza
New York, New York 10017 U.S.A.

United Nations Publications
Room A-3315
United Nations Secretariat Building
New York, New York 10017, U.S.A.
or
CH 1211 Geneva 10
Switzerland

World Bank
Publications Unit
1818 H Street, N.W.
Washington, D.C. 20433 U.S.A.

Publications Office
World Health Organization
CH 1211 Geneva 27
Switzerland
or
49 Sheridan Avenue
Albany, New York 12210, U.S.A.

World Rehabilitation Fund Inc.
400 East 34th Street
New York, New York 10016, U.S.A.

NATIONAL ORGANIZATIONS AND PUBLISHERS

Australian Council for Rehabilitation of Disabled
Acton House
P.O. Box 1937
Canberra City, A.C.T. 2601 Australia

Berkeley Planning Associates
1912 Bonita Avenue
Berkeley, California 94704 U.S.A.

Bureau of Economic Research
Rutgers University
165 College Avenue
New Brunswick, New Jersey 08903 U.S.A.

Canadian Council on Social Development
55 Parkdale Avenue
Box 3505 Station C
Ottawa, Ontario K1Y 4G1 Canada

Cornell University Press
124 Robert Place
Ithaca, New York 12936 U.S.A.

Council for Exceptional Children
1920 Association Drive
Reston, Virginia 22091 U.S.A.

Coventry Social Service Dept.
New Council Offices
Coventry CV1 5RS United Kingdom

Danish National Board of Social Welfare
Amaliegade 25
1256 Copenhagen K Denmark

Disablement Income Group
Attlee House, Toynbee Hall
28 Commercial Street
London E16 LR United Kingdom

Economist Intelligence Unit
Spencer House
27 St. James Place
London SW1A 1NT United Kingdom

Excerpta Medica
P.O. Box 211
Amsterdam, Netherlands

Ford Foundation
320 East 43rd Street
New York, New York 10017 U.S.A.

Greenleigh Associates, Inc.
30 East 42nd Street
New York, New York 10017 U.S.A.

Harper and Row
10 East 53rd Street
New York, New York 10022 U.S.A.

Heinemann Educational Books Ltd.
48 Charles Street
London W1X 8AH United Kingdom

Industrial Relations Centre
Queens University
Kingston, Ontario K7L 3N6 Canada

Institute for Information Studies
400 N. Washington Street
Falls Church, Virginia 22046 U.S.A.

Institute for Research on Poverty
3412 Social Science Building
University of Wisconsin
Madison, Wisconsin 53706 U.S.A.

Japanese Society for Rehabilitation of the Disabled
3-13-15 Higashi-Ikebukuro
Toshima-ku
Tokyo, Japan

Johns Hopkins Press
34th and Charles Streets
Baltimore, Maryland 21218 U.S.A.

Macmillan Publishing Co., Inc.
866 Third Avenue
New York, New York 10022 U.S.A.

Ministry of Health and Social Welfare
Miodowa 15
Warsaw, Poland

Ministry of Social Affairs
Zeestraat 73
The Hague, Netherlands

National Fund for Research into Crippling Diseases
Vincent House
1 Springfield Road
Horsham, Sussex RH12 2PN United Kingdom

National Institute for Social Welfare (INPS)
Rua Pedro Lessa 36 Sala 622
20030 Rio de Janeiro, Brazil

National Rehabilitation Board
25 Clyde Road
Dublin 4, Ireland

Netherlands Central Bureau of Statistics
Prinses Beatrixlaan 428
The Hague, Netherlands

Ohio State University Press
2070 Neil Avenue
Columbus, Ohio 43210 U.S.A.

Office of Health Economics
162 Regent Street
London W1R 6DD United Kingdom

Ontario Economic Council
81 Wellesley Street East
Toronto, Ontario M4Y 1H6 Canada

Oxford University Press
200 Madison Avenue
New York, New York 10016 U.S.A.

Permanent Inter-American Committee on Social Security
Apartado Postal 20532
Mexico City, 20 DF Mexico

Praeger Publishers
111 Fourth Avenue
New York, New York 10003 U.S.A.

The Disability Alliance
96 Portland Place
London W1, United Kingdom

United Kingdom Department of Employme
Research and Planning Division
Almack House
26–28 King Street
London SW1 United Kingdom

United States Department of Housing and Urban Development
1875 Connecticut Avenue N.W.
Washington, D.C. 20009 U.S.A.

United States Office of Management and Budget
726 Jackson Place N.W.
Washington, D.C. 20503 U.S.A.

United States Social Security Administration
1875 Connecticut Avenue N.W.
Washington, D.C. 20009 U.S.A.

University Centers for International Rehabilitation
Michigan State University
East Lansing, Michigan 48824 U.S.A.

University of Chicago Press
5801 Ellis Avenue
Chicago, Illinois U.S.A.

RESOURCES: PERIODICALS

Ageing International
International Federation on Ageing
1909 K Street N.W.
Washington, D.C. 20049 U.S.A.

American Rehabilitation
U.S. Rehabilitation Services Administration
330 C Street S.W.
Washington, D.C. 20201 U.S.A.

Archives of Physical Medicine and Rehabilitation
American Congress of Rehabilitation Medicine
30 North Michigan Avenue
Chicago, Illinois 60602 U.S.A.

British Journal of Preventive and Social Medicine
British Medical Association
BMA House, Tavistock Square
London WC1 H9JR United Kingdom

Contact
Christian Medical Commission
150, Route de Ferney
1211 Geneva 20, Switzerland

The Courier-Africa, Caribbean, Pacific-European Community
Commission of European Communities
200 rue de la Loi
1049 Brussels, Belgium

The Economist
25 St. James Street
London, SW1A 1HG United Kingdom

Evaluation Quarterly
Sage Publications Inc.
275 S.Beverly Hills Drive
Beverly Hills, California 90212 U.S.A.

Health Policy Quarterly
Human Sciences Press
72 Fifth Avenue
New York, New York 10011 U.S.A.

Health and Society
MIT Press
28 Carleton Street
Cambridge, Massachusetts 02142 U.S.A.

International Labor Review
International Labor Office
CH 1211 Geneva 22 Switzerland

International Rehabilitation Review
Rehabilitation International
432 Park Avenue South
New York, New York 10016 U.S.A.

International Social Service Review
(now the International Social Development Review)
United Nations Publications
Rm. LX 2300
New York, New York 10017 U.S.A.

Journal of Chronic Diseases
Pergammon Press Journals Department
Maxwell House
Fairview Park
Elmsford, New York 10523 U.S.A.

Journal of Health Policy, Politics and Law
Department of Health Administration
Duke University
6697 College Station
Durham, North Carolina 27708 U.S.A.

Journal of Human Resources
University of Wisconsin Press
Box 1379
Madison, Wisconsin 53701 U.S.A.

Mental Retardation
American Association on Mental Deficiency
5101 Wisconsin Avenue N.W.
Washington, D.C. 20016 U.S.A.

National Rehabilitation Digest
National Advisory Council for the Handicapped
P.O. Box 1
Woden, A.C.T. 2606 Australia

New England Journal of Medicine
11 Shattuck Street
Boston, Massachusetts 02115 U.S.A.

Oxfam News
Oxfam
274 Banbury Road
Oxford, United Kingdom

Readaptation
National Office of Information on Professional Placement
10 Rue de Sevres
Paris 7, France

Scandinavian Journal of Rehabilitation Medicine
Almqvist & Wiksell Periodicals Co.
P.O. Box 62
S-101 20 Stockholm 1 Sweden

Social and Rehabilitation Record
(now the U.S. Health Care Finance Review)
U.S. Health Care Finance Administration
Rm. 1E9 Oak Meadows Building
6340 Security Blvd.
Baltimore, Maryland 21235 U.S.A.

Social Security Bulletin
U.S. Social Security Administration
1875 Connecticut Avenue, Room 1120
Washington, D.C. 20009 U.S.A.

UNESCO Courier
UNESCO
Place de Fontenoy
75700 Paris, France

UNICEF News
United Nations Children's Fund
866 U.N. Plaza
New York, New York 10017 U.S.A.

Photo Credits

We thank the United Nations Photo Library for its cooperation in providing many of the photographs in this publication. All photographs not otherwise identified are United Nations photos.

Page ii - World Health Organization
iv - Norman Potter, Leonard Cheshire Foundation
vi - Dianna Mah-Jones, Edmonton, Alberta, Canada
vii - *Ich bin doch auch wie ihr*, Elizabeth Niggemeyer, Federal Republic of Germany
viii - " " "
ix - " " "
x - Diego Pedro Benzol, Barcelona, Spain
2 - Photo of girl, D. Mangurian, UN; photo of men in boat, Lech Szymanski, Poland
4 - Ray Witlin, UN
5 - Phelps K. Manning
6 - M. Hopp, UN
7 - Boy, Elizabeth Niggemeyer; Elderly woman, B. Wolff, UN
8 - Group, Francisco Molins Rabella, Barcelona
12 - Man in hut, Ray Witlin, UN
13 - Department of Social Welfare, Bureau of Vocational Rehabilitation, Philippines
14 - Ray Witlin, UN
15 - Wolff, UN
17 - Group, J. Mohr, International Labor Organization
18 - New Zealand Crippled Children's Society
23 - O. Monsen, UN
24 - Jan Corash, UN
26 - Ulreike Schleifanbaum
29 - O. Monsen, UN
37 - Norman Potter, Leonard Cheshire Foundation
41 - Terry Tullis, England
43 - *UNESCO Courier*
46 - F. Griffing, UN
47 - P. Teusher, UN
55 - Bureau of Social Welfare, Philippines
59 - Christian Vignand, Paris
65 - Dianna Mah-Jones, Edmonton, Canada
67 - Alan White and Vladimir Pavlovic
71 - M. Rothstein, UN
75 - Woman, B. Wolff, UN
Man, A. Rozberg, UN
77 - J. Sunshine
81 - Institute for Social Services (INSERSO), Spain
90 - Peter Till, *New Statesman*
92 - Netherlands Society for Rehabilitation
95 - Abraham Menashe
99 - Leo Pumanes, St. Mandaluyong, Philippines
101 - Phillip Weisbecker
103 - " "
115 - League of Red Cross Societies
119 - Japan Sun Industries
123 - Polish Cooperatives
125 - ILO
129 - "
131 - "
133 - Department of Social Welfare, Philippines
134 - D. Mangurian, UN
137 - Bjorn Myrman
141 - Workmen's Compensation Board, Ontario, Canada
143 - "
153 - Japan Sun Industries
155 - John McKay
160 - Muldoon

162 - Marta Pinter, Interfoto/UN
163 - " " " "
168 - P. Teuscher, UN
169 - " " "
175 - League of Red Cross Societies
176 - A. Jongen, UN
179 - Abraham Menashe
199 - Dietmar Gerstenberg, German Democratic Republic
200 - League of Red Cross Societies
201 - Tiedotunstoimiasto, Helsinki, Finland
203 - Pearl Mojica, Rizal, Philippines
205 - Foto Afdeling, Minerva, Denmark
207 - Nationfoto, Nairobi, Kenya
209 - Top, bottom - Foto Afdeling, Minerva, Denmark

The Economics of Disability: International Perspectives

Reader Response Form

1. I found this publication to be (check all that apply):

   - ☐ useful and informative
   - ☐ informative but not practical
   - ☐ irrelevant to my needs
   - ☐ other ____

2. I work in a/an:

   - ☐ government agency
   - ☐ organization of rehabilitation professionals
   - ☐ organization of disabled people
   - ☐ private rehabilitation facility or workshop
   - ☐ insurance company
   - ☐ medical organization
   - ☐ higher education or university
   - ☐ other ____

3. I work as a/an:

   - ☐ economist
   - ☐ senior planner/analyst
   - ☐ educator
   - ☐ administrator
   - ☐ information provider
   - ☐ researcher
   - ☐ rehabilitation service provider
   - ☐ other ____

4. Have you introduced any of the concepts or issues of the publication into the following activities:

   - ☐ policy evaluation or planning discussions
   - ☐ discussions with colleagues in your organization
   - ☐ discussions with professionals in other organizations
   - ☐ papers or other presentations
   - ☐ work with other individuals or service organizations
   - ☐ other ____

5. As a result of reading the publication, have you sought or obtained any of the references in the publication? Yes No

   Would you have any difficulty in obtaining the references if you needed them? Yes No

6. Since reading the publication, how many persons have you recommended or suggested it to: None 1-2 3-5 5-10 more than 10

7. Could you make use of other language editions of this publication?

- ☐ Spanish
- ☐ French
- ☐ Other ________________

8. I found out about this publication through:

- ☐ complimentary distribution
- ☐ review or notice in a newsletter, journal, or magazine
- ☐ a friend or colleague
- ☐ promotion material
- ☐ other ________________________________

9. For future publications, I would like to suggest the following improvements in format, contents, or distribution:

____

____

____

10. I would like to receive additional information about the following Rehabilitation International publications and activities:

- ☐ "One in Ten" Newsletter, quarterly, a publication of the Rehabilitation International/UNICEF Technical Support Program
- ☐ International Rehabilitation Review (quarterly)
- ☐ International Year of Disabled Persons Support Program
- ☐ Charter for the 80s
- ☐ International Journal of Rehabilitation Research (quarterly)

NAME AND ADDRESS ________________________________

____

____

THANK YOU FOR YOUR COOPERATION.

PLEASE MAIL TO: Rehabilitation International
432 Park Avenue South
New York, New York 10016 USA